T0341199

Disease Mapping

From Foundations to
Multidimensional Modeling

Disease Mapping
From Foundations to Multidimensional Modeling

Miguel A. Martinez-Beneito
Paloma Botella-Rocamora

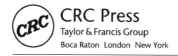

CRC Press
Taylor & Francis Group
Boca Raton London New York

CRC Press is an imprint of the
Taylor & Francis Group, an **informa** business

A CHAPMAN & HALL BOOK

CRC Press
Taylor & Francis Group
6000 Broken Sound Parkway NW, Suite 300
Boca Raton, FL 33487-2742

International Standard Book Number-13: 978-1-4822-4641-4 (Hardback)

Library of Congress Cataloging-in-Publication Data

Names: Martinez-Beneito, Miguel A., author. | Botella-Rocamora, Paloma, author.
Title: Disease mapping : from foundations to multidimensional modeling / Miguel A. Martinez-Beneito & Paloma Botella-Rocamora.
Description: Boca Raton : Taylor & Francis, 2019. | "A CRC title, part of the Taylor & Francis imprint, a member of the Taylor & Francis Group, the academic division of T&F Informa plc." | Includes bibliographical references and index.
Identifiers: LCCN 2019009770 | ISBN 9781482246414 (hardback : alk. paper)
Subjects: LCSH: Medical mapping. | Epidemiology--Statistical methods.
Classification: LCC RA792.5 .M35 2019 | DDC 614.4072/7--dc23
LC record available at https://lccn.loc.gov/2019009770

Visit the Taylor & Francis Web site at
http://www.taylorandfrancis.com

and the CRC Press Web site at
http://www.crcpress.com

To all those sad stories underlying our figures.
We hope this book could make those events a bit useful.

Contents

Preface

This book is intended to summarize our professional trajectories as statisticians, which have been mainly devoted to the study of the geographical distribution of diseases. Although our academic background is related to mathematics/statistics, most of our professional careers have been developed in extra-academic public health institutions so, currently, we do not know well if we should define ourselves as statisticians working as public health practitioners, or vice versa. Our careers have evolved surrounded by geographically referenced health data, which is not so frequent in academic profiles. As a consequence, the exploration and development of spatial statistic methods, in our case, has been frequently motivated by practical requirements of our data sets instead of a research exercise. Moreover, our working time has consisted of hours and hours running models on real data sets, up to the point that we know from memory the geographical distribution of the main causes of death in the Valencian Region, our most common region of study, and for many other studies. In this sense, we feel that our background makes us a bit different than most of the authors of previous disease mapping books, or of spatial statistics methods in general, in the literature. Our intention with this book is to share that applied view with our readers. On one hand, we seek to introduce the statistical theory required to fully understand and undertake disease mapping problems, even of the highest complexity. On the other hand, we want also to transmit the practical view required for fully interpreting the results in disease mapping studies, paying particular attention to the epidemiological side of the studies made. We hope to have succeeded in this purpose.

Besides the epidemiological perspective, the particular interest in most applied issues of the disease mapping practice makes this book, in our opinion, different than the rest of the books previously published in the literature on this topic. We would really love if the readers of this book would get their hands dirty with the data and code that we have used in this book in the same manner as we have. In our opinion this would be the most profitable way of taking advantage of its content. With this aim, we have made all the code and the data sets used in the examples available for enhancing the reproducibility of our analysis and as a pedagogic tool of very high interest. A GitHub repository (`https://github.com/MigueBeneito/DisMapBook`) has been created for hosting all the online supplementary material of the book. Thus, you can make use of the functionalities that GitHub deploys for their repositories, such as 'issues' to report to us and to everyone else as well as your feedback, errors found or doubts on each example. We promise to stay aware of the feedback that you provide us. The online material will enable readers to have direct access to most of the statistical/computing details that do not have enough room to be fully explained within the content of the book. This is a great novelty of the book, as compared to the rest of the monographs in this area, and one of its greatest strengths in our view. We strongly encourage readers always to have this supplementary material in mind and use it as frequently as they can.

We find it necessary to conclude this Preface by paying several duties to the people who were instrumental during the writing of the book. First, several colleagues have reviewed and helped us in some particular parts of the book. Jim Hodges has provided us quite enlightening feedback and shared his expertise on confounding ecological regression models. Gonzalo García-Donato has also shared his expertise and comments on prior distributions in Bayesian statistics in general and their use in disease mapping in particular. Finally, Lola Ugarte has also enlightened us with her comments on spline models in disease mapping and has also kindly shared the statistical code used for developing Example 7.3 in this book. We feel also very indebted to several people who have played a key role in our academic and professional training. In particular, we owe the warmest thanks to Herme Vanaclocha and Óscar Zurriaga for all the years shared in the professional practice of epidemiology. The little epidemiology that we could know is, for sure, just a consequence of their influence. On the statistical side, we feel also very indebted to Susie Bayarri, Juan Ferrándiz, Antonio López-Quilez and Gonzalo García-Donato. They introduced us to the foundations of statistics and how they always should be kept in mind also when developing and practicing applied statistics. We also want to thank our former PhD students, Marc Marí-Dell'Olmo, Rubén Amorós and Paqui Corpas-Burgos since their works have made us learn many of the issues contained in this book. Without any doubt, the footprint of all these researchers is very present in this book. In conclusion, we cannot forget to apologize to our families, in particular our beloved daughters (Carmen and Elena), our parents (the 'Emilios', Pepa and Fina), and our friends, for the time stolen working on this book. We hope that time was only lent instead of stolen and that we will have the opportunity to make up for that missed time in the upcoming years.

Authors

Miguel A. Martinez-Beneito has two mathematics and statistics under-graduate degrees and a mathematics PhD. He has spent his whole career working as a statistician for public health services, first at the epidemiology unit of the Valencia (Spain) regional health administration and later as a researcher at the public health division of FISABIO, a regional bio-sanitary research center. He has been also the Bayesian hierarchical models professor for several seasons at the University of Valencia Biostatistics master's program. He has mainly devoted his career to developing statistical methods for health studies, in particular for disease mapping problems. During all those years, he has always been surrounded by applied problems and tons of real data where the models developed have been constantly applied. This circumstance has given him a hybrid professional profile between statistics and epidemiology, or vice versa, if you prefer.

Paloma Botella-Rocamora has two mathematics and statistics undergraduate degrees and a mathematics PhD. She has spent most of her professional career in academia, although now she works as a statistician for the epidemiology unit of the Valencia regional health administration. Her docent duties have been often related to biostatistics courses for health, veterinary and nursing students, but she has taught also different courses for statisticians. Most of her research trajectory has been devoted to developing and applying disease mapping models to real data, although her work as a statistician in an epidemiology unit allows her to develop and apply statistical methods to health data, in general.

Part I

Disease mapping: The foundations

1

Introduction

It is quite common to find someone convinced that people in his or her town die of, let's say, cancer, more than they ought to. This is a very common belief, to a point that people do not usually question it but, on the contrary, *assert* it, convinced they live surrounded by risk sources that increase their chances of dying. Years ago, when both authors of this book did not have a clear idea what epidemiology was really about, we could not even imagine that under such a simple and common question could lie such a statistical complexity. Nowadays, we have at least learnt that answering such a question requires a thorough statistical study and the use of specific techniques is required, unless we are willing to be at serious risk of giving disparate or plain wrong answers. That collection of techniques, developed to yield reliable estimates of the geographical distribution of the risk of a disease throughout a region of interest, is usually known as 'disease mapping', the main object of interest in this book.

Disease mapping has historically evolved from two separate, but confluent, areas of research: epidemiology and statistics. Epidemiology has been defined as 'the science that studies the patterns, causes, and effects of health and disease conditions in defined populations' (Wikipedia contributors, 2018a), that is, epidemiologists are mainly interested in determining if something has an effect on the occurrence of a disease. Disease mapping practitioners are specifically interested in determining if geographical locations determine in some way the distribution of diseases and in what manner. Disease mapping is fully considered as an epidemiologic research area, in fact epidemiology provides lots of resources and methods making it possible to carry out disease mapping studies. Nevertheless, those studies find their own methodological problems when the units of study considered are small. In that case the contribution of statistics, 'the study of the collection, analysis, interpretation, presentation and organization of data' (Wikipedia contributors, 2018b), is very important. Statistics provides a plethora of methods in order to deal with the scarce information of those small areas, making it possible to solve, or at least to give a more satisfactory treatment, to the problems raised in disease mapping studies of these geographical units. In this sense, disease mapping is a paradigmatic example of the confluence of these two research areas that, separately, would not achieve such useful results. On one hand, epidemiology poses an interesting inference problem where statistical developments make sense and therefore statistics becomes a useful area. On the other hand, statistics provides alternative inference tools for estimating traditional epidemiological indicators better in settings where traditional naive tools show themselves as deficient. Therefore, disease mapping may be considered as the successful history of the confluence of these two fields of knowledge.

Not all epidemiological studies linking health and place are considered as disease mapping problems. Thus, disease mapping studies consider the estimation of epidemiological indicators for areal administrative divisions of a region of study, *lattices* from now on. That is, disease mapping is intended to deal with the observed counts of health events on sets of areal units where the small size of those units usually undertakes some specific estimation problem. Therefore, the two distinctive features of disease mapping problems are the work with areal data and the statistical problems induced by the size of the units of study. In this sense, disease mapping practitioners are like opticians who devise lenses, in this case statistical models, in order to make visible the geographical variability of the risks underlying the mentioned observed counts. The search for good 'lenses' which make it possible to surface those risk patterns as much as possible is the ultimate goal of disease mapping.

Disease mapping is just a small part of spatial epidemiology, the subfield of epidemiology in charge of studying the link between geographic locations and the occurrence of diseases, regardless of the kind of data at hand. Thus, other areas of spatial epidemiology, such as cluster detection problems (either with or without areal data), whose goal is the determination of geographical locations of anomalous risk excesses, should not be confused with disease mapping studies since their goals and methods are markedly different. On the other hand, geostatistical methods seek also to estimate the geographical distribution of geographically referenced variables, that is, the study of a spatially varying variable or process that we have observed on just a few locations. Being more precise, geostatistical problems seek to estimate the underlying risk distribution of some process as a continuous spatial surface and use the observations of that process in few geographical sites for predicting the mentioned continuous surface at every single place of the whole region of study. Thus, data in geostatistical studies is far different from those in disease mapping studies, requiring therefore completely different methods of analysis. Similarly, point processes would pursue studying risk geographical patterns according to the exact location of some known cases of some disease. Obviously, point process studies will require the use of more accurate data and specific statistical methods. Those methods will have very little in common with the methods used for disease mapping since the data for both settings are completely different.

A large bibliography has already been published on spatial epidemiology as a general topic (Alexander and Boyle, 1996; Lawson et al., 1999; Elliott et al., 2000; Waller and Gotway, 2004; Lawson, 2006; Lawson et al., 2016). Nevertheless, this book particularly focusses on the problem and statistical methods for disease mapping, i.e., our aim is to introduce the geographical analysis of health data on lattices of small areal units (see Lawson et al. (2003) and Lawson (2018) for some other references on this particular topic). As we will see, getting reasonable risk estimates in that setting may be much more difficult, under a statistical point of view, than it would seem at first glance, at least for people without an appropriate statistical background. That challenging goal is the main purpose of the journey that we are starting just now.

Example 1.1

We start this brief introduction to disease mapping with a motivating example. Let us assume that we were Valencian Region inhabitants, the Spanish region on which most of the examples in this book will be based. Let us also assume that we were concerned about the geographical distribution of the risk of oral cancer in men for this region since we have known of several deaths from this cause in our municipality or other nearby municipalities during the last few months. Municipalities are an administrative division in Spain that basically correspond to the territory of cities or towns in some other countries. The Valencian Region is a compound of 540 municipalities with a mean population of around 10,000 inhabitants, but with substantial variability between municipalities. Thus, municipal populations may vary from around 800,000 inhabitants in Valencia, the most populated municipality of this region, to Castell de Cabres, with a population of just 16 inhabitants.

As a first approach for assessing the risks for these municipalities, we could think of comparing the total number of observed deaths for each of them with those that we could expect according to their populations, for the available period 1987–2011. We could calculate those expected deaths by simply dividing the total observed oral cancer deaths in men in the Valencian Region among the municipalities as a function of the proportion of the whole Valencian population that they contain. The upper-left plot of Figure 1.1 shows the ratio between the observed and expected deaths multiplied by 100 (the Standardized Mortality Ratio, SMR, for epidemiologists) for each municipality in the Valencian Region. SMRs are one of the main epidemiological measures comparing the risk of population groups with that of a reference group, the whole Valencian Region in our case. For this map, the dark brown zones point out the places where the observed deaths have been substantially higher than those expected so therefore those municipalities are of higher risk. In a similar manner, dark green areas correspond to those municipalities with the lowest risks. Lighter colours correspond to those municipalities with milder risks. That plot does not show any clear geographical pattern, showing apparently lots of noise or unstructured variability. For this plot, low and high risk areas are scattered all around the region of study with lots of high risk municipalities placed beside other low risk municipalities. This map does not show any particularly useful risk distribution since that distribution seems to be hidden by the noise shown by the SMRs.

SMRs are epidemiological indicators quite useful to determine high risk populations in comparison to other groups. Nevertheless, these indicators are not well suited when data are scarce, as for many of the low populated municipalities in the Valencian Region. This is the main reason why the upper-left map of Figure 1.1 does not show any useful geographical pattern. Disease mapping techniques yield enhanced statistical indicators solving the problems that SMRs typically show when calculated on small areas with low populations and therefore scarce data. The main tool for improving risk estimates in disease mapping models is to assume that data corresponding to nearby locations are dependent and should therefore show similar risk estimates. In this manner, risk estimates for each municipality would take into account information also from surrounding places instead of on the observed deaths of just that location, in contrast to the previous SMRs. The upper-right plot of Figure 1.1 shows the kind of geographical patterns estimated by incorporating the hypothesis of spatial dependence on the risk estimates. Now those risk estimates are very different from those corresponding to the SMRs represented in the upper-left plot. This new map depicts a clear geographical pattern highlighting the location of very few high risk areas, in contrast to the SMR maps where many regions had high risk estimates. Most of the variability showed in the original SMR map has been filtered out for this alternative plot yielding a much more useful map accounting for the spatial dependence that data should hypothetically show.

Although the upper-right plot of Figure 1.1 shows many appealing features as compared to that in the upper-left side, both have a common problem. For having a reasonable number of deaths, in order to build two maps, we have considered a long period of study: 1987–2011. This has provided us a considerable number of deaths, insufficient for estimating municipal risks by means of SMRs, but suitable for that aim if dependence between nearby locations was considered. Nevertheless, the risk estimates derived correspond to the whole period of study considered, which is clearly too long for answering questions as the original one referred to a short period of study. Thus, in many real settings we would want to have time specific risk estimates of much shorter time length, although this could obviously introduce additional statistical problems since the corresponding data will be much scarcer. Spatio-temporal disease mapping models allow us to consider shorter time intervals by considering dependence between consecutive time intervals for each municipality. In this manner temporal dependence, as for spatial dependence in the upper-right plot of Figure 1.1, makes it possible to share information between (spatio-temporal) units of analysis and get therefore reasonable risk estimates in such an adverse setting. The lower-left plot in Figure 1.1 shows the estimated spatio-temporal risk estimates for each municipality of the Valencian Region for the period from 2010 to 2011, which is much more useful in epidemiological terms than those risk estimates in the upper row of that same

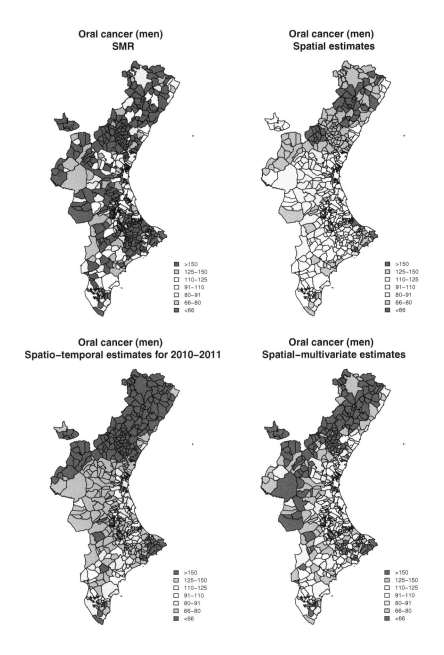

Figure 1.1
Oral cancer mortality risk estimates for the municipalities of the Valencian Region. Four estimates are shown for settings with different assumptions.

figure. This plot shows how the risks for this latest period are in general lower than for the whole original period yielding additional insight on the evolution of the risks for the whole period of study.

Finally, more enhanced risk estimates could be proposed than those already introduced. Considering dependence between different units of analysis seems to be the main tool for enhancing risk estimates, making it possible to retrieve reliable risk estimates in settings where it otherwise would not be possible. Hence, considering additional information sources and dependence between their risk estimates could improve them all. In particular, many different causes of death share joint risk factors making them show similar geographic risk patterns. If several related causes of death were jointly considered, dependence between their geographical patterns could be accounted for, yielding therefore enhanced risk estimates that would share information between diseases in the same manner that information is shared between spatial units in the upper-right plot of Figure 1.1. The lower-right plot of that same figure shows the estimated geographical risk distribution for oral cancer for a joint study of 21 diseases, accounting for dependence between those diseases. As can be appreciated, the geographical pattern depicted in that plot is remarkably more clear than for the rest of the maps in that figure. This makes evident that dependence between diseases is a secondary information source bringing substantial benefit when incorporated into disease mapping studies.

The example above has illustrated the main goal of this book. Disease mapping has emerged as a research area in statistics motivated by the problems that some traditional epidemiological indicators show in some specific settings, of particular interest in practical terms. Substantial theory, models and methods have been specifically developed to overcome those problems and, as introduced above, they allow us to derive reliable estimates in those adverse settings. The aim of this book is to introduce that theory, models and methods in order to provide a thorough view of the research field of disease mapping for the last few years.

We introduce now the structure that we will follow to achieve this goal. This book has been divided into two separate parts: Chapters 1 to 4, the Foundations of Disease Mapping, and Chapters 5 to 9, Towards Multidimensional Modeling. Part I is devised as an introduction to disease mapping for readers without a previous background in this field; indeed it has been written for people without a strong background in mathematics or statistics. Part II of the book addresses different advanced or specialized topics in disease mapping for readers with a previous knowledge of this area. Topics in this second part have been ordered as a function of their complexity, ending with multidimensional modeling, the most complex research area in disease mapping nowadays, structuring several sources of dependence altogether in a single model. Advanced readers may decide to skip the first introductory part of this book and focus directly on its second part.

Regarding Part I of this book, in the next section we will introduce some guidelines and mathematical notation that will be used during the rest of the book. Chapter 2 introduces Bayesian statistics for readers without a previous knowledge of this approach. Most of the modeling proposals in disease mapping have been made following the Bayesian paradigm so we find it necessary for newcomers to this area to have at least a minimal knowledge of this approach. Chapter 3 introduces some computing tools of widespread use between disease mapping practitioners for performing Bayesian inference. Specifically, we introduce readers to `WinBUGS`, a simulation-based inference tool, and `INLA`, an alternative mathematical tool of increasing popularity avoiding simulation. Once having introduced Bayesian inference and some computing tools for that area, Chapter 4 introduces readers to disease mapping. This chapter motivates disease mapping as a statistical problem and introduces the simplest and most common models of use in this area.

Regarding Part II of this book, Chapter 5 introduces Ecological Regression. This is a variation of disease mapping with a more inferential aim trying to determine the relationship between the risks for the spatial units and some covariate(s) that could be associated with those risks. Chapter 6 introduces some alternative spatial models to those already introduced in Chapter 4. This chapter introduces many different ways of structuring and inducing spatial dependence in lattice based data. Chapter 7 introduces spatio-temporal disease mapping models where time is also considered as an explanatory variable for risks, in addition to spatial locations. These models make it possible to consider thinner time intervals for the observed counts and therefore provide more precise risk estimates in temporal terms, such as for the left-lower plot of Figure 1.1. Chapter 8 introduces multivariate disease mapping, where several diseases are jointly analyzed. These models allow us to introduce dependence between diseases as a secondary source of dependence for risks, making it possible to share information on the risks for all those diseases, as illustrated in the lower-right plot of Figure 1.1. Finally, Chapter 9 introduces multidimensional modeling. A combination of multivariate modeling with some additional factors such as time, sex, etc. These models make it possible to formulate, for example, multivariate spatio-temporal models which could also share information between sexes, for example, if wanted. Obviously, this is the most complex kind of models formulated for disease mapping problems nowadays and the final stage of this journey.

1.1   Some considerations on this book

This book is intended to follow a very practical approach, so you will find lots of examples all over the book putting in practice the theoretical content introduced. At the end of each chapter (except for this introductory chapter) you will find some exercises devised to put in practice its content. Those exercises will generally suggest some activities related to that same chapter on an alternative data set also related to its content. These exercises will allow you to practice the topics covered without the specific guidance provided within the examples.

In addition to the written content of the book we have found it very convenient to develop additional complementary online material to enhance its practical aim. All the examples in this book have been run in R, whose code will possibly call to either WinBUGS or INLA. Thus, we have uploaded the R code for most of the examples in this book to the website https://github.com/MigueBeneito/DisMapBook, which contains the code and related material needed to run them all. By the way, in regard to the computing times of all those examples, we find convenient to mention that all of them have been run in a DELL XPS13 laptop with an i7-5500 processor. When both WinBUGS and INLA implementations of some of the examples have been possible, we have generally included both of them in the accompanying material for illustrative purposes. The R code provided for the examples has been generated and uploaded as RMarkdown documents (Allaire et al., 2018). Additionally, we have uploaded a compiled pdf document generated from running each RMarkdown file, in case you wanted to take a look at the code and outcoming results instead of executing the whole code by yourself. In our opinion, this is one of the greatest contributions of this book since it allows a closer contact of readers with the examples, which will allow them to execute and therefore to check all their details. We suggest you keep this resource very much in mind, which we are sure will provide readers with a deeper understanding of the content of the book.

Although our intention was that readers could reproduce exactly the same results shown in our examples, regretfully this is not going to be possible. The R code provided reproduces exactly our analyses made for all the examples. Nevertheless, confidentiality issues do not allow us to share the original data sets used for those examples. This has forced us to share 'fake' data, which do not match up with the original data sets, although they are very similar. Specifically, each of the data sets that we have used has a number of observed and expected health events, o_i and e_i, for each spatial unit in the study $i = 1, \ldots, I$. All the data sets available for your use have the original expected cases e_i but the number of observed health events o_i per spatial unit has been changed by o_i^*. This o_i^* has been generated in the following manner: We have sampled from a $Pois(e_i)$ distribution $\lceil e_i \rceil$ values, where $\lceil e_i \rceil$ denotes the lowest integer number higher than e_i, afterwards we have set o_i^* as the closest of those sampled values to the real o_i. In this manner, we preserve the confidentiality of the observed cases in our original data sets, particularly for those smaller spatial units for which the number of sampled values is lower. As a summary, these 'fake' data will allow you to completely reproduce our examples. Nevertheless, you may find small differences between the results that you will reproduce and those in our examples as a result of the small differences of both the original and provided data sets.

Most of the examples in this book are referring to mortality studies throughout the Valencian Region, so in our opinion it is worth including a few lines to introduce this region at this stage of the book. The Valencian Region, see Figure 1.2, is one of the 17 regions that compose Spain located at the eastern Mediterranean coast of this country. By 2017 this region had a population of almost 5 million people. This region is divided into 3 *provinces* (blue borders in Figure 1.2), and 540 *municipalities* (black borders). The points in the map denote some key municipalities of the Valencian Region. Castellón, Valencia and Alicante (blue points) are the capitals of the three provinces of the Valencian Region and Gandía and Torrevieja (green points) are large cities of this region of particular interest for the rest of the book. Finally, it is also convenient to put some attention on the variability in the population of the municipalities in the Valencian Region, also shown in Figure 1.2. In this region, 4 municipalities have more than 100,000 inhabitants and 10 municipalities have less than 100 inhabitants, so that variability is huge. Specifically we can see two areas with a particularly low population, one at the left side of the Castellón province and another one at the upper-right side of the Alicante province.

Finally, we want to define some terminology conventions for the book. In general, the term region will be used for the whole region of study, usually the Valencian Region in our examples, in contrast to each of the spatial units that compound that region of study. We will refer to those small units as spatial units, areal units, units of study, sites, etc. in contrast with *region* which will always refer to the whole set of spatial units. In the same manner, the term *period* will refer to the whole period of study considered in any spatial or spatio-temporal study while if this period is split into several separate pieces we will refer to them as time intervals or subperiods. The health events that will be studied throughout this book could be of very different types: traffic accidents, incident cases for a disease, hospital admissions or even deaths from that same cause. Without loss of generality, we will refer to all health events as deaths for the rest of this book regardless of the fact that the methods used could be equally applied to any other health events beyond deaths. The reason for this is that mortality is usually the main health event of study in disease mapping problems; indeed all the examples in this book study mortality data, surely because of the high quality and availability of that kind of data. Referring to mortality data throughout the book will make its reading easier without loss of generality.

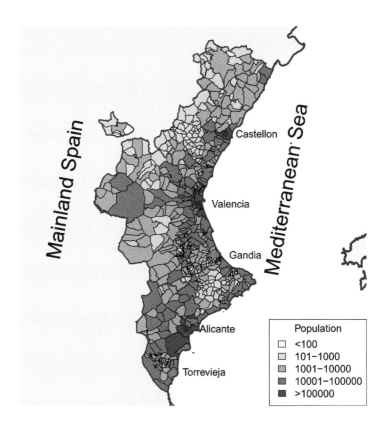

Figure 1.2
Valencian Region with its municipalities, provinces and some main cities.
Colours of the municipalities in the map represent their corresponding popu-
lations.

1.1.1 Notation

We find it convenient to describe the notation used throughout the book in a single section, so that you can use it as a reference whenever you find a notation doubt on any of the expressions used henceforth. This is the aim of this section. If you prefer, you can skip this section now and only come back if you find any particular doubt for any of the subsequent expressions. In general we have attempted to use a similar notation to that typically used in the disease mapping literature; however, we have preferred to set it in advance for the completeness of the book.

In general, Greek characters will be typically reserved for unobserved variables in statistical models, whereas Latin letters will be used for denoting observed quantities or fixed parameters. Thus, we will typically make inference just on the elements denoted by Greek letters in our models. We will use regular characters for denoting single quantities. On the contrary, we will use bold characters for denoting either vectors, usually denoted as lowercase characters $\boldsymbol{v}$, and matrices or arrays in uppercase characters $\boldsymbol{M}$. We will not make in general any distinction between vectors and matrices with a single column. We will refer to the i-th row of matrix $\boldsymbol{M}$ as $\boldsymbol{M}_{i\cdot}$ and its j-th column as $\boldsymbol{M}_{\cdot j}$. Similar notation will be used for arrays with as many subindexes as the dimension of the array. Note that, although $\boldsymbol{M}_{i\cdot}$ and $\boldsymbol{M}_{\cdot j}$ are vectors, we will frequently denote them by uppercase letters to stress that they are a part of matrix $\boldsymbol{M}$. In a similar manner $\boldsymbol{v}_{-i} = (v_1, \ldots, v_{i-1}, v_{i+1}, \ldots, v_I)$ will denote the I-vector $\boldsymbol{v}$ removing its i-th component. Similar interpretation will be followed for $\boldsymbol{M}_{-i\cdot}$ or $\boldsymbol{M}_{\cdot -j}$ that will denote matrix $\boldsymbol{M}$ removing its i-th row or j-th column, respectively. We will use $[\boldsymbol{v}_1 : \ldots : \boldsymbol{v}_J]$ to denote a matrix whose columns are the vectors $\boldsymbol{v}_j$, $j = 1, \ldots, J$, which have all the same length. Similarly, for a set of matrices $\boldsymbol{M}_j$, $j = 1, \ldots, J$ with the same number of rows, $\boldsymbol{M} = [\boldsymbol{M}_1 : \ldots : \boldsymbol{M}_J]$ would still be valid, defining a matrix composed as the binding of the columns of those matrices. If $\boldsymbol{M}_j$ has dimensions $I \times J_j$, then $\boldsymbol{M}$ will have dimensions $I \times \sum_j J_j$. Finally, we will denote as $\mathbf{1}_I$ and $\mathbf{0}_I$ the I-vectors having all its components equal to 1 and 0, respectively, and $\boldsymbol{I}_J$ will denote the $J \times J$ identity matrix. We will also denote as $1_A(x)$ the characteristic (or indicator) function, which is equal to 1 if x belongs to the set A and to 0 otherwise.

Chapters 7 to 9 in this book deal with disease mapping models of multivariate outcomes (number of observed deaths) per site. For these chapters some particular matrix operations will be required, thus you will maybe prefer to postpone the reading of the next few paragraphs until then. First, we will denote the *transpose* of a matrix $\boldsymbol{M}$, of dimensions $I \times J$, as $\boldsymbol{M}'$. We will denote as $block(\{\boldsymbol{M}_{ij}\}_{i,j=1}^{I,J})$ the *block matrix* whose (i,j)-th block is equal to the matrix $\boldsymbol{M}_{ij}$. In a similar manner $Bdiag(\{\boldsymbol{M}_i\}_{i=1}^{I})$ will denote a *block-diagonal matrix* whose i-th diagonal element is equal to the matrix $\boldsymbol{M}_i$. If $\boldsymbol{M}_i$, $i = 1, \ldots, I$ in the latter expression were substituted by scalar values $v_1, \ldots, v_I$

instead of matrices, then $Bdiag(\{v_i\}_{i=1}^I)$ would be a simple *diagonal matrix* that we will denote as $diag(\boldsymbol{v})$ where $\boldsymbol{v} = (v_1, ..., v_I)$.

Hadamard or *component-wise products* between vectors or matrices will be denoted by the operator $\circ$. Thus, for two vectors $\boldsymbol{x}$ and $\boldsymbol{y}$ of the same length, $\boldsymbol{x} \circ \boldsymbol{y}$ denotes the vector whose i-th component is given by $x_i y_i$. Component-wise products may also be used for multiplying matrices of equal dimensions in a similar manner to that used for vectors.

Kronecker products are matrix operations that will be regularly used in Chapters 7 to 9. The Kronecker product of two matrices $\boldsymbol{A}$ and $\boldsymbol{B}$, denoted by $\boldsymbol{A} \otimes \boldsymbol{B}$, is defined as the block-matrix:

$$\boldsymbol{A} \otimes \boldsymbol{B} = \begin{pmatrix} A_{11}\boldsymbol{B} & A_{12}\boldsymbol{B} & \cdots & A_{1J}\boldsymbol{B} \\ A_{21}\boldsymbol{B} & A_{22}\boldsymbol{B} & \cdots & A_{2J}\boldsymbol{B} \\ \vdots & \vdots & \ddots & \vdots \\ A_{I1}\boldsymbol{B} & A_{I2}\boldsymbol{B} & \cdots & A_{IJ}\boldsymbol{B} \end{pmatrix}.$$

Additionally, we will regularly use the *vec* operator as the linear transformation which vectorizes a matrix into vectors as $vec(\boldsymbol{M}) = ((\boldsymbol{M}_{.1})', \ldots, (\boldsymbol{M}_{.J})')'$. Thus the *vec* operator vectorizes a matrix $\boldsymbol{M}$ by stacking its columns on top of one another. In a similar manner $vec(\boldsymbol{M}') = (\boldsymbol{M}_{1.}, \ldots, \boldsymbol{M}_{I.})'$ performs a similar operation on $\boldsymbol{M}$ by stacking their transposed rows into a single column.

Besides the notation above, we find it also convenient to set here some mathematical properties that will be repeatedly used throughout the book. For example, regarding the relationship between $vec(\boldsymbol{M})$ and $vec(\boldsymbol{M}')$, note that the elements of the second of these vectors are a simple permutation of the first. As a consequence exists a permutation (orthogonal) matrix $\boldsymbol{P}$ accomplishing $vec(\boldsymbol{M}') = \boldsymbol{P}vec(\boldsymbol{M})$ (Henderson and Searle, 1979). Also related with this result we have that if $vec(\boldsymbol{M})$ had $\boldsymbol{A} \otimes \boldsymbol{B}$ as covariance matrix, then $vec(\boldsymbol{M}')$ has as covariance matrix $\boldsymbol{P}(\boldsymbol{A} \otimes \boldsymbol{B})\boldsymbol{P}' = \boldsymbol{B} \otimes \boldsymbol{A}$ (see also Expression (13) in Henderson and Searle, 1979).

Kronecker products have also some interesting properties, mainly in computational terms, such as: $(\boldsymbol{A} \otimes \boldsymbol{B})' = \boldsymbol{A}' \otimes \boldsymbol{B}'$ or $(\boldsymbol{A} \otimes \boldsymbol{B})^{-1} = \boldsymbol{A}^{-1} \otimes \boldsymbol{B}^{-1}$. Moreover, for an $I \times I$ matrix $\boldsymbol{A}$ and a $J \times J$ matrix $\boldsymbol{B}$, the eigenvectors and eigenvalues of $\boldsymbol{A} \otimes \boldsymbol{B}$ are, respectively, $\boldsymbol{v}_i^A \otimes \boldsymbol{v}_j^B$ and $\lambda_i^A \cdot \lambda_j^B$ where $\boldsymbol{v}_i^A, \boldsymbol{v}_j^B$ are the eigenvectors and λ_i^A, λ_j^B the eigenvalues of $\boldsymbol{A}$ and $\boldsymbol{B}$, respectively, for $i = 1, ..., I$ and $j = 1, ...J$. A direct consequence of this is that if $\boldsymbol{A}$ and $\boldsymbol{B}$ are positive definite, then $\boldsymbol{A} \otimes \boldsymbol{B}$ will be also positive definite since all its eigenvalues will be positive. Proofs for all these results on Kronecker products may be easily found in specific linear algebra books such as Harville (1997) or Gentle (2007).

2

Some basic ideas of Bayesian inference

In Chapters 2 and 3 of this book, we are going to introduce some background needed to suitably follow the rest of the book. Surely, advanced readers will prefer to skip all or part of these chapters. Nevertheless, both will allow readers without that background to acquire it. This will allow them to get involved in the disease mapping world or, at least, follow the remaining chapters of this book.

First, we start this chapter by stating a disclaimer. Most of the theory developed or cited throughout this book follows the Bayesian paradigm, whatever this means. We acknowledge that this is surely the main bias of this book. We do not mean at all that the Bayesian framework is the only way to proceed or carry out disease mapping studies. A lot of valuable models have been proposed for disease mapping from the frequentist approach (the alternative to the Bayesian approach). In our opinion, it is undoubtable that Bayesian models have increased their popularity and become the most used approach in disease mapping for the last few years. That is the reason (jointly with our personal bias) why we are paying particular attention to the Bayesian framework throughout the book. This chapter is not intended to be a full overview of Bayesian statistics but, on the contrary, it will just introduce the basic concepts and tools needed to follow the models to be introduced in the rest of this book.

This chapter is structured as follows: Section 2.1 introduces the basic ideas and concepts of Bayesian inference. Section 2.2 introduces Bayesian hierarchical models and random effects, the main modeling tool used in this book and for disease mapping in general. Finally, Section 2.3 introduces Markov Chain Monte Carlo (MCMC) as the main tool to carry inference out in hierarchical models, paying particular attention to convergence analysis, the process used to assess the correctness of the inference made.

2.1   Bayesian inference

Statistics deals with transforming data into knowledge. We will typically have some data available coming from a process under study, such as the number of observed deaths for different periods or geographical units, and we will try to generate from them some knowledge on the underlying process. The most usual way to do this is to assume that the available data have been generated from a statistical model, i.e., a relationship linking data to a mathematical mechanism including some random component(s). It has been said that 'all models are wrong but some are useful' (Box and Draper, 1987); under that principle, models are going to be the starting point of all our statistical analyses. Namely, our particular aim will be to convert data's noisy information about the model on knowledge about the unknown parameters underlying the corresponding mathematical relationship. This process is usually known in statistics as *inference*.

The main difference between the Bayesian and the frequentist frameworks comes from the way that the two treat the parameters of the model that we want to learn about. As unknown quantities, these parameters can be treated in two different manners: (i) as fixed, although unknown quantities, or (ii) as random variables, whose randomness accounts for the uncertainty that we have on them. The frequentist approach is founded on the first of these possibilities and so treats the parameters of the model as fixed although unknown quantities. Under this paradigm, the data usually inform us about the values of the parameters of higher likelihood, i.e., those values that would be more likely for the parameters according to the observed data. The maximum likelihood method and some related modifications are the main inference tools under that approach.

On the other hand, the Bayesian paradigm considers the parameters of any model that we may be interested to learn about as random variables. Random variables are ruled by the corresponding probability distributions that define the probability of any possible outcome of the variables, and these are going to be the main objects of interest under the Bayesian point of view. Even before having any data available, we can talk about the probability distribution of the parameters in a model ($\boldsymbol{\theta}$ hereafter); we will refer to that distribution as $P(\boldsymbol{\theta})$. That distribution, known in Bayesian terms as the *prior distribution* of the parameters, will usually reflect our ignorance of them or, in the case that we wanted to do it, will incorporate some external information, such as previous knowledge from experts' opinion (previous to the observation of the data in our experiment). Regardless of the prior information that we could have on the parameters of the model, the observed data provide us information on the most likely values of the parameters, according to the observed data. That information is summarized by the conditional distribution of the data ($\boldsymbol{y}$ hereafter) given the values of the parameters, i.e., $P(\boldsymbol{y}|\boldsymbol{\theta})$. That probability distribution of the data is usually known as *data likelihood* in the Bayesian literature. Additionally, the corresponding analytic expression of the data likelihood is known as the *likelihood function* as it coincides with the function with the same name of the frequentist approach, which quantified the most likely values of $\boldsymbol{\theta}$ according to the observed data. Once we join data's information, $P(\boldsymbol{y}|\boldsymbol{\theta})$, with the prior knowledge that we had on the parameters before observing the data, $P(\boldsymbol{\theta})$, we derive the conditional distribution of the parameters given the data, $P(\boldsymbol{\theta}|\boldsymbol{y})$, what is known in Bayesian terms as the *posterior distribution* of the parameters. Therefore, the prior distribution, data likelihood and posterior distribution are the three main objects summarizing the knowledge on the parameters of the model at any stage of the data analysis, i.e., before, during and after observing the data, respectively.

Bayesian statistics takes its name from Bayes' theorem, an elementary result of probability theory linking the conditional probability of two events $P(A|B)$ with the corresponding reverse conditional probability $P(B|A)$. Namely, Bayes' theorem states for any two events, A and B, that

$$P(A|B) = \frac{P(B|A)P(A)}{P(B)}.$$

Therefore, both conditional probabilities are linked by the marginal probabilities of the two events of interest, $P(A)$ and $P(B)$. This theorem is of high relevance for the Bayesian tools introduced above. Hence, for A being the event that $\boldsymbol{\theta}$ have some specific value and B that the observed process had $\boldsymbol{y}$ as observed values, Bayes' theorem yields:

$$P(\boldsymbol{\theta}|\boldsymbol{y}) = \frac{P(\boldsymbol{y}|\boldsymbol{\theta})P(\boldsymbol{\theta})}{P(\boldsymbol{y})}. \tag{2.1}$$

This expression shows how to derive the posterior distribution of a set of parameters from their prior distribution and the corresponding likelihood function. The posterior distribution is just the product of the information available on the parameters before observing any data and that coming from them, divided by a third factor of minor importance. In fact, this factor does not depend on $\boldsymbol{\theta}$ and therefore it is just a constant within the posterior distribution of the parameters. That is why that factor is frequently ignored in Bayesian analyses and the main relationship in Bayesian statistics (2.1) is usually stated just as:

$$P(\boldsymbol{\theta}|\boldsymbol{y}) \propto P(\boldsymbol{y}|\boldsymbol{\theta})P(\boldsymbol{\theta}).$$

The full posterior distribution of a parameter in the model is usually more than we need to know about it and, besides, it is something that is not very comfortable to deal with. Therefore, it is usual to summarize posterior distributions by means of some specific statistics such as their mean, median or mode yielding, respectively, the *posterior mean*, *posterior median* or *posterior mode* of the parameters in the model. These are just some Bayesian point estimates of the parameters, playing a similar role to frequentist point estimates of parameters, the posterior mean being the most common choice among them. Besides, posterior distributions can also be summarized by means of intervals instead of point estimates, similar to confidence intervals under the frequentist approach. Thus, given any posterior distribution and a probability α, it would be possible to build an interval covering the $100(1-\alpha)\%$ of its mass just considering all values between its $100(\alpha/2)\%$ and $100(1-\alpha/2)\%$ percentiles.

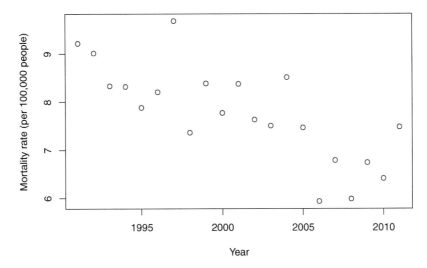

Figure 2.1
Annual oral cancer mortality rates in the Valencian Region from 1991 to 2011.

This interval is called the $100(1 - \alpha)\%$-*credible interval* of the corresponding parameter and its interpretation is pretty appealing: the probability that the corresponding parameter lies within that interval is exactly $1 - \alpha$.

Example 2.1

This example intends to illustrate the main differences between the frequentist and Bayesian analyses of a simple data set. Figure 2.1 shows the annual mortality rates (per 100,000 people) for oral cancer in the Valencian Region from 1991 to 2011. In statistical terms, these are just the observed probabilities of dying from this cause at each of those years multiplied by 100,000. Figure 2.1 suggests the existence of a linear time trend during the period of study and we are interested in assessing its statistical relevance.

First, we start by performing the frequentist analysis of this data set. In order to do that, a statistical model should be assumed and we propose to start with a Gaussian linear model. This model assumes the annual rates to be distributed as Normal observations whose means follow a linear trend as a function of its year. Remember that 'all models are wrong' and this is not an exception at all. The Normal assumption implies that both positive and negative values would be admissible for rates when actually they are not. Moreover, the linear assumption for the mean of the rates implies that at some point in the future (or at some point in the past if the trend was determined to be increasing), rates will be expected to be negative. Nevertheless, this model may be useful to explain oral cancer mortality during the period of study, or even in the close upcoming years, so we are going to consider it as a first useful approach for the analysis of this data set.

One can undertake the corresponding frequentist approach by simply making use of the `lm` function of `R`, suitable to fit linear models. Thus, we make

```
> year.centered=year-mean(year)
> RateVsYear=lm(rate ~ year.centered)
```

We have considered a centered version of the year as covariate instead of the raw year, so that the intercept of the linear model (the value of the rate for the covariate being equal to 0) has a meaningful interpretation. This analysis yields, among other things,

```
> summary(RateVsYear)
```

```
              Estimate Std. Error t value Pr(>|t|)
(Intercept)    7.75854    0.14611  53.102  < 2e-16 ***
year.centered -0.12358    0.02413  -5.122 6.06e-05 ***

Residual standard error: 0.6695 on 19 degrees of freedom
```

This means an estimated mortality rate, per 100,000 people, of 7.76 deaths for year 2001 and an annual decrease in that quantity of 0.12 deaths per year. These estimates are accompanied by the corresponding p-values, pointing out that both terms are significantly different from 0. These point estimates may also be accompanied by the corresponding (95%) confidence intervals

```
> confint(RateVsYear)
                    2.5 %       97.5 %
(Intercept)     7.4527395   8.06434706
year.centered  -0.1740793  -0.07307567
```

Regardless of the controversy on the use of p-values and confidence intervals (see, for example, Nuzzo (2014)) and the difficulties to interpret them (their correct interpretation is not as straightforward as usually assumed), these are the main tools used for summarizing the results of statistical analyses under the frequentist approach.

On the other hand, a parallel Bayesian analysis could also be made of the same data set. In that case, the data likelihood (the distribution of the data as a function of the parameters of some specific model) should be defined for the data, as well as the prior distribution of its parameters. The frequentist analysis above already considered a data likelihood since it implicitly assumed

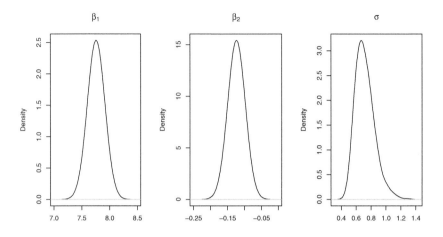

Figure 2.2
Posterior distributions of the parameters in the Bayesian linear regression model.

the data to follow independent Normal distributions around a linear function of the year. Therefore, if we wanted to make a parallel Bayesian analysis of the frequentist analysis above, we should also assume as data likelihood

$$P(\boldsymbol{y}|\boldsymbol{\beta},\sigma) = \prod_{i=1}^{n} N(y_i|\beta_1 + \beta_2 x_i, \sigma^2),$$

where x_i stands for the i-th centered year of the period of study and σ^2 the variance of the Normal distributions. For the frequentist approach, this would be enough to start the analysis, but from a Bayesian perspective we also have to define some prior distribution for the parameters of the model, $\boldsymbol{\beta}$ and σ. Since we do not have any previous knowledge on these parameters, we could assume, for example,

$$P(\beta_1) = N(0, 10^6), \ P(\beta_2) = N(0, 10^6), \ P(\sigma) = U(0, 1{,}000).$$

We will introduce the Normal and uniform distributions with more detail later; nevertheless, these prior choices reflect our scarce knowledge on these parameters. They simply put flat prior distributions (the high variance of the Normal distributions make them roughly flat) on the range of values that could have some sense for the parameters. Note that even values of β_1 lower than 0 would not have much sense in practice, but we do not care about this because those values should be penalized by the data through the likelihood function.

Once we have set the data likelihood and the prior distribution of the parameters, Bayesian inference can be made following Expression (2.1) which yields the posterior distributions for β_1, β_2 and σ shown at Figure 2.2. Details about how to derive those distributions will be given in the next chapter. Figure 2.2 shows the posterior distributions of the parameters in the model that can be also summarized with, for example, the posterior mean of the parameters, yielding: 7.758 for β_1, -0.124 for β_2 and 0.718 for σ. These values fully agree with the frequentist estimates, except maybe the point estimate of σ which is slightly higher than the frequentist value. We can also build credible intervals accounting for the uncertainty in the estimates of the parameters by simply calculating the corresponding quantiles of their posterior distributions. Thus, [7.43,8.05], [$-0.18,-0.07$] and [0.51,1.01] would be the 95% credible intervals for, respectively, β_1, β_2 and σ. The intervals for β_1 and β_2 closely agree too with the frequentist 95% confidence intervals, although the interpretation of credible intervals is much more straightforward and intuitive than that of confidence intervals. The annex online material at `https://github.com/MigueBeneito/DisMapBook` contains the code used for reproducing the results in this example.

Prior distributions are, by far, the most controversial issue in Bayesian statistics. The need of specifying a prior distribution for any parameter in the model raises lots of criticisms from the non-Bayesian world, blaming Bayesian analyses of being subjective. In defense of the Bayesian approach, we find it convenient to mention that the election of a statistical model for the data is as subjective as the election of prior distributions; therefore, that subjectiveness is also present in frequentist analyses although, we admit it, maybe to a lesser extent. We acknowledge that the choice of prior distribution of the parameters is a sensible task conditioning; in some cases, the results of the analyses and therefore lots of care should be put in this process of Bayesian analyses.

Unless we wanted to incorporate some kind of information in prior distributions (our prior knowledge, experts' opinion, etc.), we will typically want them to be as least influential as possible, so that data may speak for themselves during the inference process. Thus, it is convenient to have some notions on the definition of (supposedly) non-influential prior distributions. The choice of non-informative prior distributions may be a very technical issue and very influential in some contexts, such as objective Bayesian model selection (Zellner, 1986). Leaving aside those technicalities which are beyond this introduction, the main way to try to make prior distributions non-influential is to make them *vague*, i.e., to choose prior distributions mainly flat along, or beyond, the set of values that could have some sense for the observed data. In the example above, we have implicitly used that idea to define the prior distributions for both $\boldsymbol{\beta}$ and σ. Regarding β_1, as an example, even before seeing any data we could be sure that any mortality rate for the period of study was much lower than 1,000 or even 100 since oral cancer is not such a prevalent disease; therefore, putting a zero-centered Normal prior distribution of variance 10^6 basically implies a flat prior on the range of values where β_1 has some sense. On the other hand, the uniform distribution on σ gives equal prior probabilities to any value of this variable lower than 1,000. In this case 1,000 is intended to be a high enough value so that it does not bound in practice the posterior distribution of σ. Even before observing our data, it would not seem reasonable to think of annual rates placed farther than 1,000 units away from the regression line, that is why we have considered it as a reasonable value for the upper limit of the prior distribution of σ. Nevertheless, if we were not sure if 1,000 was a non-informative enough choice for that upper limit, we could have perfectly chosen it to be 10,000, or even 100,000 if we find these to be safer choices. In fact, a very reasonable procedure would be to repeat the analysis with all those three values for the upper limit and check that the corresponding results are not sensitive to them. In that case we would have some guarantees on the non-influential feature of these choices. This is what is usually called a *sensitivity analysis* of the prior distributions and it is a really convenient procedure in case we had some doubts on the effect of the prior distributions used.

The above example shows that there are two parallel ways to carry out statistical analyses. Although they are very different even for the concept of parameters of statistical models, their results, at least in simple studies as that in Example 2.1, usually (should) agree. Nevertheless, the Bayesian approach shows its main potential when modeling hierarchical models, as we will illustrate in the next section. Bayesian hierarchical models have been the main tool that has contributed the most to the popularization and use of the Bayesian approach, specifically between disease mapping practitioners, so they will be our main focus from now on.

2.1.1   Some useful probability distributions

Before introducing Bayesian hierarchical models, we are going to talk a bit about probability distributions. Probability distributions are ubiquitous in Bayesian statistics. They are used at the two layers of Bayesian models as defined above, i.e., for defining the data likelihood and the prior distributions of the parameters in a model. Moreover, the product arising from merging the information of both is also a probability distribution, the posterior distribution of the parameters in the model. Thus, a basic knowledge of probability distributions is essential for an adequate understanding of Bayesian models. In order to make this book self-contained, we are going to briefly introduce the main probability distributions that will be used later, regardless of the fact that at some point we can also use some more specific distributions (those specifically considering multivariate or spatial dependence) that will be appropriately introduced when required.

Table 2.1 summarises the most common univariate distributions. Namely, it shows for each distribution how it will be denoted throughout the book, its mean and variance as a function of its parameters and the most typical uses of each one of them. Bernoulli, binomial, Normal, Poisson and t distributions are the most common probability distributions to be used as data likelihood, at least in this book. Their use depends on the nature (continuous, discrete, upper bounded, presence of outliers, etc.) of the data to be modeled, as described in Table 2.1. Namely, Bernoulli and binomial distributions will be used as data likelihoods for logistic regression models for upper bounded Natural numbers; Poisson will be used for Poisson regression on unbounded Natural numbers; and Normal and t distributions (the latter in the case of wanting to account for the presence of outliers) for classical linear regression, or some more flexible alternatives, on continuous real values.

The Normal and t distributions are also used as prior distributions of variables in Bayesian models, as well as the uniform (proper and improper) and gamma distributions. Note that both Normal and t distributions are parameterized in Table 2.1 as a function of their variances; we will follow this convention throughout the book. The improper uniform, Normal, and t distributions are used as priors for variables taking values in the whole Real line, such as the parameters β_1 and β_2 modeling the mean in Example 2.1 or, in general, for the coefficients modeling the mean in any linear or generalized linear model. In this case, the improper uniform prior is always a vague choice since it will show no preference on any particular value in the Real line and has infinite variance. Nevertheless, we should bear in mind that this distribution is a bit particular since it is *improper*. This means that, in contrast to regular proper distributions, whose integral (or sum in the discrete case) is necessarily equal to 1, the integral of improper priors is infinite. So, they may be considered a degenerate case of the regular proper probability distributions.

The use of improper prior distributions is licit, provided the posterior distribution of the corresponding parameter is proper, i.e., the impropriety of the prior does not translate to the posterior distribution. This is not usually a condition easy to be proved in theoretical terms. Nevertheless, in our experience, improper posterior distributions usually show weird performances, such as bad convergence properties of the MCMC (we will explain this further in the next chapter). So, in case you found signs of that kind in models with improper prior distributions, call into question the posterior property of your results. In any case, if you intend to be vague on a variable taking values on the whole Real line, the improper uniform distribution should be your default choice. As an alternative, Normal or t distributions could also be used. The vagueness of these distributions will depend on their variance, being more vague as long as that variance grows. Hence, for these distributions it is possible to choose the amount of vagueness desired. Sometimes Normal and t distributions are used as vague (but proper) substitutes of improper uniform priors, by giving them a high variance. In that case we prefer to use, in general, the genuine improper uniform distribution since the property of Normal and t distributions, which necessarily lead to proper posterior distributions, may only hide the impropriety posterior problems that being vague with that variable could

Distribution	Notation	Mean	Variance	Suitable for	Often Used as
Bernoulli	$Bern(p)$	p	$p(1-p)$	Binary variables	Data likelihood for binary variables
binomial	$Bin(p,n)$	pn	$np(1-p)$	Natural numbers bounded by n	Data likelihood for bounded Natural values (# of successes among n trials)
gamma	$Gamma(a,b)$	a/b	a/b^2	Positive real values	Prior distribution for the precision of Normal variables
improper uniform	$U(-\infty,\infty)$	$\sharp$	∞	Real values	Vague prior distribution for Real values
Normal	$N(\mu,\sigma^2)$	μ	σ^2	Real values	Data likelihood for Real values, vague prior distribution for Real variables
Poisson	$Pois(\lambda)$	λ	λ	Natural numbers	Data likelihood for variables taking Natural numbers (typically counts)
t	$t_d(\mu,\sigma^2)$	μ	σ^2	Real values	Robust alternative to the Normal distribution
uniform	$U(a,b)$	$(a+b)/2$	$(b-a)^2/12$	Real values between a and b	Vague prior distribution for positive Real variables (standard deviations, etc.)

Table 2.1
Brief summary of the most common univariate distributions to be used throughout this book.

entail (Berger, 2006). Therefore, we prefer to have the possibility of becoming aware of those problems by using improper uniform distributions.

The distributions above may not be used as default vague choices for any parameter in a model. For example, variances or standard deviations in a model, which may only take positive values, may not use all of them as prior distributions since Normal and t distributions, for example, put positive probability on negative values, so some alternative prior distributions should be used in this case. Gamma and uniform prior distributions are commonly used instead for modeling these specific parameters. Namely, vague gamma distributions are often used for modeling precisions (the inverse of variances) of Normal variables. This is typically done by choosing both parameters of the gamma distribution so that its variance (a/b^2 in terms of Table 2.1) is high. In general this is achieved by taking low values for a and b, close to 0. As an alternative, vague uniform prior distributions are also typically used for modeling the standard deviation of Normal variables. In that case the lower bound of that distribution is taken as 0 so that it does not constrain possible low values of this parameter. On the other hand, the upper bound of this distribution is fixed to a high enough value so that it does not constrain in practice the values of the posterior distribution of that standard deviation. As an example, if our variable varies in a small scale of some few units, it will be enough to set the upper value in the distribution of the standard deviation to 10, or even 100 if we have some doubt about the suitability of the previous value. Anyway, we will talk more in depth in Chapter 4 about the use of these two prior distributions for modeling the variability of random effects.

2.2 Bayesian hierarchical models

The model in Example 2.1 fits to the following scheme: the data, by means of a statistical model, depend on a set of (unknown) variables which, in turn, depend on other fixed parameters through their prior distributions. Namely, the data in that example depend on both β and σ through the likelihood function and these depend on their own parameters through their prior distributions. The left-hand side of Figure 2.3 shows this dependence structure. Squares in that figure stand for either data or fixed (known) parameters in the model, meanwhile circles stand for (unknown) variables in the model. Arrows in Figure 2.3 denote dependent pairs of nodes, namely those variables placed at the head of the arrow depend on the variable placed at the node on its tail. Solid line arrows denote pairs of nodes linked by the likelihood function, meanwhile dotted lines denote pairs linked by the prior distribution of the variable placed at its head. Finally, y and x denote, respectively, the data and covariate in the model, i.e., in Example 2.1 the annual rates and the centered years.

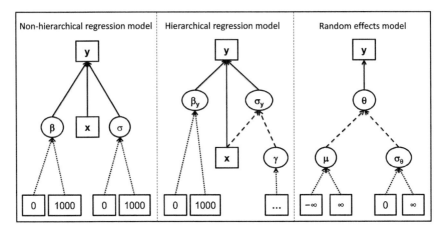

Figure 2.3
Dependence graph for several Bayesian models. Arrows stand for pairs of dependent nodes within each model.

The balance between the strength of the data and that of the prior distributions in the model makes the posterior distributions of the variables resemble either of these two factors. Frequentist models simply do not have the layer corresponding to the prior distributions in Figure 2.3. This is frequently considered a virtue of frequentist models (they do not have to bother by the sensitivity of prior distributions) but, as we are just going to see, prior distributions yield some modeling advantages to the Bayesian approach.

The modeling scheme in the left-hand side of Figure 2.3 is fairly general and lots of statistical models under the Bayesian approach, such as linear or generalized linear models, fulfill it. The modeling framework developed under the Bayesian approach goes far beyond the scheme just depicted. The layer with the prior distribution in that figure can be easily expanded so that a wider collection of models can be fitted. Namely, the mid-layer of the model, containing the variables to be fitted, could be split into several more layers where some of the variables hierarchically depend on other new variables, which finally depend on the fixed parameters of their prior distributions. This defines a very flexible modeling framework where some variables play the role of data for other variables and, conversely, some variables define the prior structure of some other variables in the model. These models, where the variables are not placed in just a single layer, but they form a complex hierarchical structure, are known as *hierarchical models*.

This new wider modeling framework makes it possible to tune models to the data's needs easily. For example, in the case of a Normal linear model where the homoscedasticity hypothesis did not hold (the variance of data around the regression line was not constant), hierarchical modeling could provide some solutions. If the variance of data was found to depend on, for example, the same covariate(s) used to explain their mean, we could model that variance as a function of that same covariate(s) and some other variables ($\boldsymbol{\gamma}$). The central column of Figure 2.3 shows the dependence structure corresponding to this model. Dashed lines in that figure correspond to the dependence relationships making the model hierarchical. Without them the model would just be a non-hierarchical model, as the model in the left-hand side of Figure 2.3. Those arrows have been drawn as dashed lines, because they can be both seen as a kind of data likelihood for $\boldsymbol{\gamma}$ and as part of the prior distribution of $\boldsymbol{\sigma}_y$.

As a second example of hierarchical model, turning back again to Example 2.1, Figure 2.1 seems to suggest that some rates show higher variability than others due to some unknown factor. In this case we could assume that the variance of every observation around the linear regression function may take two different values, depending if that rate is normal or if it is a kind of 'abnormal' rate with higher variability. In more statistical terms, the data would follow a mixture of two distributions of different variance. In that case it would not be enough to model the variability of data with a single variance, as usually done in Normal linear models. Therefore, it would be convenient to define a richer hierarchical structure where the variance of every observation depends on an unobserved binary underlying variable that classifies every year as normal or abnormal. This would clearly be another example of hierarchical model.

Thus, as just illustrated, hierarchical models make it possible to create tailored fits of any specific part of a model, adapting its performance to the data's needs. This modular feature of hierarchical models makes them particularly appealing and flexible tools. In this sense, as we read once (Baath, 2014), an appropriate parallel can be made between frequentist/Bayesian statistics and two well-known toys: Playmobil® and Lego®. Although this comparison may seem somewhat frivolous, in our opinion it perfectly reflects the main philosophy of hierarchical models. Baath points out: 'In some way, classical statistics (as it is usually presented) is a bit like Playmobil, everything is ready out of the box but if the box contained a house, there is no way you're going to turn that into a pirate ship. Bayesian statistics is more like Lego, once you learn how to stick the blocks together, the sky is the limit. That is, a frequentist linear model may be a great tool (frequently an unbeatable tool in computational terms) to analyze data, but it is not so straightforward to use it to model, let's say, the variance of another linear model. This is the reason why we adopt hierarchical models as the main proposal for developing the theory and study the examples in this book. The flexibility introduced by hierarchical models makes them a perfect tool to fit very different data sets incorporating very different sources of dependence.

Random effects are surely the main tool enabled by hierarchical models. It is hard to find a general definition of random effects because, as time has evolved, their intended use has also changed and definitions (and concepts) that could be suitable for them years ago, now would seem outdated. We will try to sketch the idea of random effects below starting with the following example.

Example 2.2

Let us suppose that we were interested in studying the prescription levels of a non-compulsory vaccine among a population of children. We expect those prescription levels to depend on the pediatrician who follows every child in the study. Pediatricians' advice may influence parents' decision on either vaccinating their children, or not. Therefore, our study assumes the following: Let V be a matrix of binary observations whose (i, j) element is equal to 1 if the j-th children of the i-th pediatrician has been vaccinated, and 0 otherwise. This corresponds to a balanced design where all pediatricians have the same number of children in the study; if this was not true, the model could be appropriately modified. We propose to model our data by means of a logistic regression as Bernoulli variables of probabilities depending on the corresponding pediatrician, i.e.,

$$v_{ij} \sim Bern(\pi_i), \ i = 1, ..., I, \ j = 1, ..., J.$$

Pediatricians' probabilities, in turn, are modeled as

$$logit(\pi_i) = \log\left(\frac{\pi_i}{1 - \pi_i}\right) = \theta_i, \ i = 1, ..., I.$$

Under a frequentist perspective, this would have been enough to carry inference out on $\boldsymbol{\theta}$ if we wanted to. Under a Bayesian perspective, we have to put a prior distribution on $\boldsymbol{\theta}$ so that inference can be performed. At this stage, a reasonable possibility would be to choose vague prior distributions for every element of $\boldsymbol{\theta}$ so that nothing interferes in the estimation of any pediatricians' effect. As pointed out in Section 2.1, this could be done by means of the following improper prior distributions

$$\theta_i \sim U(-\infty, \infty), \ i = 1, ..., I. \tag{2.2}$$

These prior distributions assume full independence for the components of $\boldsymbol{\theta}$. Moreover, the likelihood function is composed of several independent terms, each of them depending on just one component of $\boldsymbol{\theta}$. As a consequence, the posterior distribution of $\boldsymbol{\theta}$ may be expressed as a product of independent distributions corresponding to their different elements. That is, any two θ_i and θ_j with $i \neq j$ will have fully independent posterior distributions. Moreover, as the prior distribution of θ_i is completely flat for any i, showing no preference for any given value, the corresponding posterior distribution will be fully data-driven and will only depend on the data available on the patients of the i-th pediatrician.

Another alternative prior structure for $\boldsymbol{\theta}$ seems also reasonable. Since we are not particularly interested in estimating any specific pediatrician's effect (they are just a sample of pediatricians with no particular interest in any of them), the prior distributions in (2.2) may not be suitable since they were devised to estimate those effects without any external interference. Alternatively, we may consider pediatricians as random nuisance artifacts grouping the observations into clusters and making the inference on the general prescription level harder to be performed. In this case, we would not be interested in estimating specific pediatricians' effect but, on the contrary, we will pursue to incorporate and control their effect on the estimation of the general prescription level. In that case, the components of $\boldsymbol{\theta}$ would be realizations of a random mechanism inducing heterogeneity among practitioners and our model should reflect that. Thus, an alternative and more suitable prior structure reflecting this would be

$$\theta_i | \mu, \sigma \sim N(\mu, \sigma^2), \; i = 1, ..., I. \tag{2.3}$$

This prior distribution would reflect that all pediatricians' effects are random realizations of the same process, that we have assumed to be Normal, although this could be changed if needed. The Normal distribution in Expression (2.3) depends on two parameters that will be regarded as unknown since we do not find convenient to assume them fixed. Moreover, the prior distribution of $\boldsymbol{\theta}$ in (2.3) is not vague for two reasons. On one hand, we want to estimate the variability among practitioners so σ^2 should be treated as an unknown value instead of a large quantity expressing vagueness on $\boldsymbol{\theta}$. On the other hand, we do not intend to express full lack of knowledge on $\boldsymbol{\theta}$ with our prior, instead, we want to reflect that all their components have a common distribution since they are realizations of a common process which is itself unknown. These two reasons invite us to not be vague with the prior distributions of $\boldsymbol{\theta}$ but, on the contrary, to use the new prior structure that we have just proposed to learn about the corresponding underlying process.

Finally, to complete the formulation of this new prior structure, prior distributions should be given to both μ and σ^2 so that they can be estimated. It would also be admissible to put prior distributions on some transformations of these parameters since they will also implicitly define prior distributions on μ and σ^2 (by means of the change of variable theorem). Thus, bearing in mind that uniform vague prior distributions are usually put on standard deviations, we find it convenient to propose the following vague prior distributions for completing the model defined by Expression (2.3)

$$\mu \sim U(-\infty, \infty),$$

$$\sigma \sim U(0, \infty).$$

Expression (2.3) makes the model used to estimate the prescription level of the vaccine to be a hierarchical model. This seems evident according to the right-hand side of Figure 2.3, where the dependence structure of this model is shown. Namely, for this model the data depend on pediatricians' effects $\boldsymbol{\theta}$; these, in turn, depend on μ and σ^2 the unknown mean and variance of the prior distribution of $\boldsymbol{\theta}$; finally, μ and σ have their own prior distributions. That is, we can distinguish in that model three different layers, contrary to the non-hierarchical version of the model defined by the prior distributions of $\boldsymbol{\theta}$ introduced in Expression (2.2).

The example above illustrates the use of both fixed and random effects. Sometimes, we will be interested in controlling some effect in a study that cannot be modeled with a simple covariate because, basically, we do not have that variable available. In that case, what we only know about that factor is which are their levels (the groups defined by its values), but we do not have any more information on them. Nevertheless, we might be forced to include that factor in the analysis since we suspect that it may seriously condition its results. In this situation, we can model that effect ($\boldsymbol{\theta}$), in two different manners, as either fixed or random effects. *Fixed effects* modeling of a set of parameters considers them to have fully known prior distributions, independent of any unknown parameter in the model. Therefore, no inference is made on the prior distribution of $\boldsymbol{\theta}$. These priors will usually be independent and vague, although these two conditions are not necessary if they are not suitable for the data to be analyzed. One example of fixed effects modeling would be the prior modeling of $\boldsymbol{\theta}$ defined in Expression (2.2) since those prior distributions are fully known. On the other hand, a set of parameters is said to be modeled as *random effects* if a common prior distribution is used for all of them and inference is also made for that common distribution. One example of random effects modeling arises from Expression (2.3), where a common prior distribution is used, which is the main object of interest for that model. Models including random effects are usually called *mixed effects models* since they will also contain usually fixed effects, as for example the typical intercept term.

Random effects are a wonderful tool for putting in practice the aforementioned modularity of hierarchical models. They allow us to consider a submodel, within the whole model, to make inference or give a particular covariance structure to the set of parameters considered as random effects. This modularity enables hierarchical models to perfectly fit to the particular features that the data could have. However, modelers should not abuse this possibility. It is tempting to give extra flexibility to any component in the model putting a specific sub model to fit it, but this has a clear limit, *identifiability* of the parameters in the model. Identifiability is the property of some models by which they are able to learn about their parameters. Unidentifiable parameters in a model cannot be estimated because they are usually confounded with other parameters in the model playing a similar role. Therefore, identifiability is a typical problem of overparameterized models. We have often seen our students trying, for example, to define a single parameter in a model (instead of a vector of values) as a Gaussian random effect. Obviously, the underlying distribution of that variable assumed in the model will not be identifiable because you cannot reasonably estimate a distribution from a single observation, so treating that parameter as a random effect makes the model unidentifiable. Therefore, random effects should only be used for sets of variables (not for a single variable), with a similar role within the model, such as $\boldsymbol{\theta}$ in Example 2.2, otherwise it will make no sense to put a common prior distribution to all those variables. As a summary, random effects should be used with caution, only for sets of variables with a similar meaning and trying not to abuse their flexibility, bearing in mind that they are limited by identifiability.

Historically, random effects were originally devised with the meaning shown in Example 2.2; they are draws from a population and they are not of interest by themselves. Including them in the model makes it possible to induce several sources of variability on the outcome of the model, or quantify the percentage of variability explored by each of those sources. Obviously, more than one random effect could be considered within a model, yielding richer analyses and richer variance decompositions. Thus, under this primary conception, random effects are a tool mainly conceived for modeling and structuring the sources of variability underlying the data. Hodges (2013) names random effects conceived under this approach as *old-style random effects* according to its original conception.

Besides the old-style use of random effects, these have been increasingly used as a flexible way for modeling the mean of a process instead of a tool to model its variance; this is named by Hodges as the *new-style random effects*. Under this conception, random effects cannot be considered as random samples or sets of draws from a population. In fact, under this approach there will not be usually a real population, as for example pediatricians, to sample from. New-style random effects are sets of parameters in the model providing a smoothing device for the mean of a process, so they will not necessarily have a physical or real meaning. In this sense, we will now be interested in knowing the specific value of every level of the random effect since they will allow us to estimate the mean of the process that we want to estimate, although once again we will consider a common prior distribution for all of them. That prior distribution will be in this case of secondary interest as it will be just a smoothing device, penalizing anomalous values on $\boldsymbol{\theta}$ and therefore making the fit of the random effects more parsimonious. Thus, new-style random effects are devices for building parsimonious highly parameterized models, since they allow us to include a large number of parameters into our model while their common prior distribution avoids overfitting. A lot more insight on this definition of old- and new-style random effects can be found in Hodges (2013). New-style random effects will be the main modeling tool used in this book and hereafter we will find lots of examples of their use in disease mapping studies.

But, how do new-style random effects act as smoothing devices in regression studies? Random effects do not have vague prior distributions, on the contrary, they have common non-vague distributions to be estimated. This informative prior distribution constrains the estimates of the levels of the random effects, making them fit not only to data, but also to the informative distribution defined by the consensus of the random effects considered. That is, new-style random effects combine both sources of information: the data and that coming from the consensus of their components through their prior distribution. As usually said, random effects pool their strength in order to yield improved estimates, by sharing their information or, more specifically, the information on the population which they come from. Thus, any random effect estimate will not be only based on the data depending on that effect but also, indirectly, on the information of other data through the rest of random effects. In this sense, random effects will yield more parsimonious estimates than fixed effects since they are constrained by their prior distribution, and that distribution makes every estimate to be based on a higher amount of information.

We find it convenient to mention a last use of random effects of particular relevance for disease mapping. As just mentioned, the prior distribution of random effects has itself an effect on their estimates. Therefore, that prior distribution could incorporate any kind of dependence if it was considered appropriate. This makes random effect modeling as a suitable tool for modeling correlated data in general such as time series, point referenced spatial (geostatistical) data and obviously areal data. The incorporation of correlation in $\boldsymbol{\theta}$ is not possible in fixed effects models, unless that correlation was previously and fully known, i.e., it does not depend on any unknown parameter that we may want to learn of. But that scenario is a very rare exception; therefore, the main tool for modeling correlated data will be random effects. Hereafter, we will see lots of examples of how random effects are used to model correlated data throughout the rest of the book.

Example 2.3

We turn back once again to the data of Example 2.1 on the oral cancer mortality time trend in the Valencian Region. We are now interested in detecting any hypothetical non-linear component in that time trend that we could have missed in the previous analysis. We will consider now the following model: annual rates $\boldsymbol{y}$ are once again modeled as independent Normal variables given their means $\boldsymbol{\mu}$ and common variance σ, that is:

$$P(\boldsymbol{y}|\boldsymbol{\mu},\sigma) = \prod_{i=1}^{I} N(y_i|\mu_i, \sigma^2),$$

whose means have the following form

$$\mu_i = \beta_1 + \beta_2 x_i + \gamma_1 Z_{i1} + \ldots + \gamma_K Z_{iK},$$

or, expressed in a more compact, matrix-based, form

$$\boldsymbol{\mu} = \boldsymbol{X\beta} + \boldsymbol{Z\gamma}.$$

Matrix $\boldsymbol{X}$ contains the intercept and the centered year, the covariates used in the linear model of Example 2.1. The columns of $\boldsymbol{Z}$ are a set of functions belonging to a common family, used to model any non-linear variation that the time trend could show. That family of functions is usually named the *Basis of functions* in *Spline modeling* nomenclature, for example. For our particular analysis, we have defined the columns of $\boldsymbol{Z}$ as a set of Gaussian functions centered at a grid of points, the *nodes* of the Gaussian basis of functions. Thus, if a specific component of $\boldsymbol{\gamma}$ takes a positive value, respectively negative, the vector $\boldsymbol{\mu}$ will reproduce a positive, respectively negative, 'bump' around the node where the corresponding column of $\boldsymbol{Z}$ is centered. Note the convenience of the model proposed since it makes a linear-combination of non-linear functions so it is transforming a non-linear fit, which is usually problematic to be done, in a linear problem typically much more convenient from several points of view. This is the main underlying idea of models relying on bases of functions.

We have considered different numbers of elements in the basis $\boldsymbol{Z}$ to model the oral cancer time trend. In principle, it would be convenient to consider as many columns in $\boldsymbol{Z}$ as possible so that any non-linear feature (having bumps anywhere) could be reproduced at any moment of the period of study. However, considering more variables in the model than observations would introduce additional statistical problems in the analysis. So we will perform the analysis with two different choices for $\boldsymbol{Z}$. First, we will consider a $\boldsymbol{Z}$ matrix with 19 columns where every column corresponds to a Gaussian function (evaluated at each year of study) centered, respectively, from 1992 to 2010 and of standard deviation equal to 1. That is, the j-th column of $\boldsymbol{Z}$ will correspond to a Gaussian function centered at $1991 + j$, of standard deviation equal to 1, evaluated at every year of the period of study. This function will be basically non-zero only from $1991 + j - 2$ to $1991 + j + 2$, i.e., it is a quite low two standard deviations away from the mode of the corresponding Gaussian function. On the other hand, we have considered as second choice for $\boldsymbol{Z}$ a matrix with just 9 columns that correspond to Gaussian functions centered, respectively, at $\{1993, 1995, ..., 2009\}$. In this case we consider a standard deviation of 2 for these Gaussian functions since the nodes considered in this second matrix are more dispersed than those in the previous definition of $\boldsymbol{Z}$. Our intention is to assess the sensitivity of the model used to the election of these two bases of functions.

We set now exactly the same vague prior distributions for both $\boldsymbol{\beta}$ and σ as in Example 2.1. Moreover, we can model $\boldsymbol{\gamma}$ as a vector of either fixed or random effects. For the fixed effects modeling of $\boldsymbol{\gamma}$, we set the following prior distributions

$$\gamma_k \sim U(-\infty, \infty), \ k = 1, ..., K,$$

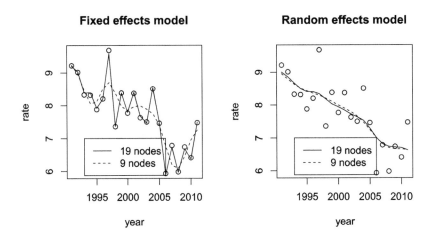

Figure 2.4
Non-linear fit of the oral cancer mortality time trend. Fits by means of both fixed and random effects for the parameters of the basis of functions are considered.

where K, the number of columns in $\mathbf{Z}$, will be either 9 or 19 depending on the basis of functions used. On the other hand, for the random effects modeling of $\boldsymbol{\gamma}$, we consider

$$\gamma_k \sim N(\mu_\gamma, \sigma_\gamma^2), \ i = 1, ..., K,$$

for some unknown values μ_γ and σ_γ^2 that we would be interested to estimate. For these parameters we choose the following vague prior distributions

$$\mu_\gamma \sim U(-\infty, \infty),$$

$$\sigma_\gamma \sim U(0, \infty).$$

Therefore, the random effects model will also make inference on the underlying distribution of this particular component of the model. That distribution is not of specific interest in our study since the random effects are not samples of some population that we could be particularly interested in. Nevertheless, that distribution plays an important role into the model, as it acts as a smoothing device yielding a parsimonious fit for the values of $\boldsymbol{\gamma}$. In contrast, the main interest in our model will be to estimate $\boldsymbol{\gamma}$ as reliably as possible since these values will determine the time trend that we seek to visualize. The random effects model improves the estimation of $\boldsymbol{\gamma}$ by allowing their components to share their information and making them share a common distribution. The vector $\boldsymbol{\gamma}$, when modeled as random effects, is a clear example of what Hodges calls new-style random effects, which are in charge of estimating the mean of the model instead of structuring its variance.

Figure 2.4 shows the fit obtained from both bases of functions modeled as fixed and random effects models. For the fixed effects modeling, both bases of functions produce very different results. Thus, the model with 19 nodes basically interpolates all the points since there are 21 points to be fitted and 21 parameters to model their means (β and γ). On the other hand, the model with 9 nodes is much more parsimonious due to its lower dimensionality (11 parameters for modeling the means, instead of 21). The main problem arising from the fixed effects modeling is how many nodes to use to fit the data since, as just shown, this is a very sensitive issue and we do not have clear criteria available to choose this number. On the contrary, on the right-hand side of Figure 2.4, random effects modeling shows a much more parsimonious behavior. Regardless of the number of nodes used, the fit obtained is closely similar, depicting subtle deviations from linearity.

Fixed effects modeling does not introduce penalty of any kind on the values of γ; therefore, as more terms are included in the model, the fitted trend reproduces the data more closely, regardless of whether these terms have a real explicative power or not. The vector γ simply takes the values that best fit the data, regardless if one specific γ_i could be completely crazy according to the values taken by the rest of the elements in γ. That is, for fixed effects modeling, the amount of variance explained by the fit is just a question of how many variables are introduced in the model. On the contrary, if γ is modeled as a vector of random effects, its prior distribution penalizes abrupt changes in the fitted trend since any γ_i should be in agreement with the rest of the values in γ, in accordance to their common prior distribution. This is a very reasonable hypothesis for many settings where the data should show smooth variations. In this case, if a new element was added to the basis of functions, it would not necessarily mean a substantial improvement in the fit, possibly avoiding overfitting of the data. Therefore, random effects modeling keeps a balance between the fit of the data and the fit of γ to its prior distribution, which is what makes the fit of this model more parsimonious than the fixed effects modeling.

The models fitted within this example have been run in `WinBUGS`, which will be introduced in the next chapter. Nevertheless, you can find the `R` and `WinBUGS` code used to undertake this analysis at the online accompanying material: `https://github.com/MigueBeneito/DisMapBook/tree/master/Example2_3`.

One last issue regarding Bayesian hierarchical models is *model selection*, which deals with the selection of the most appropriate model for fitting a data set. Model selection is a very technical field within Bayesian statistics in general, where extreme care has to be put into the choice of prior distributions (Berger and Pericchi, 2001). If an 'objective Bayesian' analysis is undertaken, model selection becomes a hard issue with lots of practical difficulties. For better or worse, some alternative criteria have been proposed in the applied literature for selecting models based on more informal criteria. Among all of these proposals, the *Deviance Information Criterion* (Spiegelhalter et al., 2002), usually known as just DIC, is the proposal of most common use in the literature. The use of this model selection criterion is not free of controversy, and several alternative criteria have been proposed with the same goal (Celeux et al., 2006; Gneiting and Raftery, 2007; Plummer, 2008; Cui et al., 2010; Watanabe, 2010). In fact, specific model selection and validation procedures have been proposed for disease mapping problems specifically (Stern and Cressie, 2000; Marshall and Spiegelhalter, 2003). However, it is not the aim of this book to discuss the particular benefits of DIC or some other criterion. Thus, when performing some model selection throughout the rest of the book we will base it on the DIC, as this is nowadays the most used criterion for this purpose, regardless of whether this is the most appropriate procedure or not.

DIC is a Bayesian analog of the frequentist *Akaike Information Criterion* (Akaike, 1973), known as AIC, so DIC is also defined as the sum of two terms. The first of them, the *deviance*, measures the lack of fit of the model; therefore, it is lower for those models that fit the data better. The second term is a complexity measure of the model, the *effective number of parameters*. Thus the DIC will be lower in those models with better fit and are less parameterized, as a consequence, those models with lower DIC will be in general preferred to those models with higher values of this criterion. The DIC is an adimensional measure, i.e., their values have only a relative meaning, since they have only sense when compared with DICs corresponding to other models. Nevertheless, as the proposers of DIC point out (Spiegelhalter et al., 2002), models with DICs within 3 units of the 'best' model (that one with lowest DIC) 'deserve consideration', models within 3 to 7 units have 'considerably less support' than the best model, and differences higher than 7 units point out the best model as being clearly better than other alternative models considered.

2.3   Markov Chain Monte Carlo computing

Without any doubt, Bayesian hierarchical models are an invaluable tool, making it possible to fit lots of models and taking any particularity of the data into account. However, such an interesting tool could be simply useless without a technique making inference possible in this setting. In fact, Bayesian hierarchical models had just a modest development until about 1990 when *Markov Chain Monte Carlo* techniques, usually known as simply MCMC, were introduced into the statistical literature (Gelfand and Smith, 1990). MCMC has undoubtedly made possible the explosive popularization of Bayesian hierarchical models.

The main inference tool for the frequentist approach is *maximum likelihood estimation* and some of its variants. Maximum likelihood estimates are those values of the parameters in a model that maximize the likelihood function, the probability of the observed data given the parameters of the model. These are the values of the parameters that are more in agreement with the observed data. Thus, for deriving the maximum likelihood estimates of $\boldsymbol{\theta}$, the vector of parameters of a model, we will 'just' have to maximize $p(\boldsymbol{y}|\boldsymbol{\theta})$ as a function of $\boldsymbol{\theta}$. In some situations, this may be a task harder than one could expect at a first glance; thus, for example, if the length of $\boldsymbol{\theta}$ is very long, let's say thousands of components, this is a particularly problematic setting. Regretfully, this is a very common setting in disease mapping studies.

Turning back to the Bayesian inference process outlined in Section 2.1, Bayesian inference on $\boldsymbol{\theta}$ is made by applying Bayes' theorem in the following way

$$p(\boldsymbol{\theta}|\boldsymbol{y}) = \frac{p(\boldsymbol{y}|\boldsymbol{\theta})p(\boldsymbol{\theta})}{p(\boldsymbol{y})}$$

the numerator of this expression is, for every value of $\boldsymbol{\theta}$, just the product of two known functions, the likelihood function and the prior distribution of the parameters, so this does not entail any particular problem to be computed. On the contrary, the term in the denominator had received little attention in Section 2.1, as it is just the proportionality constant without much importance for several mathematical purposes. Nevertheless, that term should be computed in order to fully know $p(\boldsymbol{\theta}|\boldsymbol{y})$, the posterior distribution of $\boldsymbol{\theta}$. As for any probability density function, the integral of the posterior distribution of $\boldsymbol{\theta}$ has to be equal to 1, therefore

$$1 = \int \cdots \int_{\Theta} p(\boldsymbol{\theta}|\boldsymbol{y})d\boldsymbol{\theta} = \int \cdots \int_{\Theta} \frac{p(\boldsymbol{y}|\boldsymbol{\theta})p(\boldsymbol{\theta})}{p(\boldsymbol{y})} d\boldsymbol{\theta} = \frac{\int \cdots \int_{\Theta} p(\boldsymbol{y}|\boldsymbol{\theta})p(\boldsymbol{\theta})d\boldsymbol{\theta}}{p(\boldsymbol{y})}$$

and thus,

$$p(\boldsymbol{y}) = \int \cdots \int_{\Theta} p(\boldsymbol{y}|\boldsymbol{\theta})p(\boldsymbol{\theta})d\boldsymbol{\theta} \qquad (2.4)$$

where Θ is the set of all possible values that $\boldsymbol{\theta}$ can take. Thus, in order to fully know the posterior distribution of $\boldsymbol{\theta}$, we are forced to calculate a multiple integral containing as many integrals as the length of $\boldsymbol{\theta}$. This is quite frequently a non-trivial mathematical task, particularly hard when the length of $\boldsymbol{\theta}$ is longer.

In summary, both the frequentist and Bayesian approaches find their particular mathematical obstacles, maximization and integration respectively, to carry inference out in statistical models. Both problems become particularly hard when the length of $\boldsymbol{\theta}$ is longer, a particularly common setting in disease mapping studies where we will have to estimate lots of quantities. Therefore, for both approaches, it would be very convenient to have alternative tools available that would make it possible to override the inference problems just described. Luckily MCMC provides a way to carry Bayesian inference out, overcoming the computation of the integrals in Expression (2.4).

Monte Carlo computing, in general, is a collection of mathematical methods performing hard mathematical tasks by means of simulation, i.e., drawing samples from the process of interest and using them to make conclusions. The specific goal in MCMC, which is indeed a Monte Carlo method, will be generating a sample of the posterior distribution of the variables in a model $p(\boldsymbol{\theta}|\boldsymbol{y})$, instead of deriving the mathematical expression of that posterior distribution solving the integrals therein. Statistical theory ensures that for large enough samples it would be mostly equivalent to dispose of the full posterior distribution of $\boldsymbol{\theta}$ or the mentioned sample, as any quantity of interest of that distribution could alternatively be computed as a function of the sample drawn. This is simply the main principle of statistical inference, deriving population knowledge from a random sample of that population. Thus, if we wanted to know the shape of the posterior distribution of a variable, we would just have to draw a large sample of that variable and plot it by means of, for instance, a histogram. If we wanted to estimate the posterior mean, or median, of a variable, we would just have to calculate the corresponding mean, respectively median, in our sample. If we wanted to know the probability of a variable to be higher than a specific value a, we would just have to calculate the proportion of elements in our sample higher than a. That is, whatever we want to estimate on $\boldsymbol{\theta}$, we will just have to compute its corresponding estimate in our sample and in this manner we will avoid calculating the problematic integrals in (2.4).

The term 'Markov chain' in MCMC methods is used as these do not draw independent samples of values from the posterior distribution but, on the contrary, they draw a *Markovian sample*. A Markovian sample is a set of sequential draws from a population where the probability of any value to be drawn at any step depends just on the value drawn in the previous step of the process. This sequential feature gives the term 'chain' to the sampled values, since we are drawing an ordered series of values instead of random independent draws. The main benefit of sampling Markov chains instead of independent samples of values is that, in general, the first case requires just assessing the probability of new draws in relation to the previous ones. In that comparison, the problematic $p(\boldsymbol{y})$ term of both draws cancels out and consequently the computation of that term is no longer required. This avoids the multiple integration problem that inference in Bayesian models showed.

We need to set up two issues in order to start up a Markov chain: (i) a collection of initial values $\boldsymbol{\theta}^{(0)}$ for the set of parameters to be sampled, and (ii) a mechanism that, given $\boldsymbol{\theta}^{(i)}$ for any iteration i, determines how to sample $\boldsymbol{\theta}^{(i+1)}$ depending just on $\boldsymbol{\theta}^{(i)}$, so that the Markovian property is accomplished. Regarding the initial state of the Markov chain $\boldsymbol{\theta}^{(0)}$, its values will be usually arbitrary, although we will introduce some more detailed guidelines below to generate them. Regarding the mechanism allowing us to sample $\boldsymbol{\theta}^{(i+1)}$ given $\boldsymbol{\theta}^{(i)}$, *Gibbs sampling* is by far the most common choice. The sampling of $\boldsymbol{\theta}^{(i+1)}$ given $\boldsymbol{\theta}^{(i)}$ may be difficult mainly if the length of $\boldsymbol{\theta}$ is long. For example, accept-reject methods may find difficulties for building adequate proposals

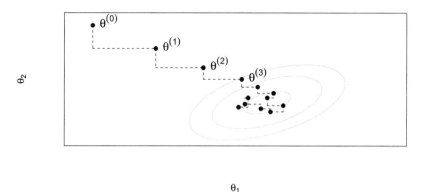

Figure 2.5
Sample of $p((\theta_1, \theta_2)|\boldsymbol{y})$ drawn by means of a Gibbs sampling algorithm.

with reasonable acceptance probabilities when the length of $\boldsymbol{\theta}$ is longer. Gibbs sampling enables to split the sampling of $\boldsymbol{\theta}^{(i+1)}$ into separate steps where, at every step, either a different component or a different block of components of $\boldsymbol{\theta}$ is sampled. Therefore Gibbs sampling makes it possible to decompose the complex task of sampling $\boldsymbol{\theta}^{(i+1)}$ given $\boldsymbol{\theta}^{(i)}$, into smaller and in principle simpler pieces.

Figure 2.5 illustrates the Gibbs sampling algorithm for simulating from the posterior distribution of the bidimensional variable $\boldsymbol{\theta} = (\theta_1, \theta_2)$. The gray ellipses show the high-density regions of the posterior probability of both parameters. As mentioned, $\boldsymbol{\theta}^{(0)} = (\theta_1^{(0)}, \theta_2^{(0)})$ is arbitrarily fixed so that the simulation has a point to start up and hence subsequent draws of the chain can be sampled. For sampling every new draw, two movements are made, one along the horizontal axis corresponding to the sampling step of θ_1 and afterwards a second step, along the vertical axis, corresponding to the sampling of θ_2. As can be appreciated, in a few simulations the Markov chain reaches the high-density region and, once there, it starts to move around that region. Note how the Markovian feature of the sample introduces dependence on the sample drawn. Thus, every iteration of the MCMC produces a value $\boldsymbol{\theta}^{(i+1)}$ nearby to $\boldsymbol{\theta}^{(i)}$. This makes it necessary to draw samples of the posterior distribution longer than could be expected so that the sample drawn was representative of the underlying posterior distribution.

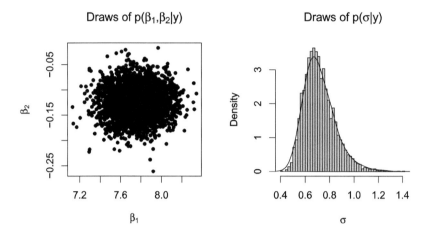

Figure 2.6
MCMC posterior draws of (β_1, β_2) (left) and histogram of the posterior draws of σ (right). The theoretical posterior distribution of σ has been overlaid on the histogram of the right-hand side of the figure.

Example 2.4

We turn back once again to Example 2.1. Due to the low dimensionality of that problem where inference was carried out for just 3 parameters, we did not require MCMC to obtain the posterior distributions in Figure 2.2. We resorted to numerical integration to calculate the integration constant $p(\boldsymbol{y})$. Nevertheless, we are now going to illustrate how MCMC-based inference could have alternatively been undertaken. The MCMC simulation in which this analysis is based was made in `WinBUGS`, which will be introduced in detail in the next chapter. However, you can find the R and `WinBUGS` code for this example at the online supplementary material.

A total of 5,000 samples were drawn from the posterior distribution of the parameters in the model. Figure 2.6 shows some results of the MCMC simulation. The left-hand side of that figure shows the sample drawn from $P((\beta_1, \beta_2)|\boldsymbol{y})$. A histogram of the values drawn for σ can also be seen on the right-hand side of Figure 2.6. The density function for σ estimated in Example 2.1 has also been overlaid on that histogram, where the close agreement between the MCMC results and those derived from numerical integration can be checked. Nevertheless, if a closer agreement was pursued, the MCMC sample could be increased as much as desired.

We have also calculated some posterior summaries of the parameters in the model from the MCMC samples drawn. For example, the posterior mean of

β_1 has been estimated to be 7.76 as the mean of the first component of the draws at the left-hand side of Figure 2.6. Likewise, we have also estimated the posterior median (7.76) and the 95% credible interval ([7.45,8.08]) for this same variable. It could also be interesting to assess the statistical 'significance' of the decreasing trend found. This could be assessed by the probability of β_2 being lower than 0 that, in turn, can be estimated by the proportion of posterior draws of β_2 in the MCMC sample that are lower than 0. Since all posterior draws of β_2 have been lower than 0, therefore $p(\beta_2 < 0|\boldsymbol{y})$ may be estimated as virtually 1. The direct calculation of any of these statistics (without the MCMC posterior sample) would require us to calculate as many integrals as there are variables in the model. On the contrary, as shown, the MCMC-based summaries are really straightforward to calculate once a posterior sample has been drawn. This makes MCMC inference very convenient, particularly when the number of variables in the model is higher.

To conclude our introduction to MCMC-based inference, we would like to mention a particular kind of algorithm that makes inference possible in very general settings. This family of algorithms is known as *trans-dimensional MCMC* and *reversible jump MCMC* (Green, 1995) is surely the most popular of these algorithms. Trans-dimensional MCMC algorithms allow sampling from models where 'the number of things you do not know is one of the things that you do not know' (Richardson and Green, 1997). Trans-dimensional MCMC can be applied for a wide variety of settings such as regression models where the model itself decides which covariates are included into the regression, mixture models with an unknown number of components, etc. As an example, in the regression setting just mentioned, trans-dimensional MCMC would move (or sample) between the different subsets of covariates of the whole original set with probabilities given by the posterior probability of every one of those subsets. Therefore trans-dimensional MCMC moves through the set of models considered, likewise as conventional MCMC algorithms move through the set of variables of a specific model. We will mention these algorithms several times throughout this book.

2.3.1 Convergence assessment of MCMC simulations

Although MCMC algorithms make it possible to carry inference out even in very complex hierarchical models, it introduces some additional practical problems that will be necessary to take care of. The assessment and checking of the absence of these problems in the samples drawn is commonly known as *convergence assessment* of the Markov chains. We are just going to briefly enumerate a collection of issues that should be kept in mind when assessing the correctness of an MCMC simulation, and we will also propose some potential solutions for each of them.

How to obtain a representative sample?

As mentioned, the values drawn with an MCMC algorithm are not independent samples from the corresponding posterior distribution but a Markovian
sample. This feature may hide some potential problems that would be convenient to discard. In the case that the posterior distribution of any of the
variables was multimodal, the Markov chain could get trapped in any of the
modes since visiting the rest of the modes would require going across low
probability regions that the Markov chain will try to avoid. This will make
the sample drawn to not be representative of the, supposedly sampled, real
posterior distribution. Likewise, if the Markov chain moves very slowly, we
could have the impression that it is moving along the full range of values of
the posterior distribution while it has just explored a small part of that distribution. Once again, this would make useless the MCMC sample drawn or,
even worse, it could lead us to wrong conclusions based on non-representative
samples.

A common solution to these problems is to simulate several independent
MCMC chains instead of just one. Running three chains is usually the default
choice for most MCMC analyses. These chains should be started at different
(preferably distant) starting points $(\boldsymbol{\theta}^{(0)})$. The performance of these chains
will make us aware of problems of the kind just mentioned. Specifically, if one
of the chains moves around a different set of values than the rest of the chains,
this could be a sign of either a slow convergence, since every chain would still
be moving around its initializing value, or severe multimodality, which makes
one of the chains get trapped in one of the modes of the distribution. On
the other hand, if chains are jumping between two or more sets of values,
this could be a sign of a multimodal posterior distribution, although with
modes not as disconnected as the previous case. These settings will invite us
to draw more values for our posterior samples than those initially expected,
or to devise a new MCMC algorithm suitable for those scenarios. If, on the
contrary, all chains considered mix up in a homogeneous manner, regardless
of their starting points, this would be a sign that all chains are visiting the
high-density region of the posterior distribution that they were expected to
explore.

How to remove the influence of $\boldsymbol{\theta}^{(0)}$?

When introducing MCMC, we mentioned that an initial set of values $\boldsymbol{\theta}^{(0)}$ was
needed to start any Markov chain. Moreover, for getting more confident on the
Markov chain to be representative of the full posterior distribution, it seems
advisable to run several Markov chains with distant starting points. Since
the starting points of the simulated chains are usually chosen in an arbitrary
manner and Markov chains generate sequences of dependent values, it may
take a while to get rid of the effect of the starting points used. The harmful
effect of the starting values seems evident in Figure 2.5 where the Markov

chain takes around 4 iterations to reach the core of the posterior distribution. These initial values have very low posterior probability and they should not be part of the posterior sample drawn, since they are just an artifact arising from the (arbitrary) location of $\boldsymbol{\theta}^{(0)}$. Therefore, it is usually convenient to remove the first samples drawn in any Markov chain to avoid this kind of artifacts. The initial samples to be removed in any Markov chain are known as *burn-in period* of the MCMC.

Regretfully, Figure 2.5 is just a synthetic example, and the burn-in period to be removed is usually much longer than just 4 draws of the posterior sample. Therefore, an obvious question arises here, how many iterations of the chain should be removed so that we get rid of the effect of the starting point of the Markov chains? One could be tempted to define a burn-in period as short as possible so that a minimum number of draws is wasted. However, that procedure is not very common. Once an MCMC process is coded and ready to be run, it is usually 'cheap' to generate reasonably large samples. Bayesians usually prefer the computer to do the dirty work (we are a bit lazy in this sense) and generate chains longer than in principle would be needed, with long burn-in periods too. Therefore, they do not have to bother too much deciding if that burn-in period is long enough or not.

Although very long chains were generated, there is a remaining question to be solved. What proportion of the chains would be convenient to be discarded as burn-in? It has been stated that burn-in periods comprising around one-half of the chains, or longer, are not reasonable (Carlin et al., 1998). Indeed, throwing away just the 1% or 2% of the chain has been claimed to be an advisable choice (Geyer, 1992). The reasoning for these short burn-in periods is that you need a long burn-in period to reach the core of the distribution sampled because the chain shows a large dependence (auto-correlation) between consecutive samples, which makes it move more slowly. In that case a long chain should also be sampled so that it is representative of the whole underlying distribution instead of exploring just a biased side of the distribution. For the rest of the book, we will usually take burn-in periods corresponding to approximately the 10% of the simulated chains, this should be enough even if the starting points of the chains were ridiculous, placed very far apart from the core of the distribution to be sampled. If this burn-in period was found to be insufficient, it would be advisable to simulate further, increasing both the length of the chains and the burn-in period in a similar proportion.

Although 10% of the chains as burn-in should suffice if the generated chains were long enough, it is convenient to have a tool for checking that all the simulations saved are already sampling the core of the posterior distribution. The *Brooks-Gelman-Rubin statistic* (Gelman and Rubin, 1992; Brooks and Gelman, 1998), usually known as simply the R-hat statistic, is an appropriate tool for this task. This statistic, for the first few draws saved of any parameter in the sample, divides the variance between chains by the mean variance within the chains, following the main idea of Analysis of Variance. If that statistic is substantially higher than 1, it would be a sign that the variance between chains is higher than that within chains. Thus, for the first iterations saved, the chains are too distant, which evidences that convergence was not already achieved. If, on the contrary, the Brooks-Gelman-Rubin statistic was close to 1, it would show that the distance between chains is in accordance with the inner variability of those chains, suggesting that convergence could already be achieved. For the rest of the book, we will require as convergence criteria that the Brooks-Gelman-Rubin statistic for all the parameters saved be lower than 1.1. In that case, we will consider that the burn-in period taken is appropriate and the draws saved are exploring the core of the posterior distribution from the very moment that they start to be saved.

How many iterations are required to simulate?

One obvious question when performing MCMC-based inference is, how many simulations (draws of the posterior distribution) should be run? MCMC simulations are afterwards used as elements of a sample that allows us to make inference on any feature of interest of the corresponding posterior distribution. Obviously, the more elements we have in this sample, the more accurate estimates we could make. However, iterating MCMC algorithms has a computationally (sometimes quite high) cost, which limits the number of samples of the posterior distribution that we can sample in practice. This number should be a compromise between these two criteria, the sample size needed to make appropriate inferences and the computational cost needed to generate them. We introduce below two criteria for determining a suitable number of iterations to be simulated.

First, we could guide the choice of that number by means of the *Monte Carlo error* of the parameters simulated, which is the error on the estimates arising from having a sample of the posterior distribution instead of fully knowing that distribution. The Monte Carlo error of any parameter is defined as the standard deviation of its estimated posterior mean (Geyer, 1992). If the MCMC sample drawn had independent values, the Monte Carlo error of any parameter would be $S/\sqrt{n}$, where S is the posterior standard deviation of the parameter (possibly estimated from the sample drawn) and n is the number of elements in the sample. Regretfully, MCMC produces dependent samples; therefore, this value should be corrected as a function of the auto-correlation of the chains (Carlin et al., 1998). Specifically, auto-correlation will increase the Monte Carlo error of any of the parameters since the chains will be of 'lower quality'. Therefore, Monte Carlo errors of parameters will usually depend on the posterior standard deviation of the parameter, the length of the chain(s) generated and the auto-correlation of the chain(s). Specific stopping criteria of MCMC simulations could be based on the Monte Carlo error of the parameters, such as requiring the Monte Carlo error of each variable in the model to be lower than 1% of the corresponding posterior mean. In that case, we would run the MCMC until those criteria are finally fulfilled.

A second alternative for setting the length of the simulation would be to base it on the *effective sample size* (Carlin et al., 1998). Let us assume that we were interested in estimating the posterior mean of every parameter in the model. If the MCMC generated independent draws of the posterior distributions, surely just 100 draws would be enough as to generate estimates of the parameters with a reasonable accuracy. A mean of a distribution should be, in general, reasonably estimated with 100 independent draws of that distribution. If we wanted to achieve a higher accuracy or to estimate some other quantities that are harder to be estimated, such as the 2.5% or the 97.5% quantiles, a higher number of values should be drawn, such as 1,000 or maybe more. This is very convenient criteria, since we can have some intuition about if a reasonable estimate can be derived, or not, from a given sample of independent values. Nevertheless, as MCMC samples are dependent, it would be convenient to know, if possible, how many independent values would our dependent sample be equivalent to. Obviously, if a chain of length n had mostly independent values, that sample would be mostly equivalent to an independent sample of length close (although slightly lower) to n. On the contrary, if the same chain showed large auto-correlation, it would be equivalent to a sample of m independent values, with m much lower than n. The effective sample size is a statistic with just this interpretation, the size of an independent sample that our Markov chain would be equivalent to. Specifically, this statistic is defined as:

$$n/\left(1 + 2\sum_{k=1}^{K^*} \rho(k)\right),$$

where $\rho(k)$ is the k-th order auto-correlation of the Markov chain, n its length and K^* a value such that $\rho(k)$ is basically 0 for $k > K^*$. In general, we will assess during the rest of the book the appropriateness of the length of Markov chains according to the effective sample size. We will typically require the effective sample size of any parameter in the model to be higher than 100, although this value could be increased sometimes if it was found not to be appropriate.

How to reduce the auto-correlation of a Markov chain?

We are sure that, at this moment, readers will have already realized that dependence on the Markov chains is a serious drawback. That dependence is usually measured by means of the auto-correlation of the Markov chains generated. Therefore, we will pursue to simulate chains with auto-correlations as close to 0 as possible. Auto-correlations of Markov chains will mainly depend on the algorithms used to generate them. The scope of this book does not allow us to change the MCMC algorithms used to sample from a model, since we will mainly rely on either tools generating their own MCMC algorithms by themselves or tools directly avoiding MCMC sampling. Fortunately we will have some other tools to try to modify the auto-correlation of the chains in case that we opt for MCMC sampling.

The first, naive but very useful, procedure for reducing auto-correlation in Markov chains is known as *thinning*. This procedure is adequate for problems where posterior samples are generated at a high speed. Since Markov chains depend on just the actual value to generate the next one, the dependence between the i-th and the j-th value of the chain will vanish as $|i-j|$ increases. As a consequence, thinning consists of saving, sequentially, just 1 out of every n draws generated, throwing away the simulations between them. This will not improve the MCMC algorithm; indeed it would be exactly the same as that used for deriving the unthinned chains, but it will certainly decrease their auto-correlation. The cost of thinning is paid by increasing the computing time of the algorithm since for generating a sample of 1,000 draws, with for example a thin of 10 steps (1 out of 10 iterations is saved), the MCMC process will have to generate 10,000 values; therefore, it should be run for a period 10 times longer. We mentioned previously that Bayesians are a bit lazy with MCMC-related issues and this is not an exception. Hence the inefficient decision of decreasing auto-correlations by means of thinning is usually taken, as its cost is assumed by computers. Therefore, this is usually an appropriate cost/effective decision. Thinning implies a second advantage that should not be overlooked; if we wanted to reach a specific effective sample size in an MCMC sample with high auto-correlation, we should save lots of iterations of the MCMC process to achieve our goal. This will cause wasting a high amount of memory in our computers that could be saved by simply thinning the simulated chains. For a thinned sample, it would be usually enough to store thousands of simulations, while for an unthinned sample achieving a similar accuracy could imply to save maybe millions of runs. This makes thinning to be a very frequent procedure in MCMC sampling in general.

Since thinning leaves the main burden of decreasing auto-correlation to computers, this discards it as an option when the MCMC algorithm used to sample from the posterior distribution is slow. In this case, throwing away a lot of costly simulations does not seem to be a clever, neither sometimes a suitable, choice. Therefore, in that case, it would be convenient to decrease auto-correlations by resorting to some alternative procedure. Since, in general, we will not have a direct control of the MCMC algorithms used throughout the rest of the book, our only chance to change the algorithms used will be to reformulate/reparameterize the model in an equivalent manner that could possibly be sampled with a different MCMC algorithm.

An example of reformulation leading to a different MCMC algorithm would be the following. Let's go back to the random effects model in Example 2.2. There, the logit of the probability for every pediatrician was modeled as Normal variables ($\boldsymbol{\theta}$) of mean μ and variance σ^2. A simple equivalent statement of that formulation would be to define those logits as $\mu + \eta_i$ where $\eta_i \sim N(0, \sigma^2)$, $i = 1, ..., I$. It is evident that $\theta_i = \mu + \eta_i$, $i = 1, ..., I$; therefore, both formulations are equivalent. However, in practical terms they are not so equivalent. In the original formulation of the model, μ appeared only at $\boldsymbol{\theta}$'s distribution and at its own prior distribution. This makes the conditional posterior distribution of μ (the distribution used to sample from this parameter by means of Gibbs sampling) to depend on, just $\boldsymbol{\theta}$ and μ's hyperparameters. On the contrary, for the second formulation, the data $\boldsymbol{V}$ depend directly on μ between other parameters. As a consequence, the conditional posterior distribution of μ in this case directly depends on the data, in contrast to the previous formulation of the model. As a consequence, the Gibbs sampling step for μ in both models will be different and these two different algorithms could show very different convergence properties. So, in case that one of these formulations did not work well (auto-correlations of their chains were very high), a reformulation of the model could alleviate the convergence problems that we are trying to get rid of.

Reparameterizing statistical models can be a very technical task if a mathematical justification of the superiority of an MCMC algorithm is pursued. Therefore those mathematical arguments in very complex models are usually left out and reparameterization becomes an empirical art more than a science. Nevertheless, a useful tool for reparameterizing models is the exploration of the *cross-correlation* of the chains sampled. Cross-correlations are just the correlations of the chains for any pair of variables sampled. Those pairs of variables with a cross-correlation particularly high (close to 1) or low (close to -1) will point out to us candidate sets of variables to be reparameterized in order to improve the convergence of the model, since they are possibly confounded with the current formulation of the model.

For illustrating the use of cross-correlations between chains, we go back to the random effects model of Example 2.2. Let us assume that the pediatrician's random effects in that model were defined as: $\theta_i \sim N(\mu_1+\mu_2, \sigma^2)$ with $\mu_1, \mu_2 \sim N(0, 100^2)$. That is, μ in the original model, has been substituted by $\mu_1 + \mu_2$. Now μ_1 and μ_2 will be just two variables adding up μ, but this is not enough to identify their values since an increase of δ units in the estimation of μ_1 can be compensated by a decrease of δ units in μ_2, and vice versa. Therefore, these two values cannot be identified within the model. This will yield a cross-correlation for these two variables very close to -1 since any increase in any of them will be compensated with a decrease in the other one; therefore, both chains will reproduce opposite paths. This lack of identifiability, or other weaker pathologies in the model's formulation, could be highlighted by means of the cross-correlation matrix corresponding to all the pairs of variables in a model.

Example 2.5

We are going back once again to Example 2.1, now to illustrate some convergence issues of MCMC-based inference. We have changed the prior distributions of β_1 and β_2 in that example to $p(\beta_1) = p(\beta_2) = t_2(0, 1,000^2)$, i.e., a t distribution with 2 degrees of freedom, mean 0 and standard deviation 1,000. We could argue that we have proposed this alternative prior because this new distribution is more robust (insensitive to the presence of anomalous observations), but this would not be true. We have changed it because the MCMC step used to sample from β_1 and β_2 in WinBUGS (the software used for this example) is less refined for the t_2 prior distribution than for the Normal prior distribution for this example where the data likelihood is also Normal.

First, we have carried out the MCMC-based analysis of the mentioned model with the t_2 prior distributions. We have run 3 separate chains, with a burn-in period of 500 iterations followed by 5,000 additional iterations per chain. All three Brooks-Gelman-Rubin R-hat statistics for β_1, β_2 and σ are equal to 1,001; therefore, the burn-in period taken seems appropriate for all of them. The effective sample sizes for these parameters are 15,000; 15,000 and 5,300; respectively. Therefore, the dependence of the chains for β_1 and β_2 is negligible since its effective sample size (leaving the effect of auto-correlation out) is equal to the size of the posterior sample drawn. On the contrary, dependence makes the effective sample size for σ lower than the number of samples drawn. Nevertheless, that effective sample size perfectly allows us to carry inference out also on this parameter. With a sample of 5,300 independent values, we can perfectly estimate the mean, median, 2.5% quantile or any other reasonable statistic that we could be interested in. The upper-left hand side of Figure 2.7 shows the *history plot* of all three chains simulated for β_1, i.e., the x-axis stands for the number of iterations saved per chain and the y-axis stands for the values sampled at the corresponding iterations. Each of the three chains has been plotted in a different level of gray; all of them are indistinguishable and are perfectly mixed, resembling independent draws of the corresponding posterior distribution. Therefore, the convergence achieved for this model is completely satisfactory.

As a second step, we have run the same model as before but with the raw year of study (without previous centering) as a covariate. First, we have run the MCMC with exactly the same specifications (iterations, burn-in, etc.) than with the centered covariate (Example 2.1). Since except for β_1 and β_2 prior distributions the new model is exactly the same as that with the centered covariate, we would expect a similar performance of the MCMC in this new setting. However, the Brook-Gelman-Rubin's R-hat statistics are now 46.3, 46.3 and 3.4 for β_1, β_2 and σ, respectively, and the corresponding effective sample sizes are 3, 3 and 4. All these convergence statistics clearly point towards a deficient performance of the MCMC simulation carried out. The upper-right-hand side of Figure 2.7 shows the history plot of the 3 simulated chains for β_1 in this new setting. Differences in the quality of the chains in this and the previous simulation are completely evident. The new chains show extreme auto-correlation and the burn-in period is clearly insufficient since none of the three chains go across any other during the simulated period.

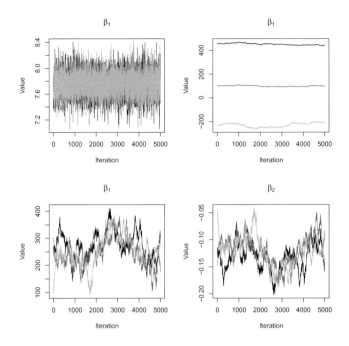

Figure 2.7
History plots of some parameters of the MCMC analyses carried out. Each line in each plot corresponds with each of the three chains simulated.

Finally, we have run once again the model with the uncentered year but with a burn-in period of 200,000 simulations, followed by further 2,000,000 simulations. Since saving such a huge amount of highly correlated draws does not seem practical, we have thinned the simulated chains saving just 1 out of every 400 simulations, thus the number of iterations saved per chain is 5,000($=2,000,000/400$), the same as in the two previous analyses. The history plot corresponding to this simulation for β_1 is shown at the lower-left side of Figure 2.7. For this new simulation, the Brooks-Gelman-Rubin's statistics for β_1, β_2 and σ are, respectively, 1.07, 1.07 and 1.00 and the number of effective simulations are 34, 34 and 15,000. Therefore, even for 2 million iterations, the convergence parameters of the MCMC indicate just a modest performance, and much more iterations would be needed to carry a reasonable inference out.

The lower-right plot of Figure 2.7 shows the history plot of β_2 for this last MCMC simulation. This plot points out some clues that may help us explain why the use of the non-centered covariate worsens the MCMC performance that much. When comparing the two lower plots of Figure 2.7, one may realize that the chains in both plots follow opposite paths, i.e., an increase in one of those variables is compensated for by a decrease in the other one, and vice versa. Indeed, the chains for both variables show a negative correlation of -0.999995 corroborating this sensation. This is telling us that both variables are closely dependent and maybe a way to make them more independent could improve the performance of the MCMC. Variable β_1 denotes the expected rate when the covariate takes 0 as value, that is the year 0 b.c. in the uncentered model. Therefore, a slight change in the estimation of β_2, the slope of the regression line, will have a large impact of β_1 since this corresponds to a year placed very far away of the observed data. An obvious way to disentangle this dependency would be to put the intercept of the regression line at the middle of the cloud of points modeled, instead of placing it at a far extreme. This is exactly what we made centering the covariate or, from a more statistical point of view, we orthogonalized the columns of the design matrix of the model. This explains the huge differences in the MCMC performance of both settings, being the use of the centered covariate much better than the uncentered one. Strategies of this kind should be kept in mind for improving MCMC performance whenever possible.

Exercises

1. The following data correspond to the number of epileptic seizures observed for a series of patients for a one-year follow-up period: {1,1,3,0,3,3,2,4,1,4}.

   - Pose a Bayesian model for estimating the annual expected number of seizures λ per patient. Assume a vague gamma prior distribution for the expected annual number of seizures having, in principle, a small influence on the corresponding posterior distribution.

   - Derive the posterior distribution of λ.

   - Calculate the posterior mean, median and mode of λ.

   - Assume now the following prior distribution (Pareto(1,1)) for λ:
   $$P(\lambda) = \begin{cases} 0 & \forall \lambda < 1 \\ \lambda^{-2} & \forall \lambda \geq 1 \end{cases}$$

   Derive the posterior distribution for this new prior and assess the practical problems that entail choosing this non-conjugate prior distribution for deriving the corresponding posterior distribution.

3

Some essential tools for the practice of Bayesian disease mapping

This chapter introduces the main tools needed to put Bayesian disease mapping in practice for those readers without previous experience in this field. These tools will be extensively used throughout the rest of the book; therefore, it is essential that all readers get used to the software introduced in this chapter.

In this chapter we are going to highlight the basic tools of the Bayesian disease mapping practitioner. These tools are going to be introduced as follows: First, Section 3.1 introduces the reader to WinBUGS, the main tool for performing MCMC inference from the Bayesian paradigm and also the main tool to be used throughout this book. Section 3.2 introduces INLA, a novel tool for carrying out inference in Bayesian models with some computational advantages as it does not rely on MCMC simulation. INLA has been the focus of attention of many Bayesian hierarchical model practitioners for the last few years, which is why we are also going to devote some attention to it throughout the book. Section 3.3 will introduce inexperienced readers to plotting maps in R, a key tool for spatial analysts. Finally, Section 3.4 introduces some additional tools and R packages of particular importance for disease mapping.

3.1 WinBUGS

WinBUGS is a software specifically designed to carry MCMC inference out in Bayesian hierarchical models. For any statistical model there are several, or more precisely, a lot of MCMC algorithms, making it possible to draw posterior samples of the parameters in that model. The specific development and coding of any of those algorithms for a particular statistical model is beyond the scope of this book, in fact there are lots of books exclusively devoted to that goal (see, for example, Gilks et al. (1996); Gamerman and Lopes (2006); Robert and Casella (2009)). Coding of MCMC algorithms is rarely a trivial task; it usually requires considerable effort and is prone to host errors. WinBUGS avoids all that process since, for a given statistical model, it develops and codes a suitable MCMC algorithm for sampling from the corresponding posterior distribution.

WinBUGS (Lunn et al., 2000) is the Windows version of the program BUGS, which is the acronym for Bayesian inference Using Gibbs Sampling. BUGS contains both a programming language suitable for coding Bayesian hierarchical models and an inner engine in charge of developing MCMC algorithms to sample from those models. The last WinBUGS version is 1.4.3, which dates back to 2007, and, regretfully, no one is currently in charge of maintaining or developing this software any longer. Nevertheless, WinBUGS keeps being nowadays a tool of current use with a large community of active users.

WinBUGS is free and can be downloaded from http://www2.mrc-bsu.cam.ac.uk/bugs/winbugs/contents.shtml. When installing WinBUGS, one should not forget to also install the patch upgrading WinBUGS to the 1.4.3 version and the key with the full license that allows running models with more than 100 nodes (data/variables). Please, pay attention to these two issues, fully described at the mentioned web page, otherwise you will have problems in the near future. WinBUGS also runs in other operating systems beyond Windows. In that case you will need some auxiliary software, such as WINE (http://www.winehq.org/) to make it work. If you search the terms "WINE" and "WinBUGS" on the Internet you will find lots of web pages describing how to set it all up in order to make them work.

There are several alternatives to WinBUGS available, such as OpenBUGS or JAGS, that can be considered as parallel implementations of the BUGS language, with their own MCMC engines. OpenBUGS is intended to be an open version of WinBUGS with slight changes and almost identical menus and appearance; therefore, most of the things that will be introduced below will also be valid for OpenBUGS. However, in our experience, even nowadays WinBUGS seems to be more efficient and robust than OpenBUGS; therefore, we will limit our focus to WinBUGS. As mentioned, JAGS is also a second alternative to WinBUGS although, in this case, with some more differences (JAGS does not have the same Windows-based look as WinBUGS). Nevertheless, both tools share most of the BUGS programming language, which is why users of one of them should be in general able to reproduce their models in the other one. Although JAGS is a serious alternative to WinBUGS that deserves to be kept very much in mind, it has serious limitations for disease mapping practitioners: it lacks specific spatial distributions, which are the basic tools for disease mapping. For this reason, we will not pay more attention to JAGS during the rest of the book regardless of its appeal to Bayesian modelers in general.

WinBUGS is a very powerful inference tool; it is able to simulate from most Bayesian hierarchical models that you could think about. WinBUGS does not limit itself to a prebuilt list of models; on the contrary, it makes available at the user's disposal a blank page so that users may write any model that one could be considering. In this sense, it is something similar to R. This freedom makes most new users of this software feel somewhat uncomfortable the first time they use it. A blank page is something very rude for someone who does not have a clear idea what to do with it. Moreover, a blank page is a place very prone to put nonsense, so extreme care should be taken when building our models in that page. As mentioned, for better or worse, WinBUGS is able to sample from almost any syntactically correct model, regardless of whether it is senseless, its prior distributions are awkwardly informative, or it does not really reproduce the statistical process underlying the data. As a consequence, it is relatively easy to produce misleading answers from WinBUGS analyses. This has made some experienced Bayesian users advise against the use of WinBUGS, mainly for newcomers in the Bayesian approach, since the simplicity in the implementation of models makes it a dangerous tool in unexperienced hands. In our opinion, this is an excessively narrow point of view, although we would suggest to be extremely cautious when using this powerful tool. In the end, although cars are indeed potentially dangerous devices, people have not refused to use them just because of that reason.

Contrarily, WinBUGS has made Bayesian hierarchical models popular for most non-specialized Bayesian users. WinBUGS lets the user take care of introducing the corresponding model there, since WinBUGS will be in charge of performing all the MCMC algorithmic stuff that non-technical users will generally prefer to leave aside. Besides, the blank page which WinBUGS makes available for building models makes it a very general tool and the perfect place to assemble the pieces of hierarchical models together. In this sense WinBUGS is the flexible tool that we need for implementing the large number of models proposed in this book.

3.1.1   The BUGS language

We are going to start this introduction to WinBUGS by describing the main features of the BUGS language. This language allows us to introduce the statistical models that we found suitable for analysing our data into WinBUGS. Although this introduction to BUGS is quite extensive, it is not intended to be a complete introduction to the whole language; specifically, we will just introduce those elements that will be later used in any of the models illustrated in the rest of the book. For those readers wanting to become WinBUGS advanced users, we strongly advise them to carefully read the user manual in the 'help' menu of WinBUGS where they will find full details on its use.

Statistical models in BUGS have three kinds of components that we will call in general hereafter *nodes*. Namely, nodes are divided in stochastic, constant and deterministic nodes. As you can already guess, when talking about Bayesian statistics, stochastic (random) nodes are the main elements of models. Everything that we want to learn of in a Bayesian model (that is, every parameter in a model) is a stochastic node, with its own prior distribution that should be specified in the model and with an unknown posterior distribution that we would like to learn of. In BUGS, even observed data are considered stochastic (although known) nodes, since they are observed draws of a random process defined by the data likelihood. Likewise, missing data are also

Distribution	WinBUGS syntax	Parameters
Normal	x~dnorm(mu,tau)	mu=mean, tau=precision
Uniform	x~dunif(a,b)	a=lower limit, b=upper limit
Gamma	x~dgamma(a,b)	a=shape, b=rate
Poisson	x~dpois(lambda)	lambda=mean=variance
Binomial	x~dbin(p,n)	p=probability, n=# of trials
Improper uniform	x~dflat()	-

Table 3.1
WinBUGS syntax for some common distributions.

stochastic nodes, since they are just (unknown) draws of the data likelihood. It is compulsory to assign a distribution to any stochastic node in a model. For the data and missing values, this distribution is the data likelihood and for any other unknown parameter in the model it will be its prior distribution. Distributions are assigned to stochastic nodes in BUGS by means of the ~ operator. Thus, variable~distribution(...) would be the appropriate syntax for assigning distribution to the stochastic node variable. Table 3.1 shows the syntax used for assigning some common specific distributions. Thus, being more precise, x~dnorm(mu,tau) will mean that the stochastic node x follows a Normal distribution of mean mu and precision (inverse of its variance) tau. Note that Normal distributions are parameterized in BUGS as a function of its precision, instead of its variance, in contrast to the convention that we will use throughout the whole book.

Constants are the second kind of nodes in BUGS. Constants are fixed and known quantities that the data, through the data likelihood, or the stochastic nodes, through their prior distribution, depend on. Specifically, covariates in regression models or the fixed parameters of prior distributions (if they are not fixed; otherwise, they would be stochastic nodes) are the clearest examples of constants in BUGS. Constants will have to be given to the model jointly with the observed data.

Finally, *deterministic components*, the third kind of elements in BUGS models, are logical functions of other nodes in the model. Since deterministic nodes typically depend on stochastic nodes in the model, they are simply transformations of stochastic variables and therefore they have their own associated distributions but, contrary to stochastic nodes, given the rest of the parameters in the model they are no longer stochastic. Deterministic nodes are defined in BUGS by means of the operator <-. As an example, we mentioned above that Normal variables in BUGS are parameterized in terms of their precision, but standard deviations are more intuitive than precisions for summarizing the corresponding variabilities. In the case of being interested in obtaining the posterior distribution of the standard deviation of a Normal variable with precision tau, we would just have to include in our model a sen-

WinBUGS syntax	Mathematical function
`exp(e)`	$\exp(e)$
`log(e)`	$\log(e)$
`logit(e)`	$\text{logit}(e)$
`step(e)`	$\{1, \text{ if } e \geq 0;\ 0,\text{ otherwise}\}$
`pow(e1,e2)`	$e1^{e2}$
`equals(e1,e2)`	$\{1, \text{ if } e1 = e2;\ 0, \text{ otherwise}\}$
`sum(v[])`	$\sum_i v_i$
`sd(v[])`	standard deviation of $\mathbf{v}$
`inprod(v1[],v2[])`	$\mathbf{v1}' \cdot \mathbf{v2}$
`inprod2(v1[],v2[])`	$\mathbf{v1}' \cdot \mathbf{v2}$
`inverse(m[,])`	$\{\mathbf{m}^{-1}:\ \mathbf{m} \text{ symmetric and positive-definite}\}$

Table 3.2
`WinBUGS` syntax for the most common mathematical functions. Variables starting with `e` stand for scalars, those starting with `v` for vectors and those starting with `m` for matrices.

tence as `StDev<-pow(tau,-0.5)`, where the `BUGS` function `pow(a,b)` stands for a^b. For writing mathematical expressions in logical functions, we have the elemental mathematical operations `+,-,*,/` available. Besides, Table 3.2 introduces the mathematical functions that will be used throughout the rest of the book. Table 3.2 is not an exhaustive list of `BUGS` functions, which can be found in the `WinBUGS` User Manual (Spiegelhalter et al., 2002).

In summary, nodes in `BUGS` are necessarily stochastic, constant or deterministic. In the first case, they will necessarily have a distribution assigned by the `~` operator; in the second case, they will have to be provided as data for the model (`NA` if some of them were a missing value); or, if they were deterministic, they will have to be assigned a mathematical expression by means of the `<-` operator. As a consequence, if one node in a `BUGS` model does not have either a value, a distribution or a mathematical expression assigned, the model will be incomplete, and obviously misspecified, producing a syntax error.

The `BUGS` language is case-sensitive, so you will have to pay attention to your uppercase/lowercase letters. Models in `BUGS` start with the word `model` and are put within curly braces, i.e., the syntax `model{...}` will contain the syntax of the statistical model that we are interested to fit. Hereafter, three dots within an expression will denote some part of a model, or an output, that is not essential for the issues discussed at that moment. Comments can be inserted within a `BUGS` syntax preceded by the symbol `#`. One of the most striking features of the `BUGS` language for newcomers is that, in contrast to for example R, when specifying a model, the order of the expressions in the model does not matter. That is, you can choose to introduce, for example, the prior distributions in your model (in whatever order) and afterwards the data likelihood; or, conversely, you can introduce the data likelihood first if you prefer it instead. WinBUGS will consider them as two exactly equivalent models.

BUGS admits the use of scalars, vectors, matrix and arrays as node containers. The algebra for this kind of objects is very similar to that used in R, thus v[1] means the first element of vector v, m[1:3,1] means the first three rows of the first column of matrix m and a[1, ,] stands for the matrix with all the elements of the three-dimensional array a whose first dimension is equal to 1. In contrast to R, most operations on vectors, matrices and arrays in BUGS have to be done element-wise, thus expressions like w<-v+1 for a vector v or mat<-m1+m2 for two matrices m1 and m2 are invalid and they have to be performed, instead, for each of the elements of the corresponding vector, matrix or array. Anyway, Table 3.2 shows some exceptions to this rule since it contains some functions operating on vectors or matrices as a whole. Thus, whenever we have to refer to a whole vector or matrix in these functions, we will have to put its name followed by empty brackets to make it clear that we are referring to the whole vector or matrix. Otherwise, if we wanted to apply that function to a subset of that vector or matrix we will have to specify the indexes defining the corresponding subset. So, sum(v[1:3]) or solve(m[,]) will be valid BUGS expression, meanwhile solve(m), for example, will not.

As a result of the number of element-wise operations used in BUGS syntaxes, the for sentence will be frequently used for defining statistical models. The syntax of this function is the same as in R, thus, for defining a loop sequence for every value of i ranging from 1 to n, one should write for(i in 1:n){...}. Therefore, for example, the vectorial expression above w<-v+1 should be coded in WinBUGS as: for(i in 1:n){w[i]<-v[i]+1}.

Example 3.1

Let us consider the following setting: for the last five observed years of Example 2.1, we are interested in estimating the (assumedly common) annual oral cancer mortality rate, per 100,000 people, during that period. We now have available the observed deaths (and populations) for each year, that we consider to follow independent binomial distributions depending on a common probability

$$o_i \sim Bin(p, Pop_i), \quad i = 1, ..., 5.$$

The only unknown value in this model is the probability of dying of oral cancer (p), that we have proposed to follow a uniform distribution between 0 and 1. The following code corresponds to the BUGS syntax reproducing that model

```
model{
 p~dunif(0,1)
 rate<-100000*p
 o[1]~dbin(p,Pop[1])
```

```
o[2]~dbin(p,Pop[2])
o[3]~dbin(p,Pop[3])
o[4]~dbin(p,Pop[4])
o[5]~dbin(p,Pop[5])
}
```

As it can be appreciated, all variables in this model, either observed (**o**) or not (*p*), have a probability function assigned, by means of the ~ operator. We can also distinguish a deterministic node, `rate`, which is just a transformation of the stochastic node *p* assigned by the <- operator. The parameters 0 and 1 of the uniform distribution of *p*, or the vector **Pop** of populations, are constants in the model. The vector **Pop**, as well as the vector of observed values **o**, will have to be given later to the model as data.

According to the considerations made on the BUGS language, the syntax above would be completely equivalent to the following, more polished, reexpression of the model

```
model{
 #Data likelihood
 for(i in 1:5){
  O[i]~dbin(p,Pop[i])
 }

 #Prior distributions
 p~dunif(0,1)

 #Derivation of the common mortality rate
 rate<-100000*p
}
```

In this new version of the model, the order of the sentences seems more logical, although the order in the previous model is perfectly valid. Comments help to read the code better and the use of the `for` function avoids having to specify the data likelihood with a lot of different sentences. Beyond this, and other similar, toy examples the use of the `for` function becomes completely necessary for, at least, specifying data likelihoods, usually comprehending lots of univariate distributions, one for each observed data. Finally, note how the data likelihood is defined element-wise. Vectorial expressions like o~dbin(p,Pop) that would possibly be valid for R are not valid within the BUGS language.

Some of the functions in Table 3.2 deserve particular comments. Thus, the `log()` and `logit()` functions are somewhat particular since they are the only ones allowed to be used at the left-hand side of the operator <-. This is because these two functions are frequently used as links for the mean in generalized linear models. Specifically, `log()` is commonly used as link function in Poisson regression models, meanwhile `logit()` is often used in logistic regression models. This particularity makes it very easy to define this kind of models since, when modeling the mean of the corresponding Poisson or logistic models, we will just have to put `log(lambda)<-` or `logit(p)<-`, respectively, followed by the suitable linear combination of variables. By the way, putting `log(lambda)<-...` instead of `lambda<-exp(...)` makes `WinBUGS` use a different sampler for the variables intervening in the right-hand side of those expressions. In general, the algorithms used for the first of these expressions are more sophisticated so that specific coding will be generally preferred. When we talked in Section 2.1 about reparameterizations of models that could make the MCMC algorithms used to change, we were talking of modifications of this kind.

Both `inprod(,)` and `inprod2(,)` functions perform the same task, the scalar product of their arguments, which obviously should be vectors. The reason for having two functions for the same task is that the second is an efficient reimplementation of the first, yielding a much more satisfactory computational performance. So, by default, we will always use the `inprod2(,)` function for computing scalar products of two vectors. Since `WinBUGS` does not have a specific function for computing matrix products, that product has to be made component-wise by means of scalar products of the corresponding rows and columns of the original matrices. Therefore, matrix products will also be computed as recursive calls to the `inprod2(,)` function.

The `step()` and `equals(,)` functions deserve also particular attention. As mentioned in Chapter 2, MCMC inference relies on a sample of values of the posterior distribution to derive whatever feature of that distribution that we could be interested in. Thus, it is very common to be interested in estimating the specific posterior probability of events concerning parameters in the model, such as, the probability that a certain parameter in the model is higher than a reference value a. In that case it would be very convenient to have a tool available yielding that probability from our MCMC sample. The `step()` and `equals(,)` functions are intended to do so. The `condition.01<-step(condition)` statement returns the value 1 for every MCMC draw where `condition` is higher than or equal to 0, and 0 otherwise. If we define `condition` as an expression being positive if and only if occurs the event of interest, then `condition.01` will contain as many ones as the number of MCMC draws accomplishing the requested condition. Thus, the mean of `condition.01` will match the proportion of MCMC draws yielding the event of interest, i.e., an MCMC-based estimate of the corresponding probability. In short, the way of estimating posterior probabilities of events within the `BUGS` syntax is by means of the `step(condition)` function, with `condition` being positive just for the event whose probability we want to quantify. The function `equals(value1,value2)` is similar to the `step` function, but is intended to be used with discrete variables. This function takes two arguments and will return the value 1 if both are equal, and 0 otherwise. Obviously `equals` does not have any sense for continuous variables since the probability that these take a specific value is 0, so this function would always return a 0 when used on continuous variables. Note that the sentence `equals(value1,value2)` could be alternatively formulated as `step(value1-value2)-step(value2-value1)`, although obviously the first sentence is more compact and easier to be used.

These guidelines should be enough to understand and reproduce all the models considered during the rest of the book. Nevertheless, besides its syntax, one model will also need the corresponding data so that it can be run. Data will be provided to `WinBUGS` outside of the `model{...}` statement. There are several different ways to send the data to `WinBUGS`, although we will only pay some attention to that more likely to be used by `R`, as supposedly required by the readers of this book. Data to be used by `WinBUGS` can be formatted as the output of a `dput(...)` statement in `R`, maybe with slight changes. That is, in the typical case that we had the data to be used in a `BUGS` model stored in `R`, we would save them as a named list in a text file by means of the `dput` function. The content of this file will be used, as described in the following subsection, by `WinBUGS` in order to run the corresponding model. This will be completely fine for scalars and vectors, but matrices and arrays will have to be transposed and slightly modified since `R` exports them column by column, while conversely `WinBUGS` reads them row by row. In case you need more details on this, you can find them in the `WinBUGS` help (`Model specification> Formatting of data>S-plus format`); nevertheless, we are not going to explain this further since, as we will see in subsection 3.1.3, this process is usually automatically done when calling `WinBUGS` from `R`.

Example 3.2

We retake once again the oral cavity cancer mortality data in Example 2.1. There, the observed deaths for every year were divided by the corresponding population and multiplied by 100,000 in order to get the mortality rates that were later on regressed against the years of study. In that example, we considered the rates to follow a Normal distribution around a linear trend as a function of the years. The Normal assumption was a statistical simplification in order to make that analysis possible, but there is no particular obvious reason (except for the statistical tradition of assuming almost everything as Normally distributed) why rates should follow Normal distributions. Instead, since we are talking about binary and supposedly independent events (oral cancer deaths), given the underlying probabilities, it seems more reasonable to model them for each year by means of binomial distributions, as a function of the available population for every year. Moreover, in Example 2.1, we modeled the rates as a linear function of the year of study, without taking much care if that linear function could become negative after some years, justified by the assumption that surely no model is true, but some of them could be useful. To fix this problem, we model now the logit transformation of the year-specific probabilities that we want to fit, instead of modeling those probabilities directly in a linear manner. This is a clear example of logit regression that fits to the available data much better than the previous linear model in Example 2.1 which, as we are discussing, does not seem very appropriate.

The syntax below corresponds to the BUGS code that can be used to carry out the logistic regression posed in the paragraph above.

```
model{
 #Data likelihood
 for(i in 1:n){
  o[i]~dbin(Prob[i],Pop[i])
  logit(Prob[i])<-beta[1]+beta[2]*(year[i]-mean(year[]))
  rate[i]<-100000*Prob[i]
 }

 #Prior distributions
 beta[1]~dflat()
 beta[2]~dflat()

 #Probability of negative association (probabilities vs. years)
 P.beta2.lower.0<-step(-beta[2])
}
```

This syntax has several interesting features. Proceeding likewise to the previous example, one may realize that o and beta are the only variables in the model, o are observed data and beta are parameters that we want to learn of. Despite the fact that logit(Prob) is a vector of unknown values, they are not stochastic nodes (given beta) but just deterministic transformations of beta. Note the valid use in this case of the logit(...) function at the left-hand side of the <- operator. Note that rate is also a deterministic node in the model. This explicit definition of rate is needed if we want to derive, as a result of the model, the posterior distribution of these quantities. Finally P.beta2.lower.0 is a deterministic node being 1 for any sampled value of beta[2] lower than 0, and 0 otherwise. The posterior mean of this node yields the proportion of posterior MCMC draws with beta[2] lower than 0, which estimates the posterior probability of $\beta_2 < 0$. Finally, note the syntax used to calculate the mean year of the period of study: mean(year[]). In this case year is followed by the [] symbol (or [1:n] would also have been valid) to denote that we are referring to a vector, since the expression year without the corresponding brackets does not have a proper meaning within the BUGS language.

There are several nodes in the previous syntax which are neither stochastic variables (they are not followed at any moment by a ~ operator) nor deterministic components (they are not followed by a <- operator), these are n, Pop and year. These, jointly with the observed deaths o, can be sent to WinBUGS in the following format: list(n=21, o=c(119, ..., 190),

Pop=c(1883726,...,2541780), year=c(1991,...,2011)), where ... denotes the corresponding 21 elements of every vector that we have omitted by questions of space. This is exactly the format produced by the dput(list(n=n, o=o, Pop=Pop, year=year),file="whatever.txt") sentence of R in order to export the corresponding objects needed by WinBUGS.

Besides the model syntax and data, WinBUGS needs a third element to sample from the posterior distribution of the parameters in the Bayesian model. Any MCMC algorithm determines how to sample the next elements in the chain given the current ones; however, the algorithm needs some starting values to initialize the Markov chains and, therefore, making it possible to sample the following values of the chains. Hence, WinBUGS needs for every chain that has to sample from, an initial value for any variable in the model. If we do not provide those values, WinBUGS is able to sample them directly from the prior distribution of these variables in the model. However, in some cases (when using very vague or even improper flat prior distributions), this is not a good idea because directly generating from some prior distributions could yield disparate initial values that could make the chain take an excessive time to achieve convergence, or even make WinBUGS crash and reporting a numerical error. Moreover, if some of the prior distributions are improper uniform, it will be compulsory to initialize that variable by ourselves since otherwise WinBUGS will not be able to sample from that prior distribution. Therefore, as a general guideline, it is a safe procedure to give the initial values of the chains to be simulated to WinBUGS, at least the initial values of the variables having vague, or improper, distributions.

As previously mentioned in Section 2.1, the different chains to be run will be typically initialized at different (if possible distant) places. The format required for these starting values is just the same used for putting the data into WinBUGS, i.e., a named list with the different starting values to be used by each chain. A different list should be set for any of the chains to be run. Initial values are usually generated by sampling each variable from a sensible probability distribution taking values in the range of values of that variable. By this we do not mean that we need a prior accurate idea of the values that will take each variable. On the contrary, we mean that if a variable is used to model the logarithm of something, we should avoid initializing that variable with, for example, a U(−1,000, 1,000) distribution since it will generate disparate values in the original scale of the variable, surely leading to numerical errors. We advise you to pay attention to this issue since it will save you lots of hours searching the origin of errors in your model.

3.1.2   Running models in `WinBUGS`

First of all, we would like to remind you that for the rest of this section and, of course, the rest of this book, it is necessary to have `WinBUGS` (with the license key and the update to the 1.4.3 version) correctly installed. If you have not installed it yet, now is surely a perfect moment to do it following the instructions that you will find at `http://www2.mrc-bsu.cam.ac.uk/bugs/winbugs/contents.shtml`. If your operating system is not Windows, you will find lots of web pages showing how you should proceed to install `WinBUGS` on your computer.

Once we have introduced how to code Bayesian models in `BUGS`, we are going to see now how to run them in `WinBUGS`. As it can be seen at Figure 3.1, `WinBUGS` has the typical look of any Windows-based program. You can find the menu bar at the upper side of the `WinBUGS` window, where you will find all that you may need in order to run your model and to explore the corresponding results. In this bar, you can find the usual menu options (`File`, `Edit`, `Help`) and also other more specific options of `WinBUGS` (`Model`, `Inference`, `...`). At the lower side of the window, you will find the *status bar*, also an important part of `WinBUGS`. This bar shows information on the problems found (if any) when running a model or, on the contrary, you can check here if everything is correct at any stage of the running process. Pay attention always to this bar as it is very useful, mainly when `WinBUGS` crashes and reports some error. At the left-hand side of Figure 3.1 you can find the license window that always comes out when `WinBUGS` is launched. You will not typically have to pay attention to that window and you can even close it if it bothers you.

In Figure 3.1, you will also find a window (*compound document* following the nomenclature of `WinBUGS`) with the syntax of the model described in Example 3.2, the data needed to run it and initial values for initializing all 3 chains that we want to run. These components can be arranged in whatever order in a compound document and including comments if you find it convenient. `WinBUGS` is once again very flexible in this sense. Moreover, a single compound document can contain several models (with the correspondent data and initial values) if you wanted to.

Once you have all the components needed to run a model in a compound document, you may proceed to run it. The instructions needed to run a model can be summarized as follows. Provided you follow these guidelines carefully you will avoid lots of problems that can make you hate `WinBUGS` unnecessarily, so try to be scrupulous when reproducing them in your model. If, at any stage of the following procedure, you find some error you should start the process again from the beginning, once its cause has been fixed. Therefore, the steps required to run any model are:

1. Open the `Model>Specification` menu. Then the right-hand side window in Figure 3.1 with the name 'Specification Tool' will appear. This is the main window needed for indicating which is your model, data and initial values to `WinBUGS`.

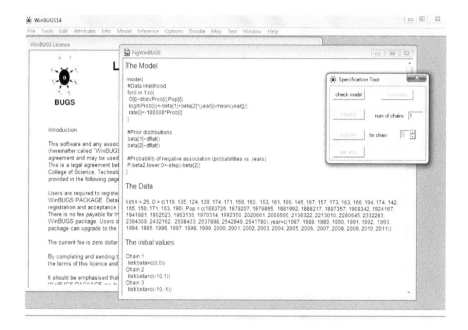

Figure 3.1

The `WinBUGS` program, general aspect. The syntax in the main window corresponds to the model developed in Example 3.2.

2. In your compound document, double-click on the `model` statement at the beginning of the syntax of your model so that this word is highlighted. Once selected, go to the 'Specification Tool' window and click the 'check model' button. This will check if the syntax of your model is correct and if it corresponds to a reasonable statistical model. If everything is correct the status bar will show the message 'model is syntactically correct', otherwise it will show a different message pointing out the syntax issue that produced the error. In that case, read the message with care and pay attention to where the cursor is placed within the model syntax (it will usually move to the place causing the error). This information will generally provide very useful clues on how to fix any error.

3. Double-click on the `list` statement at the beginning of your data and once highlighted go to the 'Specification Tool' window and click the 'load data' button. Once again, if everything is fine, the status bar will show the message 'data loaded' or, otherwise, it (and the position of the cursor in the compound document) will usually show useful information for fixing any possible error.

4. Introduce the number of chains of the posterior distribution that you want to simulate on the 'num of chains' cell of the 'Specification Tool' window and afterwards click on the 'compile' button. At this stage, that may take a bit long for very complex models, `WinBUGS` determines the variables that it has to sample from and checks if it has got everything needed to sample from them. If everything is fine, the status bar will show the message 'model compiled'.

5. At this stage we will introduce the starting values of the chains so that `WinBUGS` may start to simulate from them. For the first chain, we will double-click on the `list` statement containing the corresponding starting values and will click the 'load inits' button of the 'Specification Tool' window. If everything is fine, the status bar will show the message 'chain initialized but other chain(s) contain uninitialized variables' or 'this chain contains uninitialized variables', depending if all the variables in that chain have been initialized or not. We will have to repeat this process for the rest of the chains to be simulated. Once all the initial values have been introduced in `WinBUGS` for each chain and if everything is fine, we can have two different messages on the status bar. First, if all variables have been correctly initialized, the status bar will show the message 'model is initialized' pointing out that `WinBUGS` has everything ready for sampling values from the model. If, on the contrary, not all the variables have been initialized during this process, the messages 'chain initialized but other chain(s) contain uninitialized

variables' or 'this chain contains uninitialized variables' will remain in the status bar, pointing out that there are some variables still to be initialized. In that case, click the 'gen inits' button in the 'specification tool' window and `WinBUGS` will sample a value from the prior distribution of any uninitialized variable. In this case you should bear in mind that if `WinBUGS` has to sample from a vague or improper flat prior, this could introduce some problems in the simulation. If the 'gen inits' process works correctly, `WinBUGS` will show the message 'initial values generated, model initialized' and will be ready to start to simulate from the proposed statistical model.

6. At this stage `WinBUGS` is ready to sample from the introduced statistical model. We will need now the 'Update Tool' window that can be launched from the `Model>Update` menu, in order to draw samples. Hereafter we will no longer need the 'Specification Tool' window, so you can even close it if you find it convenient. In the 'updates' cell of the update tool, you will have to put the number of simulations that you want to draw and afterwards you will have to push the update button. The iteration cell displays the number of iterations made and it is refreshed during the MCMC sampling as a function of the number appearing at the 'refresh' cell, that can be modified at your own convenience. This updating process can be done as many times as wanted. Thus, the habitual procedure is to simulate a number of draws as burn-in period; afterwards, start saving the variables of interest (as described in the next step) and update the number of simulations that we want to save of these variables. This will avoid saving the iterations of the burn-in period, that we will typically want to discard from our posterior sample. If at the end of the simulation we feel that the sample drawn is not large enough because of its bad convergence, it is possible to simulate further draws by clicking as many times as desired on the 'update' button. The 'thin' cell, which allows thinning the drawn sample by the quantity contained there, is of particular interest for the sampling process. That is, if this cell is set to some value n, only 1 each n iterations will be saved. This will make the new simulations show lower auto-correlations and reduce memory requirements.

7. To save, monitor, plot, etc. the variables of interest in our model, we will need the 'Sample Monitor Tool' (Figure 3.2) that can be launched at the menu `Inference>Samples`. To start saving the draws of any of the variables in a model, after the burn-in period, we will have to introduce its name in the 'node' cell of the 'Sample Monitor Tool'. If `WinBUGS` recognizes it as a valid name of a node in the model, the 'set' button will be highlighted and you should click on it so that the subsequent draws of the MCMC for that node start to be stored. Regardless of whether the node to be stored is scalar,

vector, matrix or array, it is not necessary to put the corresponding brackets after the name of the node, unless you want to store only a specific selection of the node that you will have to put inside the brackets. You will have to repeat this process for any of the variables that you want to save and therefore to monitor. When you have told WinBUGS to store all the desired variables, you will have to update as many iterations of the MCMC as you want to save, turning back again to the update tool previously used to sample the burn-in period.

8. Finally, once you have saved the simulated values of the variables of interest, the 'Sample Monitor Tool' makes it possible to monitor them. For example, if we select one of the variables in the 'node' cell, or all of them by putting * in that cell, and click on the 'history' button, we will produce a history plot of the saved iterations as those illustrated in Figure 2.7. In case of finding in the previous history plot that your burn-in period was too short, you can expand it, increasing the value of the 'beg' cell by as many units as you want. On the other hand, maybe you will be interested in plotting the posterior distribution resulting from the sample drawn, in that case you can do it by means of the 'density' button. If, however, you wanted some summary statistics of the saved variables, you can retrieve them by clicking on the 'stats' button of the 'sample monitor tool'. Figure 3.3 shows an example of the summary that you may obtain of a set of variables by means of this tool. For any of the variables considered, you can see in that summary the posterior mean, posterior standard deviation and 2.5%, 50% (posterior median), 97.5% posterior quantiles of the variables among other statistics. In general, this will be usually a reasonable overview of the posterior distribution of the variables.

Following the outlined procedure, you should be able to make inference on most Bayesian hierarchical models that you could think about. You just have to code the model that you have in mind and WinBUGS will be in charge of sampling the corresponding posterior draws of the variables in that model. In the description of the procedure made just above, we have not intended to be exhaustive with the different possibilities that WinBUGS offers. Indeed, WinBUGS has implemented its own convergence checks, specific plotting tools for visualizing the distribution of a variable or the joint distribution of any two of them, etc. We encourage readers with a particular interest in developing their own statistical models to give the WinBUGS manual a thorough reading. Your WinBUGS programming skills will really improve and it will allow you to get the best results from this program.

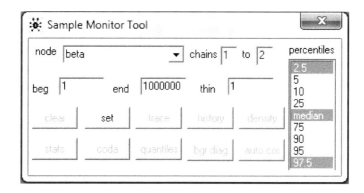

Figure 3.2
The 'Sample Monitor Tool' of WinBUGS, used to control (save, plot, summarize, etc.) the variables of interest in our model.

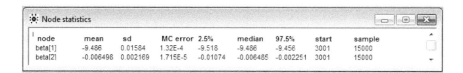

Figure 3.3
Summary statistics of the variables of interest as provided by WinBUGS.

The reason why we are not more exhaustive in our description of WinBUGS is that, paradoxically, we will not usually follow the procedure above for making inference of our models. As we will see soon, we will make use of some specific R packages that call WinBUGS and will execute all the previous steps automatically without requiring us to repeatedly click the sequence of buttons described. However, in our opinion, it is important for you to know how to run models directly in WinBUGS since the error reports that the mentioned R packages show when they find an error are very cryptic. In those cases, being capable of launching the model in WinBUGS on your own will usually help you determine the stage where the error is produced (charging the data, charging the initial values, compiling the model, etc.) and therefore to debug your model.

Error handling is the WinBUGS aspect that most users of this program frequently complain of. Although WinBUGS can be very harsh and cryptic when reporting errors, time has shown us that it usually provides some useful clues for figuring out where the error comes from. As mentioned, the information shown in the status bar is the key for knowing if everything is right at any stage of the introduction of the model into WinBUGS. If at any of these stages suddenly something does not work as expected, surely the step just made (introduction of the data, initial values, etc.) will be responsible for the error. Moreover, frequently the error in the status bar is also accompanied by the placement of the cursor wherever WinBUGS finds that the error comes from. If you pay attention to these two issues, it will be much easier to find errors at the model introduction/compilation phase. We strongly advise you to take a look at Exercise 2, at the end of this chapter, for improving your skills in the detection and treatment of WinBUGS errors.

Although models can be correctly coded in WinBUGS and accepted as valid models, errors may also be produced in the running phase, when sampling values of the posterior distribution. In the running phase, errors are notified by means of a trap window providing some details on the specific error. These windows are usually disconcerting since they show a huge amount of information that we have never found useful except that contained in the second line of these reports. We acknowledge that the information in this second line is also usually cryptic, but sometimes it is useful, for example if that line says something as enigmatic as 'GraphFlat.StdNode.Sample' we can infer that maybe there is some trouble with one of the nodes having an improper vague (dflat) distribution (did you initialize all the values with an improper vague distribution?); on the contrary, if the mentioned second line shows 'Math.Sqrt', WinBUGS may be having trouble calculating the square root of a scalar or a matrix (are you sure that all your square roots in your code are of positive scalars? Are all your precision matrices in your model positive definite?). Finally, you should also pay attention to the exact moment when the trap window is launched. If it is launched in the precise moment when WinBUGS starts to simulate values, the error will be possibly caused by some aberrant initial value of the chains, so it would be convenient for you to review the values used as 'inits' of the chains or, even more important, those values that you have not initialized for yourself. If on the contrary the trap is launched at the middle of the MCMC sampling when some values have already been sampled, the error will be surely caused by a numerical overflow, i.e. the values sampled lead to an extremely high or low value. In this case the history plot of the values saved could provide some insight about what combination of variables may be causing the numerical problem. You will have to take particular care with those terms defined in a logarithmic or logit scale, such as `log(alpha)<-u`, since an even moderate value for u could yield an extremely high or low value for `alpha`, causing some numerical overflow.

This intensive introduction to `WinBUGS` may make it seem like a tricky program, its use more an art than science. In this sense, we acknowledge that user friendliness was not a priority in the development of some aspects of this program. Nevertheless, `WinBUGS` is a powerful program, making it very easy to sample from lots of Bayesian hierarchical models. The burden of introducing slight modifications in a model is very low when working in `WinBUGS`; we just have to change the syntax of the model. This is a huge advantage in comparison to the full coding of the MCMC algorithm for new models. So, we agree that `WinBUGS` is an improvable tool, but it is in turn a very powerful inference program that deserves to be given a chance. Do not miss it.

3.1.3 Calling `WinBUGS` from `R`

Although `WinBUGS` is a wonderful inference tool, it is a pain to reproduce the scheme described above every time that you want to run a model. Think about making a simulation study where a model should be run lots of times for lots of different data sets; we would have to spend hours or days in front of our computer repeating that process. Also, let us assume that you had to run a model on 50 different data sets which takes around one hour (per data set) to run. This could be perfectly done in a single weekend, but it would require you to spend the whole weekend in front of your computer launching models every hour. If we had a recursive mechanism that could call to `WinBUGS` instead of executing it by hand ourselves, then we would save lots of hours in front of our computers doing the mechanical work of launching `WinBUGS` models.

Nowadays it is quite common, at least for this book's readers, to use `R` for data analysis. `WinBUGS` users commonly import their data into `R`, tidy them up and store them there for data analysis, visualization, etc. As a consequence, `R` has become the control centre for lots of data analysts where they make most parts of the data analysis process, without having to directly handle other applications (databases, GIS, etc.), they simply connect to them from within `R` and this application centralizes all the work. Therefore, it would be convenient to have an R package which could call to `WinBUGS` (send it tasks) and do all the tasks mentioned above on its own. This is exactly the goal of the `R2WinBUGS` package of `R`. Hereafter, everything that we will say regarding the `R2WinBUGS` package will be referring to the 2.1-21 version, the latest version at the moment of writing this book. Therefore, posterior upgrades of this package could make some of the code shown eventually fail; nevertheless, R2WinBUGS is a very stable package with few changes in time. In fact, at the moment of writing this book the 2.1-21 has been the latest version for more than three years. Therefore, we do not foresee big changes for this package in the future.

By far, the most commonly used function in R2WinBUGS is bugs. A call to bugs automatically makes the following tasks:

- Exports the data, model and initial values of the chains from R to WinBUGS (by means of intermediate text files) so that the MCMC simulation may be run there.

- Runs the model, with the data and initial values sent to WinBUGS. The bugs function automatically performs the tasks described at the previous subsection that will no longer have to be done by ourselves (you will see WinBUGS to be opened and closed as it is required by the bugs function).

- Turns back the results of the MCMC run in the previous step to R (once again by means of intermediate text files) and carries out some convergence checks and summarizes all the results.

The bugs function has several compulsory arguments needed to make it work. The first compulsory argument, data, is a named list containing all the data needed by the model in order to be run, i.e., the list of data that we sent manually to WinBUGS in the previous subsection. Be careful because the names of the elements in the list have to match exactly those used in the corresponding BUGS model. The second compulsory argument, inits, contains the initial values used to initialize each of the chains to be run. There are two main ways to specify these initial values, first, as a list where any of its elements (as many as chains to be run) is itself a named list with the initial values for one of the chains. The elements of the lists with the initial values will have to be named again with exactly the same names as those used in the model so that WinBUGS knows how to assign those values to the variables. The drawback of this procedure is that if we have to initialize a lot of values, we will typically have to manually generate all of them, which can be a burdensome task. The second, more convenient and frequent, way is to define the inits argument as an R function able to initialize the required values with random values. For example, let us assume that our model required the initialization of a vector theta of 500 components and that they could be reasonably initialized with random values of a standard Normal distribution. In that case, we could define inits.func=function(){list(theta=rnorm(500))}, set inits.func as inits argument and bugs will call that function as many times as needed to initialize all the chains to be run. Although this seems a more complicated way to initialize the chains, it is the more convenient one. We advise you to get used to it. The third compulsory argument for bugs is parameters.to.save, this argument is a vector with the names (all of them within quotation marks) of the variables to be saved and brought back to R.

The argument `model.file` is not compulsory since it takes as default `"model.bug"` as value. This argument sets the model, or `R` object, that contains the model to be run. Since it is quite usual to call to several models in a single `R` session, using `model.bug` as default file is not a good option. It is preferable to store each model in a different file, or `R` object, and call explicitly to the corresponding option, at least that is our usual way to proceed. If the argument for `model.file` is a file, that file should contain just the `WinBUGS` syntax of the corresponding model with the format `model{...}`. Alternatively, the `WinBUGS` syntax of the model could be stored, and given to `bugs`, as an `R` object. For the last few years, with the generalization of the use of `RMarkdown` documents, and for improving the reproducibility of statistical analyses this later option has become more popular. In this manner, the `WinBUGS` models used in an analysis are stored in the same document used for that analysis. For storing a `WinBUGS` model in `R` in order to be called by `bugs`, we should make, for example,

```
> whatever = function(){...}
```

where the syntax of the model, without the starting `model{` and ending `}`, should substitute the three dots in the previous expression. If the model is stored into a file `model.file` should be set equal to that file, between quotes. If that file is not stored in the working directory of `R`, we should include the full path to the corresponding file into the `model.file` argument. If the model was stored as an `R` object, it should be set equal to that object without additional quotes.

Besides the compulsory arguments, `bugs` have a series of optional arguments that allow us to control different issues of the simulation. We will just describe the use of the more frequent optional arguments. The arguments `n.chains`, `n.iter` and `n.burnin` correspond, respectively, to the number of chains, iterations (per chain) and iterations in the burn-in period (per chain) to be simulated. The `n.burnin` argument should be subtracted from the total `n.iter` iterations simulated per chain, and it has as default value `n.iter`/2, although according to the comment made in Section 2.3 it would be surely more efficient to set this argument to a lower value such as `n.iter`/10. The `n.thin` argument sets the thinning value for the simulated chains. It is fixed by default in such a way that the posterior sample size saved of all variables has around 1,000 values. However, `n.thin` allows us to change this performance. These parameters allow a perfect control of the simulation specifications from `R`.

Finally, there are some other arguments that allow us to control how `WinBUGS` is run, beyond the MCMC specifications already mentioned. An important argument is `debug`, that has `FALSE` as default value, which makes `bugs` to call `WinBUGS` and once the simulation has finished, `WinBUGS` is shut down. This is usually an appropriate procedure, but if an error is produced during the simulation, it would be better for `WinBUGS` to remain still opened once it has finished since, as mentioned above, `WinBUGS` provides useful clues that may help find the origin of the error. The value `TRUE` of the `debug` argument makes exactly that, to keep open WinBUGS once it finishes so that we can explore there whatever we find convenient. The DIC argument determines if the Deviance Information Criterion for model selection will be computed or not for the model run. WinBUGS will calculate by default this criterion (DIC=TRUE), although the calculation of DIC in WinBUGS is highly inefficient for some models (we will explain this further later), in which case it would be better to set DIC=FALSE and calculate it afterwards in R, once the simulation process has concluded. The bugs.directory argument should contain the directory where WinBUGS is installed on your computer, the default value of this argument is 'c:/Program Files/WinBUGS14/'. If you do not have WinBUGS installed there, you should change accordingly this argument or, otherwise, the bugs function will not be able to launch WinBUGS, producing an error. Finally, there are a series of arguments (useWINE, WINEPATH, ...) needed to use the bugs function in other operating systems instead of Windows. We advise the users of those operating systems to search the web for more information about how to set up those parameters in order to make bugs work. There are lots of web pages explaining this.

As previously mentioned, bugs retrieves to R the results generated by WinBUGS and bugs builds an R object of class bugs with those data and some other elements that it generates. bugs objects are basically named lists with a determined structure. For any bugs object, its sims.list, sims.matrix and sims.array components will be of particular importance. These elements contain, in different formats, the simulations of the variables retrieved from WinBUGS. Thus, sims.list is a list with a component for any of the elements in the parameters.to.save argument of the corresponding bugs function call, all of them containing the posterior draws saved by WinBUGS. sims.matrix will arrange the same posterior draws in a matrix where the rows correspond to different iterations of the Markov chain and the columns to different variables in the model. sims.array will arrange the posterior draws in an array similar to sims.matrix, but where the rows are now split in two different dimensions corresponding to chains and simulations within each chain. So the dimensions of sims.array correspond, in this order, to the number of saved simulations (within chains), chains and variables saved. Any bugs object contains also a mean component with the posterior means of all the variables in the parameters.to.save argument of the corresponding bugs function call. mean is also a named list with as many elements as the length of parameters.to.save.

bugs objects have also a useful summary component which contains a matrix mimicking the information in Figure 3.3 for all the retrieved variables. Every row in that matrix corresponds to a different variable and every column to a different posterior statistic of the variable. Besides the information retrieved from WinBUGS, bugs also calculates two convergence statistics that will make the convergence assessment of the simulation easier to be carried out: the R-hat statistic of Brooks-Gelman-Rubin and the effective sample size, n.eff in terms of the bugs output, already mentioned in Chapter 2. We remind you that the R-hat statistic assesses the suitability of the burn-in period and it is advisable that this statistic for all the variables in the model was close to 1, such as for example lower than 1.1 for all the variables. On the other hand, the effective sample size assesses the adequacy of the sample size drawn from the posterior distribution, and the higher this value for all the variables in the model the better. We will in general require the sample size for any retrieved variable to be higher than 100, regardless of whether we may require a longer value at some specific setting. When calling to a `bugs` object from the command line of `R`, it will return the information stored in the `summary` component of that object, which provides a general overview of the results of the model.

We are sure that hereafter the `R2WinBUGS` package will become an essential tool for making your spatial analyses and that you will rarely use `WinBUGS` directly, unless you want to debug a previous call of the `bugs` function ending with an error. We also want to mention a second package that is very convenient for calling `WinBUGS` from within `R`. The `pbugs` package (available at `https://github.com/fisabio/pbugs`) implements a parallelized version of the `bugs` function. You can install this package by simply installing first the `R` package `devtools` if you have not previously installed it and afterwards typing `devtools::install_github("fisabio/pbugs")`. As you know any `bugs` call will typically run several chains (3 by default) of the corresponding model. As when `WinBUGS` was developed, parallel computing and multicore computers were not in general use; therefore, all the mentioned chains are simulated in just a single core of the computer regardless of the number of cores that it has. As a consequence, `WinBUGS` is not able to take advantage of the several cores that current computers usually have. The `pbugs` function, of the package with the same name, basically decomposes a call to the `bugs` function with `n.chains` chains into `n.chains` calls to `WinBUGS`, any of them with just one chain. As a result, `n.chains` separate `WinBUGS` instances are launched, any of them running a separate chain in a separate core and therefore taking advantage of the multicore capabilities of current computers.

The `bugs` of `R2WinBUGS` exports the data to `WinBUGS`, then simulates there the corresponding MCMC samples and finally gets back the results to `R`. `pbugs` does exactly the same job, with the single difference that the mid-task, previously carried out by a single `WinBUGS` instance is now split into as many parts as chains are run. As a result, `pbugs` may speed up the simulation process of one model up to a factor close to `n.chains`. Nevertheless, this factor will depend on the proportion of time spent by `WinBUGS` in comparison with the whole time spent by `bugs` in order to complete the whole simulation and the rest of the tasks that it has to carry out. Thus, the gain in using `pbugs` for running models with a short computing time (which takes just a few seconds) is very low since for these models the time transferring the data between `R` and `WinBUGS` or for computing convergence diagnostics of the simulated variables can be as high as the time taken by `WinBUGS` to complete the simulations. On the contrary, for models taking a long time to run (hours or even days), that will be quite common in the rest of the book, the computing time may be substantially decreased (in a proportion close to $1/n.chains$) since most of the time spent by `bugs` is consumed by the simulating period of `WinBUGS`. It can really make a big difference for a model to run in 8 hours instead of 1 day which will make, for sure, your work much more productive.

The syntax of the `pbugs` function is devised so that any call to the `bugs` function may be executed in parallel by simply putting a `p` character before the corresponding `bugs` call. That is, if `bugs(...)` is a valid syntax for executing a model in `WinBUGS`, `pbugs(...)` will do exactly that call, but making use of as many cores (if these were available) as chains are run. Likewise, the object generated by a `pbugs` call is hardly distinguishable of the object that would be generated from the equivalent call to the `bugs` function so, in this sense, the call to `pbugs` is transparent.

Example 3.3

We are going back to Example 3.2. We are now going to see how to call the model developed there from within R. First, we store the data needed to run the model as a named list:

```
> data=list(n=21, o=c(119, ..., 190), Pop=c(1883726,...,2541780),
            year=c(1991,...,2011))
```

Afterwards, we create an R function for initializing the variables in the model. Since we do not want these values to be too extreme, in order to avoid computational problems, we define that function as:

```
> inits=function(){list(beta=rnorm(2,mean=0,sd=5))}
```

instead of putting a higher standard deviation that would make the distribution vaguer and, therefore, the values generated more extreme. Among the parameters in the model of Example 3.2, we will be particularly interested in retrieving the annual rates, since they are the main object of interest of the model, the parameters `beta` of the linear model and the 'significance' of `beta[2]`, so that we can know the statistical relevance of the linear time trend of the risks. Thus, we define:

```
> param=c("beta","P.beta2.lower.0","rate")
```

With this, we would have all the compulsory arguments needed by the `bugs` function. Moreover, we have also created an R object `model.logist` with the syntax of the model described in Example 3.2. We have run the model with a total of 3,000 iterations with 10% of them used as burn-in. The posterior sample drawn has about 1000 values. The syntax needed to run the model with such requirements is the following:

```
> resul=bugs(data=data, inits=inits, parameters.to.save=param,
            n.iter=3000, n.burnin=300, model.file=model.logist)
```

The model is executed by running this sentence and its results are retrieved to R. Those results are saved in the object `resul`, of class `bugs`. If we wanted to explore the structure of the object just generated, we could make

```
> names(resul)
```

obtaining the following

```
 [1] "n.chains"         "n.iter"          "n.burnin"
 [4] "n.thin"           "n.keep"          "n.sims"
 [7] "sims.array"       "sims.list"       "sims.matrix"
[10] "summary"          "mean"            "sd"
[13] "median"           "root.short"      "long.short"
[16] "dimension.short"  "indexes.short"   "last.values"
[19] "isDIC"            "DICbyR"          "pD"
[22] "DIC"              "model.file"      "program"
```

we encourage you to explore these components by executing this model as it comes in the accompanying online material. The `summary` component of `resul` will be the one that you will typically be more interested in. You can print that component by simply executing `> resul`, in that case you will see the following at your R console:

```
Inference for Bugs model at "Logist.txt", fit using WinBUGS, 3
chains, each with 3000 iterations (first 300 discarded),
n.thin = 8 n.sims = 1014 iterations saved
                 mean  sd   2.5%   25%   50%   75% 97.5% Rhat n.eff
beta[1]          -9.5 0.0  -9.5  -9.5  -9.5  -9.5  -9.5    1  1000
beta[2]           0.0 0.0   0.0   0.0   0.0   0.0   0.0    1  1000
P.beta2.lower.0   1.0 0.0   1.0   1.0   1.0   1.0   1.0    1     1
rate[1]           8.2 0.3   7.8   8.0   8.2   8.4   8.8    1  1000
rate[2]           8.2 0.2   7.7   8.0   8.2   8.3   8.7    1  1000
...
rate[25]          7.0 0.2   6.6   6.9   7.0   7.1   7.4    1  1000
deviance        232.3 1.9 230.3 230.8 231.7 233.2 237.4    1   670

For each parameter, n.eff is a crude measure of effective sample
size, and Rhat is the potential scale reduction factor (at
convergence, Rhat=1).

DIC info (using the rule, pD = Dbar-Dhat)
pD = 2.0 and DIC = 234.3
DIC is an estimate of expected predictive error (lower deviance
is better).
```

This summary is quite comprehensive and generally you will not need anything else to explore in a model. At the first lines of this output, you can see a brief summary of the simulation carried out (number of iterations, chains, etc.). Afterwards you can see a brief summary of the variables retrieved from the model. Please, pay particular attention to the last 2 columns of this table, corresponding to the convergence assessment of the simulation. This is the first thing that you will have to do once a model has been run, since they inform us about the validity of the rest of the results shown in the summary. All the values at the Rhat column are exactly 1 so the burn-in period chosen seems to be enough. Almost all the values at the n.eff column are well above 100 which means that the number of simulations sampled seems appropriate. The only variable that has a low value at the n.eff column is P.beta2.lower.0. This variable is a simple transformation of beta2 whose convergence is completely correct, so this would not be so worrisome. Moreover, if we take a look at the values sampled from P.beta2.lower.0 (taking a look for example at the sims.list component of resul), we can check that all its values are exactly one, because beta[2] has been lower than 0 for all the simulations. As a consequence, the weird value of the n.eff column for P.beta2.lower.0 is just a consequence of its lack of variability due to the high probability of beta[2] being lower than 0, instead of a symptom of bad convergence. Therefore, we consider the convergence assessment of the simulation just run to be satisfactory.

Regarding the results of the simulation, we see that the posterior mean of the intercept of the proposed logistic model is -9.5, and the coefficient corresponding to the effect of the year is 0, with 95% credibility interval [0,0]. Obviously this summary does not yield enough digits to correctly explore the results. As an alternative, we could resort to the summary component of resul in order to explore the summary in more detail. In that case, if we make

```
> round(resul$summary,3)
```

we would obtain a more precise summary where the posterior mean of beta[2] is -0.007, with 95% posterior credibility interval [-0.011,-0.002]. This result is much more informative and in agreement with the posterior probability of beta[2] being lower than 0, that is estimated as 1 by P.beta2.lower.0. The annual rates have also been estimated from the model, ranging their posterior means from 8.2 deaths per 100,000 people at the first year of study (1991) to 7.0 deaths in 2011. The summary of variables ends with some results for the deviance. This variable is the fit measure in which DIC is based. It is quite important to assess the convergence of this variable since it can be considered as a global measure of convergence of the model. Convergence of the deviance does not mean full convergence of the model, but lack of convergence for this variable could mean a global lack of convergence that could not be evident from an individual exploration of the variables in the model.

At the end of the above summary, we can see the value of the DIC achieved by the model. This value is adimensional, i.e., it only makes sense when compared with some other models. Nevertheless, the pD value shown (effective number of parameters) *effective number of parameters* informs us about the complexity of the model. For our model, the estimated number of parameters is exactly 2, which matches the number of parameters involved in the fit (beta[1] and

n.iter	3,000	30,000	300,000	3,000,000
bugs	3.63	7.90	60.12	610.84
pbugs	4.04	5.52	27.20	245.28
ratio	1.11	0.70	0.45	0.40

Table 3.3
Time spent (in seconds) by the `bugs` and `pbugs` functions to run the model above, with different numbers of iterations. Ratio denotes the proportion of time spent by the `pbugs` function as compared to that taken by `bugs`.

`beta[2]`). But this result is not always true, for random effects models for instance, as we will see in the next chapter.

Table 3.3 shows a comparison of the computing times spent by the `bugs` and `pbugs` functions for the model above with different numbers of iterations. The model has been run for 3 chains with `n.iter` equal to 3,000; 30,000; 300,000 and 3,000,000 with both functions in a 4-core laptop running on Windows 7. The results of these runs did not show appreciable differences since the effective sample sizes with 3,000 iterations already took the highest possible value that they could take. Nevertheless, this exercise illustrates the different computational performance of the `bugs` and `pbugs` functions.

Times for any of the columns in Table 3.3 should be about 10 times higher than those same times in the previous column, but that relationship does not hold that much, mainly for those columns placed at the left of the table. This is because not all the time spent by both functions is used for simulating values from the posterior distribution. Launching `WinBUGS`, transferring data between `WinBUGS` and `R` and creating the corresponding `bugs` object also consume time in calls to the `bugs` and `pbugs` functions, and that time may be considerable with respect to the computing time of the posterior distributions when the latter is lower. The `pbugs` function also spends some time creating a cluster of cores for making computations in parallel and launching 3 different `WinBUGS` instances. This makes `pbugs` take even longer than `bugs` when running the model with 3,000 iterations, since the time saved for making computations in parallel does not compensate for the time spent to perform the extra tasks made by the `pbugs` function. Nevertheless, as long as the time taken to draw the posterior sample grows (higher number of iterations), the ratio of the computing times taken by the `pbugs` and the `bugs` functions converges to $1/\texttt{n.chains}$. Regretfully, computationally intensive (and therefore long) problems are very common for disease mapping practitioners, so the `pbugs` package should be, in principle, a very useful tool for all those interested in this research field.

3.2   INLA

The acronym *INLA* stands for Integrated Nested Laplace Approximation, the approach proposed by Rue et al. (2009) for performing Bayesian inference in a wide class of hierarchical models which avoids the use of MCMC simulation. Instead, INLA takes advantage of substantial numerical approximations and integration methods that make it possible to approximate also the marginal posterior distributions of the parameters in the corresponding model. The avoidance of MCMC simulation in INLA yields, on one hand, a significant improvement in computing times for many models and, on the other hand, avoids the typical convergence problems of MCMC methods, which are one of the most problematic issues of that inference method.

INLA can be applied to make inference on any hierarchical model fitting within the following framework:

- **Data likelihood:** The observed data $\boldsymbol{y} = \{y_i : i = 1, ..., I\}$ should be conditionally independent given an underlying field $\boldsymbol{\phi} = \{\phi_i : i = 1, ..., I\}$ and $\boldsymbol{\theta}_1$, the parameters of the corresponding distribution. Each of the original observations y_i should depend on just the corresponding ϕ_i and $\boldsymbol{\theta}_1$; therefore, the likelihood function should be of the form

$$\boldsymbol{y}|\boldsymbol{\phi}, \boldsymbol{\theta}_1 \sim \prod_{i=1}^{I} P(y_i|\phi_i, \boldsymbol{\theta}_1), \tag{3.1}$$

for $P()$ a suitable distribution such as Normal, Poisson, etc. not necessarily belonging to the exponential family. Moreover, we will also assume that the parameter η_i, an additive predictor which is a function of covariates, random effects, etc. is related to ϕ_i by means of a link function g so that $g(\phi_i) = \eta_i$.

Some generalizations of the data likelihood have been considered, making it possible to fit a larger collection of models within INLA (Martins et al., 2013). Among these, it is possible to have different likelihood functions for the different observations, that is, to have $P_i()$ instead of $P()$ in expression (3.1), or making the probability of any observation y_i depend on a (sparse) linear combination of elements of $\boldsymbol{\eta}$, instead of on just η_i.

- **Latent field:** Besides the data likelihood, INLA also assumes the existence of a latent field $\boldsymbol{\psi} = \{\psi_j : j = 1, ..., J\}$, with $J \geq I$. This part of the model is usually known as the *process layer* of the model (Cressie and Wikle, 2011). The first I elements of $\boldsymbol{\psi}$ will be just the vector with the linear predictor $\boldsymbol{\eta}$, whereas the rest of the elements in $\boldsymbol{\psi}$ will be a collection of auxiliary parameters, used to give $\boldsymbol{\eta}$ its particular structure. INLA assumes a particular restriction on $\boldsymbol{\psi}$ for the models fitted. Specifically, INLA imposes $\boldsymbol{\psi}$ to follow a multivariate Normal distribution

$$\boldsymbol{\psi}|\boldsymbol{\theta}_2 \sim N_J(\boldsymbol{\mu}(\boldsymbol{\theta}_2), \boldsymbol{Q}^{-1}(\boldsymbol{\theta}_2)), \tag{3.2}$$

for $\boldsymbol{Q}$ a suitable precision matrix and $\boldsymbol{\theta}_2$ a set of hyperparameters for $\boldsymbol{\psi}$.

Despite this Normality restriction, expression (3.2) is fairly general and can accommodate lots of models. For example, it contains any model with

$$\eta_i = \alpha + \boldsymbol{Z}_{i\cdot}\boldsymbol{\beta} + \sum_{k=1}^{K} f^{(k)}(u_{ik}, \boldsymbol{\gamma}_k), \ i = 1, ..., I, \tag{3.3}$$

provided $\boldsymbol{\psi} = (\boldsymbol{\eta}, \alpha, \boldsymbol{\beta}, \boldsymbol{\gamma}_1, ..., \boldsymbol{\gamma}_K)$ follows a multivariate Normal prior distribution, which is a mild assumption. In the linear expression above, $\boldsymbol{\beta}$ is used to linearly model the effect of the covariates $\boldsymbol{Z}$ on $\boldsymbol{\eta}$. The expressions $f^{(k)}()$, for $k = 1, ..., K$, stand for a set of smooth functions, with parameters $\boldsymbol{\gamma}_k$, used to model the non-linear relationship of $\boldsymbol{\eta}$ and the covariates $\boldsymbol{u}_{\cdot k}$. These terms could be used, for example, to model the effect of a categorical variable as a random effect or the smooth effect of a numeric variable as we will see in some examples in Chapter 5. Expression (3.3) considers $\boldsymbol{\eta}$ to be a deterministic function of the rest of the parameters in $\boldsymbol{\psi}$, so strictly speaking it is not a random variable. Nevertheless, it could be considered instead to follow a Normal distribution of high, known precision around the linear function defined in (3.3). This would make the vector $\boldsymbol{\psi}$ accomplish the Gaussian requirement in (3.2).

- **Rest of parameters:** The model is finally completed by putting a prior distribution on the rest of the parameters of the model, that is, choosing $P(\boldsymbol{\theta})$ for $\boldsymbol{\theta} = (\boldsymbol{\theta}'_1, \boldsymbol{\theta}'_2)'$. Although this is not theoretically needed by INLA, it is computationally very convenient for the length of $\boldsymbol{\theta}$ (denoted by L) to be small, let's say at most 5. The speed of INLA will severely depend on that length making it prohibitive fitting models with large values of L.

Although INLA is able to run only those models fitting the scheme just above, this is not a big limitation. The amount of models comprised within this framework is huge. It is worth mentioning that the vast collection of Generalized Additive Models (GAM models) are a subset of the framework just defined and GAMs already contain most of the models commonly used in current statistical analyses. Thus, beyond its application to disease mapping, that we will introduce in detail in the next chapters, INLA has been already used for a vast variety of purposes: survival analyses, geostatistical models, stochastic volatility models, generalized dynamic linear models, change point analyses with dependent data, point processes, age-period-cohort models, etc. (Martins et al., 2013). Therefore, we are not talking about a disease mapping specific inference tool but about a fairly general inference device.

We are not going to talk in depth about the underlying mathematical theory below INLA. A deep understanding of INLA requires a strong background in numerical methods, which is well beyond this part of the book. However, we are going to give here a brief explanation of the ideas underlying INLA in order to make it easier to understand the meaning of several of the parameters involved in the fitting of INLA models. Roughly speaking, INLA instead of estimating the full posterior distribution of the parameters in a model ($P(\boldsymbol{\psi}, \boldsymbol{\theta}|\boldsymbol{y})$), it just estimates the marginal posterior distributions

$$P(\psi_j|\boldsymbol{y}) = \int P(\psi_j|\boldsymbol{\theta}, \boldsymbol{y})P(\boldsymbol{\theta}|\boldsymbol{y})d\boldsymbol{\theta}, \; j = 1, ..., J$$

and

$$P(\theta_l|\boldsymbol{y}) = \int P(\boldsymbol{\theta}|\boldsymbol{y})d\boldsymbol{\theta}_{-l}, \; l = 1, ..., L.$$

For most applications, knowing these distributions would be enough since we are frequently more interested in the marginal distributions of the variables in the model than in other issues concerning their joint distribution. Both expressions of $P(\psi_j|\boldsymbol{y})$ and $P(\theta_l|\boldsymbol{y})$ entail their own integrals with regard to $\boldsymbol{\theta}$ that have to be done numerically. Multivariate integration is a computationally intensive task, becoming prohibitive as the number of integrals to be done grows. This is why the speed of INLA highly depends on the length of the vector of hyperparameters $\boldsymbol{\theta}$, as we mentioned previously. Several integration methods could be used in INLA for performing this numerical integration, the final speed of the algorithm and its reliability may highly depend also on that method. The integration method will be one of the options that we will typically have to set when making inference with INLA. On the other hand, the integrands for both $P(\psi_j|\boldsymbol{y})$ and $P(\theta_l|\boldsymbol{y})$ are composed of two functions that we do not really know. Both, $P(\psi_j|\boldsymbol{\theta}, \boldsymbol{y})$ and $P(\boldsymbol{\theta}|\boldsymbol{y})$, are themselves the result of integrating out (or fixing) some parameters in the full posterior distribution. Therefore, these two functions are numerically approximated, since the numerical integration of the parameters, if possible, would not be affordable (they would usually integrate lots of parameters). Thus, this approximation is the second main ingredient of INLA, which is typically performed by means of *Laplace Approximation* (Tierney and Kadane, 1986) and gives name to this method. As for the integration methods, more alternatives to Laplace approximation are available, yielding also different computing times and reliability of the results. The choice of one or the other of these approximation methods will be based on the balance between these two aspects.

INLA, as an inference method, owes much of its popularity to the software developed by the authors of this method (Martino and Rue, 2008). An efficient implementation of INLA requires great expertise in numerical methods and coding, beyond the scope of most potential users. Thus, the authors have developed, and made publicly available, a set of routines for putting in practice the theory contained in INLA. These routines have been programmed as a stand-alone C program. To make the use of these routines more friendly, an R package, INLA, has been also developed to run them all from R. You can find full information on INLA at the web page http://www.r-inla.org, indeed you will not find the package INLA at CRAN, the usual repository for R packages, because of its dependence on the stand-alone C program mentioned above.

The routines in `INLA` are particularly tuned to take advantage of the hypothetical sparsity of Q, the precision matrix of the latent field ψ. Thus, the sparser is Q, the more efficient will be `INLA`. This makes `INLA` particularly suited for fitting spatial models, where the spatial arrangement of the region of study makes Q sparse. `INLA` can also be used for models without a sparse structure of Q, although in that case it will not take any advantage of this particular feature.

3.2.1 INLA basics

We are going to introduce now the basics of `INLA` that will allow us to use this package for fitting many of the models that will be introduced hereafter. `INLA` has lots of arguments and parameters that make it possible to tune almost any issue involved in the numerical fitting of any model. Moreover, `INLA` has also lots of options allowing us to derive goodness-of-fit statistics, validation or model selection criteria such as DIC, among others. However, we will restrict this introduction to show the essential use of `INLA` since a full overview needs a whole book by itself (Blangiardo and Cameletti, 2015).

Since `INLA` cannot be found in CRAN, its installation is a bit different to a typical `R` package. For installing `INLA` (as described in `http://www.r-inla.org/download`), you will have to type in `R`:

```
> options(repos=c(getOption("repos"),
        INLA="http://www.math.ntnu.no/inla/R/stable"))
> update.packages("INLA", dep=TRUE)
```

This will install in your computer the last stable version of `INLA`. This code also installs the stand-alone `C` program fitting INLA, so once you install the `R` package `INLA`, you will not have to take care of downloading anything else. For executing the examples and all the `INLA` code in this book, we have used the 3.5 version of the package, compiled in July 2018. Although `INLA` is in continuous development, and it is not as stable as `R2WinBUGS`; we do not expect drastic changes between this and subsequent versions of `INLA`. However, just in case, you can find a (supposedly permanent) copy of this version of `INLA` at `https://inla.r-inla-download.org/R/stable/bin/`. You may find lots of additional resources on INLA at the web page `http://www.r-inla.org/`, which hosts the project maintaining the package. You may search at this website whatever you may want to know about `INLA`.

Once you have `INLA` installed, to start a working session first you will have to type

```
> library(INLA)
```

like any other typical package in `R`. The main function in `INLA` used to fit models is `inla`. The syntax of this function is the typical syntax of any `R` function used for fitting models like `lm`, `lme` or `glm`, indeed `inla`'s syntax is based on `glm`'s syntax.

The `family` argument of `inla` controls the likelihood layer of the model that we are fitting. This argument may take as value any of the pre-built likelihood functions that `inla` has implemented. This collection of families is quite large and it can be listed by typing `inla.list.models("likelihood")` within R. In case you were further interested in some of the likelihoods listed, as for example `poisson`, you could retrieve more information by typing `inla.doc("poisson")`, which launches the help documentation corresponding to the term contained as argument. Among these likelihood options we highlight the `gaussian` and `poisson` families that will be the only ones used throughout this book. The first of them, the default option, corresponds to a Normal additive model, where the mean is modeled by means of an additive structure containing both linear and non-linear terms. The `poisson` option corresponds to a Poisson generalized linear mixed model, where the logarithm of the expected value is modeled as an additive structure of linear and non-linear terms.

The main argument of `inla`, modeling the process layer of the model, is `formula`. The value of this argument is an object of class `formula` that puts into R the linear predictor in Expression (3.3) corresponding to our model. The `formula` argument will be something of this form

```
> form = y ~a +b +a:b +a*b +f(id1,model1,...)
            +f(id2,model2,...) +...
```

where the terms a, b, $id1$ and $id2$ in this expression must be columns of the data.frame (or elements of the list) `data`, which jointly with `formula` are the only compulsory arguments of the `inla` function. Obviously, not all the terms on the right-hand side of the previous expression are compulsory and a typical `formula` argument will have just some of those terms, with as many linear or non-linear terms as required. The terms `a+b+a:b+a*b` are responsible for the linear fixed effects' specification of covariates `a` and `b`. The expressions `a:b` and `a*b` have the regular meaning in R formulas: interaction of both variables and main effects+interaction, respectively.

The terms of the form `f(...)` in the `inla` formula will account for the $f^{(j)}()$ terms in Expression (3.3), modeling the non-linear effect of one of the variables in our data set. Note that the `f` function can only model smoothing devices depending on Gaussian random effect. Although this is restrictive, there are lots of smoothing devices within that family such as unstructured random effects, random walks, auto-regressive processes, random effects with spatial structure, etc. The syntax of the `f` function has a single compulsory argument, the covariate whose effect is going to be modeled. This may be an index enumerating the individuals in our data set in which case a different value will be fitted for any of those individuals. The second (non-compulsory) argument is a fixed vector of weights of the same length than the covariate. The `f` function adds to the linear predictor a term of the form

$$weights_i \cdot f(covariate_i)$$

where the subindex i indexes individuals. Therefore, the weights vector can make individuals with the same value of the covariate to have different effects, which could be useful in some occasions. The weights vector has, by default, all their components equal to one. Both the covariate and the weights vector (if explicitly given) will have to appear necessarily as first and second arguments of the `f` function, respectively, without any argument name preceding them.

A third important argument of the `f` function is `model`, which controls the dependence structure of the corresponding random effect. The default value for this argument is `model="iid"`, which assumes every value of the covariate to have a different (and independent, given the common variance) random effect. Leaving aside the spatially structured random effects, which will be introduced in the next chapter, other interesting alternative values for this argument are `model="rw1"` and `model="rw2"`, which model the values of the random effect as random walks of first and second order, respectively. Likewise, `model="ar1"` and `model="ar"` models the random effects as auto-regressive processes of first and of p-th order, respectively, where p can take different integer values. The option `model="z"` can be used for including random effects in the linear predictor with the classical form $Z\gamma$, where Z is a fixed matrix with I rows and as many columns as levels in the covariate. In this case γ stands for a zero-centered vector of random effects with design matrix Z. This model can also be used for general design matrices where the columns of Z correspond to some basis of functions. In that case, the coefficients associated with that design matrix will have a random effects structure, as already illustrated in Example 2.2. Finally the options `model="generic0"`, `model="generic1"` and `model="generic2"` allow us to define random effects with general covariance matrices. We will introduce these models in the following chapters as we require their use. You can find a list of models available for the `f` function in `inla` by typing `inla.list.models("latent")` into R. If you wanted further information on some of these models, as for example the `iid` model, you can retrieve it by typing `inla.doc("iid")`.

So, once we have introduced how to set the data likelihood and process layer for models in `inla`, we are going to focus now on the remaining aspect of those models, prior distributions for the rest of the parameters in the model. The `hyper` arguments of `inla` are used to define the prior distributions of the elements of the vector of parameters $\boldsymbol{\theta}$. These arguments may be placed at different locations of the `inla` function, having therefore different meanings. We remind that $\boldsymbol{\theta}$ was formed as $\boldsymbol{\theta} = (\boldsymbol{\theta}_1', \boldsymbol{\theta}_2')'$ where $\boldsymbol{\theta}_1$ contains all the parameters in the likelihood function apart from ϕ, and $\boldsymbol{\theta}_2$ contains the parameters of the variables contained in the linear predictor $\boldsymbol{\eta}$. For example, for a model with the `family="gaussian"` option, $\boldsymbol{\theta}_1$ will be just the parameter used by `inla` to control the variability of the data likelihood. On the contrary, for the option `family="poisson"`, $\boldsymbol{\theta}_1$ will not contain any parameter since the only parameter in the data likelihood is modeled by the linear predictor. For any model that you used as data likelihood, it would be convenient for you to take a look at the INLA help (see comment above on the `family` argument), since the variables in $\boldsymbol{\theta}_1$ may not be parameterised in an obvious way. For example, for a Gaussian model, the variability of the likelihood is parameterized in INLA as a function of its log-precision, instead of the standard deviation, variance or precision which could seem more natural choices. The log-precision is a more convenient parameter from a computational point of view, with a more computationally friendly posterior distribution, that is why INLA uses it to model the variability in the data. We should be very clear on which parameter we are modeling before proposing any prior distribution.

The prior distribution of the parameters in $\boldsymbol{\theta}_1$ is controlled by means of the control.family argument of inla, which is in charge of controlling any issue concerning the likelihood function. The value of this argument should be a named list whose hyper component should be filled with the information on the prior distributions of the elements in $\boldsymbol{\theta}_1$, if they were not going to take the default values. This hyper argument is also a named list where each element corresponds to any of the parameters in charge of setting the corresponding prior distribution. To assign a prior distribution to a parameter, we should put its name inside the mentioned hyper list and assign it a list of the form: short.name=list(prior=...,param=...), where short.name should be replaced by the name of the corresponding variable, prior should be filled with the desired prior distribution and param with its corresponding parameters. Thus, for example, we could put a Gaussian distribution on the standard deviation of the data likelihood, truncated to positive values, of mean 0 and precision 0.01 (Gelman, 2005b), by including

```
control.family=list(hyper=list(prec=list(prior="logtnormal",
                     param=c(0,0.01)))))
```

within the corresponding call to inla (take a look at the documentation at inla.doc("logtnormal") for more details on this prior choice).

We can find the names of the parameters of any likelihood function, as prec in the previous case, by launching its help documentation by means of the inla.doc() function. You can find that name at the short.name argument in that document, its default prior at the prior argument and its hyperparameters at the param argument. Thus, according to the information retrieved by inla.doc("gaussian"), for example, we can check that for a Gaussian likelihood, the only parameter in $\boldsymbol{\theta}_1$ is the log-precision, which inla refers to as simply prec and takes a log-gamma as default distribution of parameters 1 and $5 \cdot 10^{-5}$. This is equivalent to the usual choice of a gamma prior distribution, with the same parameters, on the corresponding precision. A list of the available prior distributions in INLA can be found by typing inla.list.models("prior") and further information on any of these priors can be found by using the inla.doc() function. In general, we advise to always set your own prior distributions since the default prior proposals in inla may not be adequate for a general use. In any case, if you use the default prior distributions of inla, you should have previously assessed that they are suitable for your data and the sensibility to that choice.

Obviously, `INLA` does not preimplement the use of any prior distribution that we could think of, but in case we needed a distribution that was not implemented, `INLA` allows us to code it by ourselves. To make it, we will have to use the `expression` prior of `INLA`. One example of its use, which we will repeatedly use throughout the book, would be for defining an improper uniform prior distribution on the positive real line for the standard deviation of a Gaussian distribution. First, we should translate that distribution to an equivalent distribution on the log-precision, the parameter used to model the variability in Gaussian distributions, by making

$$P(\log(\tau)) = P(\sigma) \left| \frac{d\sigma}{d\log(\tau)} \right| \propto 1 \cdot \left| \frac{d\exp(-\log(\tau)/2)}{d\log(\tau)} \right| \propto \exp(-\log(\tau)/2).$$

Leaving aside the impropriety of this distribution, which INLA copes with by simply omitting the proportionality constant on this distribution, we can implement this in `INLA` by defining in R

```
sdunif="expression:
        logdens=-log_precision/2;
        return(logdens)"
```

which basically computes the log-density function corresponding to the $\log(\tau)$ distribution just derived. Thus, hereafter, if we want to use an improper uniform prior distribution on the standard deviation of a Gaussian likelihood, we would just have to include the argument

```
> control.family=list(hyper=list(prec=list(prior=sdunif)))
```

into our call to `inla`, obviously, once executed the definition of the `sdunif` function above. Please, note that `sdunif` goes without quotation marks in the `control.family` expression above, in contrast to every prebuilt prior distribution. We do not give more details on the use of the `expression` option since we will just use it to set improper uniform prior distributions on standard deviations, as shown above. However, you can find full details on its use at the documentation of the `INLA` package (`inla.doc("expression")`).

As for now, we have introduced how to set prior distributions for the parameters in $\boldsymbol{\theta}_1$, but we will also have hyperparameters in $\boldsymbol{\theta}_2$ for which we may want to set specific prior distributions. In that case, as described above for `control.family`, we would have to add a `hyper` argument with the corresponding options within the `f` functions that require the specification of a particular distribution. Thus, the `hyper` argument will have a different meaning for `inla` depending on its particular location.

So, with this, we would have everything needed ready for introducing our model in `INLA`: the specification of the likelihood, process and prior layers of our model. `inla`, in exchange, returns an object of class `inla`, which is a named list with lots of components. The main elements within `inla` objects are the summaries of the variables in the model. Thus, the components `summary.fixed` (for the fixed effects in ψ), `summary.hyperpar` (for $\boldsymbol{\theta}$), summary.linear.predictor (for $\boldsymbol{\eta}$) and summary.fitted.values (for $\boldsymbol{\phi}$) contain some of those useful summaries. The first I rows of the summary.random component of inla objects correspond to the contribution of all the random effects in the model to the linear predictor $\boldsymbol{\eta}$. The rest of their rows correspond to the fit of the different levels of the random effects fitted in the model. These summaries show a brief collection of statistics: posterior mean, standard deviation, 2.5%, 50% and 97.5% quantiles and posterior mode by default, for any variable in the model. inla objects have much more components than the summaries just described but, for now, they are enough for exploring the results of any call to inla.

We finally show some useful inla options for tuning the calls to this function. For example, the option control.compute=list(dic=TRUE), which is FALSE by default, should be included in any call to inla if we want it to compute the DIC model selection criterion. In that case we may find the corresponding DIC static in the dic component of the corresponding inla object. A second interesting option when calling inla is the following: control.predictor=list(compute=TRUE,cdf=0). The first of these arguments, compute=TRUE (the default value of this argument is FALSE), makes the values of the linear predictor $\boldsymbol{\eta}$ and fitted values $\boldsymbol{\phi}$ to be calculated. Otherwise, the summary.linear.predictor and the summary.fitted.values elements of the corresponding inla object would be returned as empty. Second, the argument cdf=0 computes for any component of the linear predictor its posterior probability of being lower than 0, that is, its cumulative distribution function at this point. You will have these probabilities as an additional column at the summary.linear.predictor component of the generated inla object. This value of the cumulative distribution will be extensively used in the following chapters. The option control.fixed=list(cdf=0) calculates the corresponding cumulative distribution function but on the fixed effects of the linear predictor. These values are useful for assessing if the fixed effect corresponding to a covariate may be considered "significantly different" from 0. Finally, it is worth mentioning that inla objects have their own plot and summary methods providing interesting information on the models fitted.

Example 3.4

We now turn back to the data in Example 2.3 on the temporal evolution of oral cancer mortality. There, we modeled that time trend by means of a non-linear function. We are now going to fit that model with INLA. As explained in Example 2.3, the model fitted can be viewed as a random effects model with the year modeled as a combination of functions. The random effects of the model will be the coefficients of a linear combination of several Gaussian functions centered at different places and evaluated at every year of the period of study. The random effects term can be put as $\boldsymbol{Z\gamma}$, for $\boldsymbol{Z}$ being a matrix whose columns correspond to each Gaussian function and their rows to the years under study. The vector γ contains Gaussian random effects for smoothing the impact of the large number of parameters that this term contains. This scheme fits into the design-matrix-based `"z"` random effects model of `INLA`. Therefore, the random effects model with 9 nodes in Example 2.3, could be fitted with `INLA` as

```
> base9 = matrix(nrow=21,ncol=9)
> for(j in 1:9){base9[,j] = dnorm(1:21,1+j*2,2)}
> data = data.frame(rate=rate,year=year-2001,id.node=1:21)
> form1 = rate ~ year + f(id.node,model="z",Z=base9)
> result1 = inla(form1,data=data,control.compute=list(dic=TRUE))
```

Figure 3.4 (left) shows the fit just made (dotted curve). The solid curve corresponds to the fit of the non-linear model with `WinBUGS` at Example 2.3. Both lines should show a closely similar fit, but they are not so close, in fact the non-linear component in the model fitted with `INLA` does not seem to have any effect since the trend fitted reproduces basically a straight line. Although both implementations correspond to the same model, we have not specified in `INLA` any prior distribution for the hyperparameters of the model, so `INLA` uses its default prior specifications and maybe this can be making a difference. According to the information in `inla.doc("gaussian")` and `inla.doc("z")` the default prior distributions for the precisions of both the data likelihood and the random effects in the non-linear term are $Gamma(1, 5 \cdot 10^{-5})$ distributions. This means that the prior mean for these two precisions is $1/(5 \cdot 10^{-5}) = 20,000$, which coincides also with their prior standard deviations.

To see what can be happening, we ask for a summary of the results of the model fitted with `INLA`

```
> summary(result1)
...
Model hyperparameters:
                                         mean        sd
Precision for the Gaussian observations  2.457 7.587e-01
Precision for id.node                18604.889 1.836e+04
...
```

We have removed some columns of this output above as they are of minor interest. The precision of the data likelihood (the `Gaussian observations` term) takes a low value, accounting for the presence of substantial residual error. On the contrary, the precision for the random effects is quite large, which cancels its effect out. It seems surprising that so few data may completely discard this term of the model. Moreover, it is also quite surprising to find the posterior mean and standard deviation so close to the same prior parameters of that precision, when these values were arbitrary. This suggests that the vague default prior distribution for this precision may be more influential than it could be initially expected. To check this, we run the same model with `INLA`

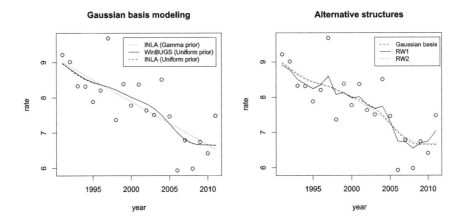

Figure 3.4

Left: Non-linear smoothing of the oral cancer mortality time trend. Model fitted with both `WinBUGS` and `INLA` and variability (for the `INLA` implementation) modeled with a $Gamma(1, 5 \cdot 10^{-5})$ prior distribution on the precision and a uniform distribution on the standard deviation of the random effects. Right: Oral cancer mortality time trend modeled with different smoothing devices: Non-linear fit with Gaussian basis and first-/second-order random walks.

but with a $Gamma(2, 5 \cdot 10^{-5})$ prior distribution, which is even vaguer than the previous one. The syntax for this new model is

```
> form1.b= rate ~ year + f(id.node,model="z",Z=base9,
                   hyper=list(prec=list(param=c(2,0.00005))))
> result1.b=inla(form1.b,data=data,
                   control.compute=list(dic=TRUE))
```

The posterior mean of the precision of the random effects for this new model moves to 38929.4 evidencing the sensitivity of this precision parameter to this gamma vague prior choice. In order to make a fair comparison with the `WinBUGS` implementation, we fit now that exact same model in `INLA`. We do this by putting an improper uniform prior distribution on the positive real line for the standard deviations of both the likelihood and the random effects term in this manner

```
> sdunif="expression:
>         logdens=-log_precision/2;
>         return(logdens)"
> form2 = rate ~ year + f(id.node,model="z",Z=base9,
                   hyper=list(prec=list(prior=sdunif)))
> result2=inla(form2,data=data,
                   control.compute=list(dic=TRUE),
                   control.family=
                   list(hyper=list(prec=list(prior=sdunif))))
```

with this prior distribution the posterior mean of the precision of the random effects is now 3.12 and its 95% credible interval [0.02, 20.76]. Therefore, the posterior distribution is now highly asymmetric, and puts considerable mass on their lower values, those putting more variability on the random effects term. In any case the precision now seems to learn from the data, in contrast to the vague gamma prior distribution, which advises for the use of the uniform prior distribution as a much more appropriate alternative. We will talk more in depth about the choice of prior distributions for parameters controlling the variability of random effects in the next chapter. The left side of Figure 3.4 shows also the fit corresponding to this model (dashed line). The curve fitted now clearly matches with that fitted with WinBUGS (solid line). This is not surprising since they correspond to the fit of exactly the same model with different softwares. The slight differences between these two curves are supposedly due to Monte Carlo error of the MCMC simulation. Nevertheless, the differences in terms of computing time are evident, WinBUGS spends 8.3 seconds to get the results when called from the bugs function and 6.0 seconds when called from pbugs (for n.iter=10000 iterations with n.burnin=1000, which yields satisfactory convergence statistics). On the other hand, INLA takes just 2.2 seconds to fit the same model with the default simplified Laplace strategy. Nevertheless, the fairest comparison within these softwares would be between INLA and pbugs since the first also uses parallel computing techniques to fit its models.

The right side of Figure 3.4 shows the fit obtained using other alternative smoothing devices. The non-linear fit with Gaussian basis in this plot (dashed line) corresponds to the INLA fit with a uniform prior distribution on the standard deviation (also the dashed line in the left side of the plot). As an alternative, we have also fitted with INLA two random effects models, fitting a different random effect for each observation, one with a first-order random walk structure (RW1) and another one with a second-order random walk (RW2). These dependence structures account for the temporal dependence that the data could show. The syntax used for fitting the RW1 model is

```
> form3 = rate ~ f(id.node,model="rw1",
                hyper=list(theta=list(prior=sdunif)))
> result3 = inla(form3,data=data,
                control.compute=list(dic=TRUE),
                control.family=
                list(hyper=list(theta=list(prior=sdunif))))
```

The syntax used for the RW2 model is exactly the same but substituting "rw1" by "rw2" in the expression for the formula of the model.

The right side of Figure 3.4 shows substantial differences for the different smoothing models compared. Although the non-linear fit with Gaussian basis and RW2 models show quite similar fits, the RW1 model depicts a much more rough trend, evidencing the effect of the dependence structure used. At this moment we just know that these fits are different but we do not have any clue pointing out which of them could be better, we could have some insight on this by means of the DIC criterion. We can get the DIC for the Gaussian basis model by simply typing `result2$dic$dic`, the same for the rest of models. The DIC for the Gaussian basis model is 48.4, 44.7 for the RW1 model and 48.6 for the RW2 model. Therefore, although no big differences are found between these three models in terms of DIC, the extra-smoothing of the Gaussian basis and RW2 models does not seem to yield any benefit.

Before concluding this introduction to the `INLA` basics, we find it convenient to pay some attention to two `inla` arguments. These are the `strategy` and `int.strategy` arguments that are set as sub arguments of the option `control.inla`. These are set as `control.inla=list(strategy=...,` `int.strategy=...)` where this expression is itself an argument of `inla`. The option `strategy` can take any of the following values: `"gaussian"`, `"simplified.laplace"` or `"laplace"`, being `"simplified.laplace"` the default option. This argument controls the approximation method used, as described at the beginning of this section. These three arguments are ordered in increasing level of numerical burden and reliability so, if you want to get a rapid fit, use the `strategy="gaussian"` option, but if you want a safe and reliable answer, use the `strategy="laplace"` option instead. Likewise, the option `int.strategy` is in charge of controlling the integration methods used for integrating θ, as also described at the beginning of this section. This option can take 1 of 6 different arguments, being `"auto"` the default option. You have to know that these two options may have important consequences on the fitting speed of models in `INLA` so you can tune them in order to make your model either more rapid or to yield more reliable results. There is not a clear guide to choose these arguments, in fact, there are very simple settings where the default options yield unsatisfactory results (see Exercise 1 at the end of this chapter). Our advice would be to try `INLA` with the most reliable options that your data, model and available time allow you.

Nowadays, although both `WinBUGS` and `INLA` have their own limitations, `WinBUGS` is able to fit a wider collection of models than `INLA`. `WinBUGS` cannot be used in general in those situations where we are not certain which model is better to fit the data at hand. This would require the use of trans-dimensional MCMC. Although `WinBUGS` has a module for reversible jump MCMC, this is very modest, with hardly any potential use. A second limitation of `WinBUGS` is that it has implemented a closed collection of distributions and going beyond them is not so easy, if possible. The third, and main limitation of `WinBUGS` is computational. MCMC methods are, per se, slow and `WinBUGS` is not an exception. This limitation with the current emergence of big data sets is a particularly dramatic problem, jeopardizing the use of `WinBUGS` in lots of current data sets. In this sense `INLA` is an interesting alternative to `WinBUGS`, making it possible to apply lots of Bayesian hierarchical models to large (or even huge) data sets. Nevertheless, INLA has a large, but closed, collection of prebuilt latent layers which we are limited to use. Moreover, WinBUGS has a full programming language for hierarchical models, making it possible to program most of the hierarchical models that we could think of, with lots of hierarchy levels if we wanted in contrast to INLA. Thus, in summary, either of these two alternatives has its own advantages, making it particularly suited for some settings and we should have both in mind, depending on the model and data set to be analyzed.

3.3 Plotting maps in R

Plotting maps is an essential activity in disease mapping studies. The models used typically return one (or several) risk estimate(s) for each of the units under study that will have to be summarized or plotted in some way. Obviously, tables will not be a sensible option when the number of geographical units is high because of the total volume of data to represent and because they ignore the geographical arrangement of data. Hence, mapping results of spatial analyses seems the only valid option available.

Disease mapping results are usually plotted by means of *choropleth maps*. These are maps composed of the boundaries of each geographical unit in the region of study. The area within each of these boundaries is shaded or coloured as a function of a variable of interest. Therefore, the first thing that we will need for plotting a choropleth map is a digital boundary file with the geometric shape of the units of study that we are going to represent. There are lots of web pages where you may download those files, such as http://geocommons.com/. National statistical institutes are also alternative sources for obtaining cartography files, thus we downloaded the Valencian Region cartography repeatedly used in this book from the Spanish Statistical Institute. Hence, the first thing that you should do in case of wanting to make a disease mapping study on a certain region is to get the corresponding digital boundary file to represent the results that you will obtain.

Boundary files can be stored in very different formats. We will just describe how to import and handle cartographies in *shapefile* format, surely the most common format for storing and sharing this information. In case you want to import boundary files in a different format, you will have to use a specific R package for this purpose such as rgdal, namely the readOGR function of this package. Bivand et al. (2008) is an excellent reference describing how this package can be used for this task and describing much more details on digital boundary files, Geographic Information Systems (GIS) and everything related to handling georeferenced information.

Shapefile is the file format originally used by ArcVIEW^{TM}, a popular GIS currently commercialized as ArcGIS^{TM} desktop by ESRI^{TM}. This format is composed of at least 3 files, the `whatever.shp` file which contains the geometric shapes that make up the map that we want to plot, the `whatever.shx` file, with an index of the shapes in the previous `.shp` file and the `whatever.dbf` file, a DBF III file (the file format of Dbase^{TM} databases) that stores some attributes for each geographical unit contained at the `.shp` file. These three files would be enough for drawing choropleth maps of the region corresponding to the shapefile. However, in some cases it would be interesting R to know how to project the objects contained in the shapefile within the globe Earth by means of its *coordinate reference system* (CRS). This would allow us, if wanted, to overlay several shapefiles in a single plot since referring all of them to a common reference system would make it possible to know the relative position of their objects. Moreover, knowing the CRS of a shapefile would also make it possible to superimpose it to background geographical information in Google^{TM} Maps or Google^{TM} Earth, for example. The CRS of a shapefile, which is optional, would be stored as a separate `whatever.prj` file. If we did not have this file available, and the CRS information was needed, we would have to retrieve it from the source where we obtained the shapefile and set the CRS by ourselves in R once we imported the shapefile. We are not going to give more details on this since, throughout the book, we will be typically interested in plotting maps in order to show the geographical distribution of the risks derived from our model regardless of the geographical context. Keep in mind that if we were interested in relating our results with the geographical context of the region of study, setting the CRS of our shapefiles would be a very useful tool.

The `readOGR` function of the `rgdal` package is particularly useful for importing shapefiles into R. The `readOGR` function has two compulsory arguments: `dsn` and `layer`. Basically, `dsn` will contain the path, within quotes and without a backslash at the end, to the directory where the shapefile is stored. If the shapefile was placed on the current working directory, it would be enough to set `dsn="."`. The argument layer should contain the name of the shapefile, without the `.shp` extension at the end and within quotes. A typical problem when importing shapefiles is that their elements may be stored in a different order than we would like. For example, municipalities could be stored in increasing order of their latitudes and we may want to have them ordered by the administrative code of the municipalities. In that case, we advise sorting the spatial units in the desired order just after importing shapefiles in order to save us lots of headaches. For example, a typical importing procedure would be the following. With

```
> Carto=readOGR(dsn=".",layer="muni")
```

we would import the shapefile `muni` stored in the current directory. Once imported, we can see the attributes of each of the spatial units imported (municipalities) by typing

```
> head(Carto@data)
```

In the output, a typical view of the first lines of a data.frame, we could check if the spatial units are ordered, or not, according to the administrative code of the municipalities (CODMUNI); otherwise, we could sort them according to this variable by making

```
> Carto=Carto[order(Carto@data$CODMUNI),]
```

It will be convenient to sort the cartography in the same order used for storing the observed deaths. Otherwise, we could easily plot by accident the information of each geographical unit in the polygon corresponding to other units, producing plots that do not reflect at all the geographical distribution of the variable to be shown. Taking care of this issue will save you lots of errors and misleading interpretations of wrong maps.

readOGR returns an object of class SpatialPolygonsDataFrame. This is a class defined at the sp package of R for containing spatial objects composed by sets of polygons. SpatialPolygonsDataFrame are composed of several components (slots), namely, for the Carto object defined above these are Carto@data, Carto@polygons, Carto@proj4strings, Carto@bbox and Carto@plotOrder. The first of them, the data slot contains a data.frame with the information stored in the DBF file accompanying the .shp file. The polygons slot is a list whose components are, in turn, a set of polygons composing each entity stored (in our case municipalities) in the original shapefile, so any of these entities may be composed of several polygons. Every one of these components of polygons has also different slots containing information on the total area enclosed by the polygons, the coordinates delimiting them, an ID, etc. The proj4strings slot contains, if available, information on the CRS used to project the coordinates of the polygons. The bbox slot contains the coordinates of a bounding box, plus a margin, containing all the polygons in the shapefile that will be useful for plotting them. Finally, the plotOrder slot contains a vector pointing out the order in which the polygons will be plotted.

If the original shapefile did not contain a set of polygons, but other geographical entities such as point risk facilities, it could also be read with the readOGR function but, in contrast, the result of the imported shapefile would be saved in objects of other different classes. Thus, when importing a shapefile composed of a set of points, readOGR will return an object of class spatialPointsDataFrame. Likewise, readOGR could be used for importing shapefiles composed of segments (such as the course of a river) which will return an object of class spatialLinesDataFrame. These objects have similar structure to the spatialPolygonsDataFrame objects; however, we will not pay them as much attention as the polygonal objects since the latter will be the ones that we will use for plotting choropleth maps. The rgdal package has also a function (writeOGR) for exporting the spatial objects just introduced. Once we have imported a shapefile into R the most convenient option for its subsequent use in this program is to store the corresponding spatial*DataFrame object into R workspaces. The

SpatialPolygonsDataFrame with the boundaries of the Valencian Region stored in `https://github.com/MigueBeneito/DisMapBook/tree/master/Data/VR.Rdata` of the supplementary material is simply that.

`spatial*DataFrame` classes have their own plotting methods. Thus, `plot(Carto)` will make a simple plot of the digital boundary file imported above. In choropleth maps, the polygons are coloured or filled as a function of a variable of interest. For colouring the units in a `spatialPolygonsDataFrame` object, we will have to give a `col` argument to the `plot` function. This argument will be a vector of the same length as the number of units in the spatial object, with the colours to be used for filling each of those units. For plotting choropleth maps, a colour palette should be defined with the colours to be used to fill the polygons. A useful way to do this is by executing `pal=gray((1:n)/(n+1))`, for a suitable value of n. This creates a palette for plotting n different groups, everyone with a different level of gray, ranging from black (the first of the n colours) to white (the n-th colour). Thus, for drawing a choropleth map, we should make `plot(Carto,col=pal[which.colour])`, where `which.colour` is a vector determining which group (out of the n available groups) each geographical unit belongs to.

The `plot` function for spatial objects in R admits lots of options as usual in `plot` functions in general. An interesting option is the `add` argument, by default equal to `FALSE`. When set to `TRUE`, this function plots the corresponding object overlaying the actual plot, which makes it possible to superimpose the information corresponding to different spatial objects, such as the polygons of some geographical units and some additional point sources. Additionally, the `plot` function for spatial objects admits the usual arguments of plot functions in general, such as `pch`, `cex` for points or `lwd` for lines or polygons, to cite just a few. Finally, a useful function for plotting choropleth maps is `legend`. This function is used to plot legends with the colours or symbols used in choropleth maps, which is a useful complement given the amount of information stored in them. We suggest you read the help documentation for this function since you will typically use it quite often when plotting your own maps.

Example 3.5

Figure 1.2 shows a customized map of the Valencian Region. We are going to review how that map was created. You can find the code with more detail in the accompanying material of the book. This map is composed of three different layers of spatial objects, originally stored as shapefiles: the division of the Valencian Region into its 540 municipalities, plotted as black lines; the division of the Valencian Region into its 3 provinces, plotted as blue lines; and third, the geographical limits of the whole of Spain, plotted as a thicker blue line. All three shapefiles come also with the accompanying material of the book. We import the municipal boundary file with these sentences:

```
> Muni=readOGR("../Data/Carto","muni")
> head(Muni@data)
> Muni=Muni[order(Muni@data$CODMUNI),]
```

The first two lines of this code allow us to explore the variables in the data.frame linked to `Muni` and thus to know the name of the variable that we want to use for setting the ordering of the municipalities. Namely, in the third of these sentences, we order the municipalities as a function of their municipal codes, the usual order used also for municipal data in most information sources. The shapefiles with the boundaries of the provinces and the whole of Spain are imported likewise.

In order to colour the municipalities in the Valencian Region as a function of their populations, we first have to set a palette of colours, in our case we have made it by making `palette=brewer.pal(5,"YlOrBr")`, which sets a palette ranging from yellow to brown, with 5 different tones (we will introduce more in depth this function of the `RColorBrewer` library just after this example). Afterwards, we cut the variable containing the populations into 5 different categories with the sentence

```
> cuts=as.numeric(cut(PopMuni,c(0,100,1000,10000,100000,Inf)))
```

where `PopMuni` is a vector with the populations of the municipalities in the Valencian Region, ordered by their municipal codes. Finally, we set the vector of colours corresponding to each municipality as `colours=palette[cuts]`. Plotting the municipalities with the colours just defined is as easy as making `plot(Muni,col=colours)`, and plotting the provinces and country layers would be similar, without the `col` argument but with the option `add=TRUE` so that these plots are overlaid to the previous plot.

Finally, we have also plotted the legend of the figure by means of the following syntax

```
> legend(x="bottomright",
        legend=c("<100","101-1000","1001-10000","10001-100000",
                ">100000"),
        fill=palette, title="Population")
```

Plotting maps may seem an easy task once you know the R functions needed to do it. However, plotting sensible maps deserves some considerations. First, the palette of colours used for filling the polygons in choropleth maps may seem an arbitrary choice; indeed it is, but some guidelines should be borne in mind for that election. The R package `RColorBrewer` allows you to easily use some appropriate colour palettes for plotting maps. Thus, a call to `display.brewer.all()` displays the range of palettes available in this library with their corresponding names. Once you choose one of these palettes at your convenience, the function `brewer.pal` will be used to build a specific colour palette for its use. This function has 2 arguments n, containing the number of different colours that you want to include in your palette and name, the name of the palette (between quotation marks) that you may have chosen from the call to the display.brewer.all function.

Regarding the choice of colour palettes, it is important that you consider the type of variable that you are intending to plot. Namely, you should distinguish between plotting qualitative or quantitative variables. In the first case, no particular ordering of the colours would be needed, so any rainbow-like palette would be appropriate in this case. These palettes are known as *qualitative* and are those placed in the second block of the plot produced by the display.brewer.all function. These palettes would be appropriate for plotting, for example, the predominant racial or confessional group for each geographical unit in a region of study since, for these, it is difficult to set some kind of ordering for the groups to be plotted.

For quantitative variables we have two sensible choices, *sequential* and *diverging* palettes. Sequential palettes are placed within the first block of those plotted with the display.brewer.all, meanwhile the diverging palettes are those shown at the third of these blocks. Sequential palettes should be used for ordinal/quantitative variables ranging from low to high without any reference value of particular meaning. These palettes often use monochromatic scales differing in the lightness or darkness of the colors. Namely, when needing a sequential scale, we often use the YlOrRd palette, whose colours differ gradually in the amount of red or yellow that they contain. We can set that palette with 5 different colours, by making brewer.pal(5,"YlOrRd") as in the previous example. When using sequential palettes, it is not convenient to use more than 5 or 6 colours, since otherwise the different colours cannot be clearly distinguished in the corresponding choropleth map.

Diverging palettes are used for ordinal/quantitative variables having a central reference value that we may want to identify, such as temperature in Celsius degrees. In this case, we may want to colour the regions having 0°C in white, for example, and put positive temperatures in one chromatic scale (for instance reds of varying darkness) different than the scale used for negative values (for example blues). For diverging palettes, we often use the BrBG palette which ranges from brown to white and from white to green, in this case white could be used for the reference value of the scale. Diverging palettes allow the use of a higher amount of colours since they really merge two sequential palettes converging at the reference (central) colour. Thus, the command brewer.pal(7,"BrBG")[7:1] would set a Green-White-Brown palette with 7 different colours. The [7:1] term in this last expression puts the green colours for the lower values of the palette, and therefore of the corresponding variable, which seems more natural for representing risks. The web page http://colorbrewer2.org, maintained by the developer of the RColorBrewer package, shows on real maps the different scales in this package and introduces some considerations such as the use of printer-friendly palettes, colourblind safe or photocopy safe scales, aspects that are usually unnoticed by novel producers of choropleth maps. So, we advise you to use one of the palettes available in this package since they are supposed to be reasonable choices, based on sound arguments and studies (Brewer et al., 1997; Harrower and Brewer, 2003) instead of just personal and arbitrary preferences.

One last issue about drawing choropleth maps is the way in which the variable to be plotted is cut so that their values are assigned to one of the colours in the palette. In our example above, we have used *fixed cuts* (the cuts are set to some fixed values, usually with a particular meaning) for plotting the population in each municipality. This is usually a convenient option, mainly when several maps have to be plotted, as these cuts make it possible to use a common scale for all the maps; indeed fixed cuts are often used in mortality atlases (Martínez-Beneito et al., 2005; López-Abente et al., 2006; Borrell et al., 2009). However, fixed cuts have some drawbacks because they do not adapt to the data plotted. This could mean, for example, that all the geographical units were plotted with a single colour of the palette used. An obvious alternative is to base the cuts of the variable on its quantiles, that is, if a palette with 5 colours is going to be used, we will split the original variable according to its 20, 40, 60 and 80% quantiles. These cuts define 5 groups with roughly the same units for any of them. The main drawback of using quantile-based cuts is that the comparison between different choropleth maps is hard to be made since each map has its own cuts. Moreover, if the original variable is highly asymmetric, some of the cuts (mostly around the mode of the distribution) may be very close, defining narrow groups with irrelevant differences compared to its adjacent categories, in contrast to fixed cuts, which are placed defining meaningful groups with meaningful differences among them.

An alternative to fixed and quantiles-based cuts is *Fisher-Jenks* cuts. These are chosen so that the intra-class variance for the resulting groups is minimized. Consequently, the range of values used to define these groups tends to be homogeneous avoiding groups with excessively large or short ranges. Nevertheless, this class of cuts shows again the problem of comparability among maps corresponding to different diseases. Since the cuts are data-dependent, they will be different for any different map making comparisons among them hard. We personally use fixed cuts for most of our choropleth maps since comparability of different maps is an important issue, mostly for producing mortality atlases where several different causes of mortality are studied. Nevertheless, we acknowledge that the scale used for some fixed cuts cannot be adequate for all data sets, yielding plots that do not display any information of interest. Thus, quantiles and Fisher-Jenks cuts are two alternatives to fixed cuts that should be borne in mind for using them in some particular contexts.

R has a specific package for setting and handling cuts of continuous variables in choropleth maps, the `classInt` package. Namely, the `classIntervals` function in this package can be used to cut a continuous variable into several disjoint intervals. The main arguments for this function are `var` which is used to set the variable to be cut, n that sets the number of intervals in which the original variable is going to be split and `style`, which sets the style to be used for building the intervals. The options `fixed`, `quantile` (the default option) and `fisher` for the `style` argument, set the different types of cuts that we have described, although the `classInt` package has implemented some other different alternatives that you can consult in the help documentation. The option `style="jenks"` performs an alternative implementation of the Fisher-Jenks cuts (compatible with the implementation made of these cuts in some GIS programs); however, few differences should be expected with respect to the `fisher` option. In case of using the option `style="fixed"`, the option `fixedBreaks` should also be specified. This argument should be a vector of n+1 components with the limits of the intervals (including the extremes of the scale) to be used to categorize the variable of interest. The `classIntervals` function admits more arguments, mainly for customizing the labels of the new variable. Nevertheless, for us, the main use of these labels will be to set the text in legends of choropleth maps, which can also be customized in the `legend` function as done in the example above. Thus you can opt for either of these two alternatives.

Once you have classified the values of the variable to be plotted into the corresponding intervals, with the `classIntervals` function, the `classInt` package has also a function for assigning colours to the values of the original variable as a function of the interval that they belong to. Thus, `findColours`, with main arguments `clI` and `pal` makes that assignment. Namely, `clI` will contain the object resulting from calling to `classIntervals`, that is the original vector divided into intervals, and `pal` will contain the palette to be used (with as many colours as intervals in the `clI` argument) for assigning colours to the intervals. Hereafter, we will use these two functions of the `classInt` package for cutting variables to be used in choropleth maps and handling the colours used to plot the corresponding variables.

3.4   Some interesting resources in R for disease mapping practitioners

Models that incorporate the spatial dependence of the geographical units have to know in some manner their geographical arrangement. The `spdep` package of R has some specific functions to handle this issue. The previous sections have shown how R imports files containing the boundaries of a region of study and stores them into specific spatial objects as `SpatialPolygonsDataFrame` objects in R. A usual way to incorporate the geographical arrangement of the region of study into spatial models is by means of a list of pairs of geographical units which are close to each other, i.e., the list of neighbours corresponding to the region of study. Specifically, the `spdep` package has the `poly2nb` function for this purpose. The only compulsory argument to `poly2nb` is `pl`, which should contain the `SpatialPolygonsDataFrame` object whose neighbours we want to determine. By default, `poly2nb` reads the boundaries of all the geographical units and sets as neighbours all two pairs that share at least one of their borders. In that case both units are said to be *adjacent* regions. This function returns an object of class `nb`, which is a list with its i-th component being a vector that contains the adjacent units of the i-th geographical unit. In case of wanting to edit the set of neighbours returned, `nb` objects easily allow for this possibility by removing or adding the desired pairs of neighbours. The `nb` objects have their own `summary` method, which is an interesting tool to detect unexpected errors. For example, this summary returns the number of geographical units without neighbours. In case that the original cartography contained some kind of error, this is an easy way of becoming aware of it, since the number of isolated units is a value that can be visually checked with just a plot of the region of study.

The `poly2nb` function has also an interesting argument `snap`, which is the minimum distance between the boundaries of two geographical units so that they may be considered neighbours. By default, this value is set as a function of the precision used by R for storing floating point numbers, that is, almost 0 in practice. In principle, putting a low value for `snap` higher than 0, 1 for example, which would mean considering two units as neighbours if they are not placed more than 1 meter away, should not induce great changes in the corresponding `nb` object. If it does, this could highlight some problem in the original boundary file. For example, one of the shapefiles that we used once showed several "islands" (regions without neighbours), when a plot of the cartography showed no island. When putting the option `snap=1`, the islands suddenly disappeared. We finally realized that the polygons corresponding to the islands had been edited in a GIS and afterwards the whole shapefile was saved again. The working precision of the machine where this task was done was different than that in the machine where the original shapefile was created. As a result, the polygons edited had some few digits less than their neighbours (which had not been edited) and with the default value of `snap` they were not matched as neighbours. Thus, comparing the `nb` objects generated for different values of `snap` can be a safe procedure to assess the neighbours generated from a `SpatialPolygonsDataFrame` object.

As a related comment, we would like to warn about handling cartography files. The importation and handling of these files is a usual source of unexpected errors. The amount of information stored in shapefiles (or any other GIS files format) may easily hide unexpected problems that will not be easy to notice. So, when having a first contact with a boundary file, we advise you to be extremely cautious with the importation and assessment of its information. If you finally find that information appropriate, with a right ordering of the units, with exact coincidence between adjacent units, etc., then store it in an Rdata file for posterior use, instead of importing it from scratch every time you need it. This will save you lots of problems in the future.

Thus, nb objects are those in charge of storing information about the geographical arrangement of the region of study. However, they do not have the format needed by WinBUGS or INLA to use this kind of objects. However, the spdep package has specific functions for converting nb objects to these formats. Namely, the nb2WB function, which has a single argument, the corresponding nb object, converts it to a suitable format to be used by WinBUGS. Likewise, the nb2INLA function converts nb objects to a suitable format to be used by INLA. The nb2INLA function has two arguments, file which contains the file for saving the pairs of neighbours in the format required by INLA, and nb which contains the corresponding nb object to be converted to INLA format. The nb2INLA function returns a file with .graph extension which would typically be placed in the working directory of your analysis.

Example 3.6

The VR.Rdata file contains a SpatialPolygonsDataFrame object with the municipal boundaries of the Valencian Region and the set of neighbouring pairs of municipalities saved in two different formats: as an nb object and with a suitable format to be used by WinBUGS. We are going to see now how these objects were generated. The VR.cart is a ShapePolyDataFrame object, which is simply the result of importing the muni shapefile in https://github.com/MigueBeneito/DisMapBook/tree/master/Data/Carto, ordered as a function of the municipal codes, as made in Example 3.5.

The VR.nb object can be obtained by executing VR.nb=poly2nb(VR.cart), once the spdep package is loaded. A summary of this object shows that there are a total of 3094 pairs of neighbours in VR.cart and all the municipalities have at least 1 neighbour, which seems good news. Nevertheless, the Valencian Region has an "island" at its western side composed of several municipalities placed some few kilometers away from the rest of the region. To avoid potential problems, we decided to define the closest municipalities of the island and of the rest of the Valencian Region as neighbours: Ademuz and Aras de Alpuente. Once searched, we find that those municipalities in the VR.cart@data object are, respectively, the 277th and 317th polygons in VR.cart. Thus, the following syntax is executed to set them as neighbours

```
> VR.nb[[277]]=sort(c(VR.nb[[277]],as.integer(317)))
> VR.nb[[317]]=sort(c(VR.nb[[317]],as.integer(277)))
```

Once the VR.nb object is modified, we convert it to an appropriate format to be used by WinBUGS by simply executing VR.wb=nb2WB(VR.nb).

This code explains how to generate all the objects saved in the VR.Rdata file from the muni shapefile. Also, https://github.com/MigueBeneito/DisMapBook/Data contains a file VR.graph with the neighbouring municipalities of the Valencian Region in a suitable format to be used by INLA.

This file has been generated by simply executing `nb2INLA(VR.nb, file="/Data/VR.graph")`.

We also find it interesting to mention two more R packages for performing advanced displays of choropleth maps: `RGoogleMaps` and `plotKML` . These two packages make it possible to plot choropleth maps into Google Maps and Google Earth, respectively, instead of into R graphics devices. This allows us to visualize and explore with detail the geographical context of the information displayed in any choropleth map and therefore make its interpretation easier. Obviously, for using these packages, our `SpatialPolygonsDataFrame` object should have a valid CSR so that it can be exactly projected on the geographical background provided by both Google Maps and Earth. We are not going to give more details on the use of these packages since they will not be of general interest to most readers of this book. However, we find it convenient that you bear them in mind in case you need a more advanced display of the geographical information that you generate. More R packages also perform similar tasks to `RGoogleMaps`, such as `leaflet` or `plotly`. These packages allow you to plot interactive choropleth maps over cartographic services. This makes it possible to explore the information in the choropleth maps in its particular geographic context. These are quite useful tools allowing us to explore the results in our analyses in a much more detailed way.

Finally, we would like to conclude this chapter with a brief review of 'The Basic Toolkit of the Disease Mapping Practitioner', as stated throughout the chapter. This tool kit should include R, `WinBUGS` and several R packages. Among these, `R2WinBUGS` and `pbugs` will allow us to call `WinBUGS` from within R. Moreover, `rgdal`, `maptools`, `sp` and `spdpep` will be used for importing/handling spatial objects in R and `RColorBrewer` and `classInt` will be useful for drawing convenient choropleth maps. If we would like to plot these choropleth maps within Google Maps or Earth in order to improve their interpretability, we could do it with `RGoogleMaps` and `plotKML`, respectively. Finally, `INLA` allows us to call the stand-alone INLA C routines from within R. In our opinion, 'The Basic Toolkit of the Disease Mapping Practitioner' is something, hereafter, you should have installed on your computer.

Exercises

1. Let us assume the following vector `y=c(1,rep(0,9))` to represent 10 independent draws of a Bernoulli random variable y. Let us assume that we wanted to estimate the probability of y being equal to 1 by means of a logistic regression model depending on simply an intercept term.

- •Fit a frequentist logistic regression model with the `glm` function of R. According to this model, estimate $P(y = 1)$ as the anti-logit of the intercept term obtained.

- •Fit a Bayesian logistic regression model with `WinBUGS`. Estimate $P(y = 1)$ for each iteration of the MCMC so that you can derive its posterior distribution. Compare the frequentist and Bayesian estimates obtained for $P(y = 1)$, do they coincide? Compare the frequentist and Bayesian estimates reported for the intercept of the logistic regression model, do they coincide? Do you find any explanation for the differences found on these estimates?

- •Fit a Bayesian logistic regression model with `INLA`. Use both `"gaussian"` and `"simplified.laplace"` options for the `strategy` argument of `INLA`. Do these new estimates of $P(y = 1)$ and the intercept coincide with any of those derived from the `glm` function or `WinBUGS`? Which of those estimates (`glm` or `WinBUGS`) would you expect to coincide with the `INLA` estimates?

- •Set now the safest option `strategy="laplace"` in `INLA` and fit once again the logistic regression. Compare the estimates of the intercept and $P(y = 1)$ derived now with those previously computed and draw your own conclusions.

2. At the web page `https://github.com/MigueBeneito/DisMapBook/tree/master/Exercises`, you will find a `WinBUGS` file (`FlawedModels.odc`) with a series of `WinBUGS` models and the corresponding data sets and initial values needed to run them. All those models have some particular bug that makes `WinBUGS` crash. Pay attention to the different warnings/errors that `WinBUGS` report and the placement of the cursor when errors are reported in order to find the corresponding bugs and guess how to fix them.

3. Use the R package `R2WinBUGS` (or `pbugs`) for running some of the flawed models in the previous exercise. Pay attention to the additional difficulties posed by `R2WinBUGS` for debugging `WinBUGS` code.

4. Use `pbugs` in order to make inference on the models proposed in Exercise 1 of the previous chapter.

5. The file `ValenciaCity.zip`, available at the online supplementary material repository of `GitHub`, contains a shapefile, with all the related files, corresponding to Valencia City census tracts. The original file, available at the web page of the Spanish National Institute of Statistics, has been modified in order to match the data that will be used for the next chapters. Calculate the adjacency matrix corresponding to that shapefile. Convert that information to a format usable by `WinBUGS` and `INLA` in order to use that matrix in the

exercises of the next chapters. Save these objects so that they can be used in the future, since they will be useful for the exercises in the next chapters.

6. Draw a choropleth map in R with the shapefile imported in the previous exercise. Colour each census tract according to the number of dwellings per census tract (variable n_viv in the shapefile). Choose an appropriate colour palette for this variable of the RColorBrewer library of R.

4

Disease mapping from foundations

In the previous two chapters we have introduced Bayesian statistics and some computational tools of current use for the practice of disease mapping. With this background, we are now in an optimal position for starting our journey through the field of disease mapping. In this chapter we are going to introduce the basics of this research area.

Section 4.1 starts by introducing some epidemiological risk measures that will be extensively used later as a basis of disease mapping studies. A good understanding of those risk measures will shed light on the underlying statistical problem that arises when working with small areas in disease mapping studies. Section 4.1 also motivates disease mapping as a statistical problem that will focus our attention for the rest of the book. In Section 4.2 we introduce some methods for dealing with small areas, but based on the assumption of conditional independence between observations. Finally, Section 4.3 in this chapter starts introducing some basic distributions that will enable us to incorporate the assumption of spatial dependence on the observed data. This section ends with an explanation of the use of those distributions for modeling disease mapping problems, paying particular attention to the Besag, York and Mollié model (Besag et al., 1991) that has been (and surely continues to be) the reference proposal in the disease mapping literature.

4.1 Why disease mapping?

This section is going to introduce the statistical problem underlying and motivating disease mapping. First, we introduce some risk measures of current use in epidemiology and, therefore, in disease mapping. This introduction will not surely be necessary for those readers with a previous background in epidemiology, but it will help readers with a stronger background in statistics and without epidemiological background to understand, from a statistical point of view, the epidemiological ideas and motivation of disease mapping.

4.1.1   Risk measures in epidemiology

Epidemiology is mainly concerned with measuring the occurrence of health events in populations (Segen, 2002), whose individual probability is called the *risk* of the corresponding disease between epidemiologists. Having a collection of sensible risk measures is of outstanding importance for doing epidemiologic studies. Naive risk estimates could lead us to conclude naive conclusions, such as that places with more deaths are those where the most people live or those with an older population. Those conclusions will be obviously valueless from an epidemiological perspective and could be hiding some important risk factors that could be otherwise evidenced with more sensible risk estimates.

There are different kinds of events that we may be interested in. For example, we may want to know the amount of new cases of a disease taking place in a region during a time window. This is what epidemiologists call the *incidence* of the disease. Incidence measures are very useful for monitoring the progression of disease epidemic outbreaks, such as influenza or Ebola, in which case we would be interested in knowing the daily or weekly number of new cases in order to quantify the strength of the epidemics as time goes by. On the other hand, the amount of new cases of a disease during a period may not be as important as the total number of cases in the same population at a specific date, regardless whether these cases are new or not. This concept is known as the *prevalence* of the disease and is particularly useful for chronic diseases, where people have the disease for all their life. Prevalence measures are useful for estimating, for instance, the cost of a disease for a health system. Finally, if we were mostly interested in the most adverse health event produced by a disease, the number of deaths produced, instead of just the raw number of cases, we would be talking about the *mortality* of the disease. Usually, due to data availability, the most common epidemiological indicator in disease mapping studies is mortality. Therefore, as already mentioned in Chapter 1, when exposing the theoretical and practical issues that will be introduced during the rest of the book, we will talk about mortality, regardless of the fact that everything exposed could be also applied to other epidemiological concepts.

The most common mortality risk measures are (annual mortality) *rates*. If a population is divided into I units of study, such as different ethnic groups, several spatial units (municipalities for instance), etc. the annual mortality rate for the i-th unit is defined as $r_i = o_i/p_i$, where o_i are the observed deaths for that unit during the period of study and p_i are the number of follow-up years of the people in that unit during that period. That number of follow-up years is usually measured in terms of *person-years*. The person-years for a rate are usually calculated as the number of people in a population multiplied by the years of the period of study. Nevertheless, if individual information for the number of follow-up years was available, it could be used for deriving more accurate estimates of this quantity. Annual mortality rates, or simply rates, estimate the probability of death for a person in some unit of study during a follow-up year. Usually, rates are multiplied by a factor, such as

100,000, in which case they are interpreted as the annual deaths for every 100,000 people. This indicator is of great interest for estimating the risk of either a whole population or subgroups of that population. In our case we will typically be interested in estimating the risks for a series of population subgroups arising of the geographical division (census tracts, census wards, counties, municipalities, etc.) of the whole population under study. Rates could be useful estimates for those risks, making it possible to compare mortality for every spatial unit in our study.

Although rates are useful in some settings, epidemiologists rarely pursue the estimation of the risk for a certain population group as a final goal. That isolated risk rarely has a particular interest, as we do not have a reference value to compare it with. As a consequence, epidemiologists are usually interested in comparing the risks for several groups of a population, in our case geographical units, with the corresponding risk in the whole population. This comparison will make it possible to determine which unit(s), if any, show some risk excess in comparison to the whole population.

The *rate ratio* is an epidemiological indicator of particular interest for comparing the relative risks of two populations, that is the quotient of their risks. The rate ratio for two populations is defined as the ratio of the corresponding (annual mortality) rates. Rate ratios are mostly used for comparing the risks of specific units of study against that of the whole population in the study. In that case, the rate corresponding to the whole population is usually placed at the denominator of the rate ratio. Therefore, a value higher, respectively lower, than 1 of a rate ratio will mean a higher, respectively lower, risk for the corresponding unit than for the whole population. More in detail, if we denoted by $o_* = \sum_i o_i$, $p_* = \sum_i p_i$ the total observed deaths and person-years for the whole region of study, and $r_* = o_*/p_*$ the corresponding overall rate, the rate ratio for the i-th unit of study is defined as

$$R_i = \frac{r_i}{r_*} = \frac{o_i/p_i}{o_*/p_*}, \ i = 1, \ldots, I. \tag{4.1}$$

This rate ratio estimates the relative risk of unit i in comparison to the whole population. Expression (4.1) can be alternatively viewed as

$$R_i = \frac{o_i}{p_i \cdot r_*}, \ i = 1, \ldots, I.$$

The denominator in this expression is the product of the persons living in unit i by the probability of death for the whole region of study. This is the expected deaths in unit i if people there died in the same manner as in the whole population, according to the overall rate r_*. In fact, the denominator in this expression is usually denoted as e_i and is referred to as the *expected cases* for that unit. Therefore, the rate ratio for unit i can be alternatively viewed as the quotient between the observed and expected cases in that population assuming, for calculating e_i, that people in that unit die in the same manner as the whole population. From here on, we will refer to R_i as simply a *mortality ratio*.

Although mortality ratios are appealing indicators for detecting units of study with risk excesses, they are in some manner naive risk indicators. For example, if the mortality ratio in a unit points out a risk excess, it could be due either to a legitimate risk excess in the people living there or just to the composition of its population. Thus, for instance, if we found a high breast cancer mortality ratio for some unit whose population was composed of a higher proportion of women than the rest of the region of study, the mortality ratio would not discern whether that proportion is the factor causing the risk excess found, or not. Consequently, mortality ratios may depict sometimes misleading views of the distribution of the risk in a population, reproducing other exogenous (possibly demographic) factors instead of the risk distribution that we want to visualize. This demographic effect in mortality ratios is usually due to the age composition of the units available, which can make substantial differences in rate ratios, regardless of the risk of the units of study. Consequently, we will be typically interested in controlling the potential effect of the age composition of the population of every unit of study.

The main way for controlling the effect of a confounding factor when risks are estimated is to consider comparable populations with regard to that factor. That is, if we wanted to estimate the risk of a disease, controlling the effect of the age composition of that unit, we could calculate the previous mortality rates for a particular age group, such as people from 50 to 60 years old. Therefore, the observed cases and population would only take into account people in this age group. This would yield the corresponding *age-specific rate*, or ratio, if divided by the corresponding age-specific rate for the general population. Age-specific rates control the effect of age since the population for each unit will be 'equally old', so age-specific rates will not show any confounding age effect. Nevertheless, age-specific mortality rates have a clear drawback; the amount of information used to calculate them is much lower and if the age band is made wider (so that the amount of people considered is increased), then the populations compared would no longer be so comparable. Moreover, the use of several age-specific rates instead of a single overall rate for the whole population is also a second drawback since handling and summarizing all the age-specific indicators is not as easy as doing it for an overall rate. In order to solve this issue, we resort to *standardizing* rate ratios.

Let us assume that we had our population divided into age groups, such as quinquennial groups, and let us denote by r_i^t the age-specific mortality rate corresponding to the t-th age group and i-th unit. Similarly, let us denote r_*^t the age-specific mortality ratio for the whole population. In that case, the *standardized mortality ratio (SMR)* for the i-th unit of study is defined as

$$SMR_i = \frac{\sum_t p_i^t \cdot r_i^t}{\sum_t p_i^t \cdot r_*^t} = \frac{\sum_t o_i^t}{\sum_t p_i^t \cdot r_*^t} = \frac{o_i}{\sum_t p_i^t \cdot r_*^t}.$$

Both numerator and denominator in this expression are weighted sums of age-specific rates, with weights given by the age composition of the i-th unit of study. Standardization induces the same age compositions in numerator and denominator making both rates comparable in demographic terms. As a consequence, the noncomparability of numerators and denominators of (un-standardized) rate ratios, due to the different age compositions of the corresponding populations, is no longer an issue for standardized ratios.

Regarding the SMRs denominator, note that each of the summands is the age-specific expected cases for unit i, assuming that the age-specific mortalities for that unit were those of the whole population. Therefore, that denominator can be once again interpreted as the number of (age-standardized) expected deaths for unit i. Hence, the interpretation of unstandardized mortality ratios as the quotient of observed and expected cases for the corresponding unit, also holds for SMRs, but now for a standardized version of the expected cases, which makes numerator and denominator demographically comparable. Consequently SMRs interpretation is exactly the same as that introduced above for the mortality ratios: SMR_i values higher than 1 will stand for a risk excess in unit i, while values lower than 1 mean a lower risk for the population in that unit.

In a similar manner that rates are frequently multiplied by 100,000, SMRs are frequently multiplied by 100 in the epidemiologic literature, making 100 the reference (neutral) value for risks, instead of 1. We will indistinctly use both conventions for the reference level of SMRs, since both scales are very different and the results in one scale will be hardly confounded with the other scale. There is no mathematical advantage for multiplying SMRs by 100, but by doing that we will match the usual epidemiological convention so, in our opinion, both options have their own advantages.

As mentioned, SMRs are estimates of the relative risk of any municipality, controlled by age, whose effect we want to leave aside. Standardization is essential in epidemiology since confounding factors modifying risk estimates, such as the age composition of populations, are present all around. Consequently, the use of standardized mortality ratios in epidemiological studies is, by far, much more frequent than that of the corresponding (non-standardized) mortality ratios. However, SMRs are far from perfect. For example, for two populations accomplishing that the age-specific rates for the second population (r_2^t) are proportional to the corresponding rates of the first population $(r_2^t = \lambda r_1^t)$ we would expect the same relationship to hold between both regions $(SMR_2 = \lambda SMR_1)$, but this does not hold in general. The populations used for weighting the age-specific rates for SMR_1 and SMR_2 are different which will make the proportionality on the SMRs fail. As a consequence, SMR_i is useful for comparing the risk in unit i with the reference population, but not for comparing the risk of that unit with some other units in the study.

Note that SMRs could be easily generalized for incidence and prevalence of diseases. In that case the corresponding ratios are known as standardized incidence ratio (SIR) and standardized morbidity ratio. In a similar manner, we have defined SMRs above using as reference population the whole population in the study (the set of all units of study considered). Nevertheless, this definition could be easily generalized for other different reference populations by using overall age-specific rates corresponding to that reference population of interest. This is just a question of the benchmark population that we want to compare our rates with. If we used the whole population in the study as reference population, rates are said to be *internally standardized* while for any other reference population, rates are said to be *externally standardized*. Interestingly, for internal standardization $e_* = \sum_i e_i = \sum_i p_i(o_*/p_*) = (o_*/p_*)\sum_i p_i = o_*$, so the SMRs will be in general centered around 1. For external standardization, the SMRs will not be necessarily centered around 1. Indeed if the region of study has a risk higher than the region of study, they will be centered at a value higher than 1 and it could be even possible that all the SMRs could be higher than 1.

There are far more risk measures in epidemiology beyond SMRs. Age specific rates (Dean et al., 2001), life expectancy at birth (Congdon, 2002) or hazards in survival studies (Banerjee and Carlin, 2003) are examples of epidemiological indicators that have been also objects of study in the disease mapping literature. However, SMRs have traditionally been by far the most studied epidemiological indicator in geographic studies. This is why we are introducing just SMRs in this section, as they are more than enough to make a wide overview of the methods used in disease mapping.

4.1.2 Risk measures as statistical estimators

From an epidemiological perspective, a reasonable model for estimating the risk for some disease for some unit of study would be the following

$$o_i|\theta_i \sim Bin(\theta_i, p_i).$$

From a frequentist point of view, the formulation of the model would be completely done and any estimator of θ_i would estimate the risk for the disease in unit i. Elemental statistics would show that the Maximum Likelihood Estimate (MLE) of θ_i is equal to $r_i = o_i/p_i$, so the rate for unit i would be equal to the MLE corresponding to this model. In a similar manner, from a Bayesian point of view, the model above would need a prior distribution for θ_i so that inference could be done. An $U(0,1)$ prior distribution for θ_i would seem a reasonable prior distribution for this parameter. In that case, Bayes' theorem would show that the posterior distribution for θ_i would be a beta distribution of parameters $o_i + 1$ and $p_i - o_i + 1$, which has its mode at $r_i = o_i/p_i$. Thus, rates can also be viewed as a Bayesian estimator (posterior mode) of a reasonable model proposal for estimating the risk of the disease.

On the other hand, if we pursued to make inference on the relative risk of a disease for some unit of study, in comparison to the whole region of study, we could consider the observed cases for that unit to follow the model

$$o_i|\theta_i \sim Pois(e_i \cdot \theta_i). \tag{4.2}$$

where the expected cases e_i account for the risk in the whole population and θ_i modifies those expected cases as a function of the particular risk of that unit. We will be typically interested in estimating θ_i since it will inform us about the existence of some factor increasing ($\theta_i > 1$) or decreasing ($\theta_i < 1$) the risk in the i-th geographical unit, in comparison to the whole population in the study. Once again, the MLE for θ_i for this model would be $R_i = o_i/e_i$, which we showed was equal to the rate ratio corresponding to the i-th unit of study. If e_i had additionally been age standardized, the previous MLE would be equivalent instead to the SMR of that unit of study. In a similar manner, we could consider a Bayesian model for estimating the relative risk θ_i. In that case it would seem reasonable to propose an improper $U(0,\infty)$ prior distribution for θ_i, which would yield a gamma posterior distribution for θ_i of parameters $o_i + 1$ and e_i, respectively, which has as posterior mode $R_i = o_i/e_i$. Thus, rate ratios can also be viewed as Bayesian estimators (posterior modes) of reasonable models for estimating relative risks.

Therefore, as a summary, rates, rate ratios and SMRs, as typically defined in classical epidemiology, can be viewed as simple estimates of the probability (risk) and relative risk of death. Moreover, the statistical models leading to rates and rate ratios as statistical estimators are extremely simple, assuming no complex or questionable hypothesis, in principle. Nevertheless, this view of rates and rate ratios as statistical estimators should make us think that there would be lots of complementary risk and relative risk estimators, as many as reasonable models we could formulate for estimating these variables. As a consequence, viewing rates and SMRs as statistical estimators corresponding to particular models should make us treat them as no holy grail, being the ultimate goal of our inference, besides their omnipresent use in classical epidemiology. Many other risk and relative risk estimators could be derived, possibly with better statistical properties. The statistical properties of those estimators will mostly depend on the adequacy of the corresponding model for fitting the available data, so they will vary for the corresponding models that we could pose.

One advantage of viewing rates and rate ratios as statistical estimators is that the corresponding models could yield additional information of interest on those estimates. For example, as every statistical estimate, SMRs have their own variability that could be appropriately derived, from a frequentist perspective, according to the model in (4.2). For doing that, it is common to assume the numerator of the SMR as a stochastic quantity, in this case following a Poisson distribution, and the denominator as a fixed deterministic quantity. This is not such a restrictive assumption since the value in the denominator is based on much more information than the numerator, the whole population of study if internal standardization is done. Consequently, the variance of SMR_i can be derived as

$$Var(SMR_i|\theta_i) = Var\left(\frac{o_i}{e_i}|\theta_i\right) = \frac{Var(o_i|\theta_i)}{e_i^2} = \frac{\theta_i e_i}{e_i^2} = \frac{\theta_i}{e_i}, \quad (4.3)$$

hence, the variance of SMR_i is inversely proportional to the number of expected deaths in that unit.

The above expression of the variance of SMR_i is sometimes used to derive confidence intervals for θ_i, although this can be done in several different manners. For example, we could use a Gaussian assumption for SMR_i; therefore, a $100 \cdot (1 - \alpha)\%$ confidence interval for the corresponding relative risk would be:

$$[SMR_i + z_{\alpha/2}\sqrt{SMR_i/e_i}, SMR_i + z_{1-\alpha/2}\sqrt{SMR_i/e_i}],$$

for $z_{\alpha/2}$ and $z_{(1-\alpha/2)}$ being the corresponding quantiles of the Normal distribution. Nevertheless, the Gaussian assumption would not be surely suitable for small populations, what could yield confidence intervals with negative values, for example. Thus, a second credible interval could be derived by assuming Normality on $log(SMR_i)$ (see, for example, page 148 of Clayton and Hills (1993)); in that case, a confidence interval for θ_i at the $100 \cdot (1 - \alpha)\%$ can be defined as:

$$\left[SMR_i \exp\left(\frac{z_{\alpha/2}}{\sqrt{o_i}}\right), SMR_i \exp\left(\frac{z_{1-\alpha/2}}{\sqrt{o_i}}\right)\right]$$

An exact confidence interval avoiding any Gaussian approximation may be derived by just assuming the number of observed deaths to follow a Poisson distribution. In that case, a $100 \cdot (1 - \alpha)\%$ confidence interval for θ_i can be derived as

$$\left[\frac{\chi_{2o_i}^2(\alpha/2)}{2e_i}, \frac{\chi_{2(o_i+1)}^2(1 - \alpha/2)}{2e_i}\right]$$

where $\chi_n^2(x)$ denotes the x-quantile of the chi-squared distribution with n degrees of freedom (see for example page 63 in Esteve et al. (1994) or page 631 in Fleiss et al. (2003)).

Similar credible intervals could be obtained for the relative risk θ_i under a Bayesian approach. We know analytically the posterior distribution, of each θ_i under the Bayesian models assumed above, so a $\alpha\%$ credible interval can be easily derived by calculating the $\alpha/2$ and $1-\alpha/2$ quantiles of the corresponding posterior distribution for θ_i. If no analytic expression was known for that posterior distribution, the $100 \cdot (1 - \alpha)\%$ posterior credible interval for θ_i could be also derived by MCMC sampling with WinBUGS, for example, or with INLA, alternatively.

Example 4.1

We are going to illustrate now how to calculate in R the internally standardized *SMR*s for the oral cancer mortality data in men for the 540 municipalities of the Valencian Region. To do it, we have three R objects available: first, Obs.muni, a vector with the 540 observed oral cancer deaths for each municipality; second, the Obs.age vector, with 18 quinquennial age-specific deaths (from 0-5 to higher than 85 years) for the whole Valencian Region and third, the Pop matrix with 540 rows and 18 columns, containing the population for every combination of municipality and age group. In case of having a matrix with the same structure as Pop, but containing the observed deaths, both objects Obs and Obs.age could be calculated as simply summing the values for every row and column of that matrix with, for example, two calls to the apply function of R. The numerators of the *SMR*s are simply the elements of the vector Obs.muni. In order to compute the denominators, we first need the age-specific rates for the whole Valencian Region, that can be calculated as

```
> Rates.VR=Obs.age/apply(Pop,2,sum)
```

For each municipality, we will have to multiply (scalar product) these reference age-specific rates by the corresponding vector of age-specific populations. Since those vectors of populations are just the rows of matrix Pop we can make

```
> Exp.muni=as.vector(Pop%*%matrix(Rates.VR,ncol=1))
```

which yields the expected deaths for each municipality assuming the age-specific risks to be the same as those for the whole Valencian Region. Finally, the *SMR*s (using the epidemiologic agreement of setting 100 as basal value) for the set of municipalities considered can be calculated as

```
> SMR.muni=100*Obs.muni/Exp.muni
> summary(SMR.muni)
  Min. 1st Qu.  Median   Mean 3rd Qu.    Max.
  0.00    0.00   68.57  90.83  119.50  3977.0
```

It can be checked that lots of the *SMR*s (194 out of 540) have 0 as value, corresponding to all those municipalities with no observed deaths. The municipality with higher risk has an *SMR* of 3977.0, a risk 40 times higher than expected!! Such a high risk should make, in principle, epidemiologists pay very close attention to that municipality.

We can also calculate confidence intervals for the *SMR*s computed above. Thus, we can calculate the 95% confidence interval based on the Normality assumption of the log-*SMR*s in the following way

```
> IC.norm=cbind(SMR.muni*exp(qnorm(0.025)/sqrt(Obs.muni)),
                SMR.muni*exp(qnorm(0.975)/sqrt(Obs.muni)))
> head(IC.norm,5)
        [,1]      [,2]
```

```
  0.000000      NaN
  3.346725 168.6643
 60.978706 974.8975
 61.311280 980.2146
 99.032440 293.7238
```

The upper extreme of the confidence interval for the first municipality cannot be calculated since it has 0 observed deaths and therefore the expression for deriving that extreme requires us to divide by 0. On the other hand, we can calculate the Poisson-based confidence intervals that do not show this problem. We could calculate those confidence intervals in the following way

```
> IC.pois=100*cbind(qchisq(0.025,2*Obs.muni)/(2*Exp.muni),
                    qchisq(0.975,2*(Obs.muni+1))/(2*Exp.muni))
> head(IC.pois,5)
        [,1]       [,2]
   0.0000000 411.0394
   0.6015167 132.3747
  29.5276827 880.7602
  29.6887250 885.5638
  90.8120692 291.6501
```

As can be appreciated, in our case, there are substantial differences between both intervals for each municipality. This is a consequence of the low number of deaths observed for most municipalities; therefore, the Normal approximation is evidently inappropriate for our data, with such small units of study. In that case, as evidenced, the underlying assumptions made for each model or for deriving some estimators are particularly sensitive on the final results.

Finally, analytic credible intervals could be derived for the relative risks assuming the Bayesian model mentioned above. These could be calculated by doing

```
> IC.Bayes=100*cbind(qgamma(0.025,Obs.muni+1,Exp.muni),
                     qgamma(0.975,Obs.muni+1,Exp.muni))
> head(IC.Bayes,5)
       [,1]       [,2]
   2.821078 411.0394
   5.754563 132.3747
  75.422190 880.7602
  75.833538 885.5638
 100.415200 291.6501
```

The upper limits of these intervals coincide with those of the exact confidence intervals, in contrast to the lower limits. Some other Bayesian models maybe could yield models with a greater agreement with the frequentist intervals. Although as we have seen, frequentist intervals, which are based on different assumptions, do not fully agree either. Therefore, this makes clear again that the results of even these naive analyses are quite sensitive to the assumptions made, at least when the number of observed and expected cases in the SMRs are low.

4.1.3 Disease mapping: the statistical problem

Disease mapping may seem at first glance as a trivial task. If we were interested in determining which are the units with higher mortality in a region of study, we could just map the observed deaths for every unit, with the R packages mentioned in the previous chapter, and visualize which of them show a higher number of deaths. However, if someone was so incautious, he will soon realize that, unsurprisingly, those units with a higher number of deaths are precisely those most populated. Hence, drawing maps with such a naive statistical indicator does not reproduce at all the risk of the disease that we intend to visualize. Consequently, if we want our analyses to show the true underlying risk of the disease under study, we will have to draw more elaborated risk estimators.

As mentioned, mortality rates control the effect of the size of the population for every unit since observed deaths are divided by the corresponding population. However, if we wanted to detect the risk excesses in a region of study, we should compare the mortality rates with a reference rate so that we can determine if they are above or below that reference. In that case, SMRs are particularly suitable indicators since they perform exactly that goal, comparing the rate of any unit with that expected if that unit had exactly the same risk as the reference population. Moreover, SMRs filter out the effect of the age composition of the population of every unit or whatever factor whose effect we wanted to remove. Therefore, mapping the SMRs of all the units composing the region of study seems a good starting point for the exploration of the geographical distribution of mortality. In fact, SMRs are one of the more frequent epidemiological indicators for assessing risk excesses either in geographical regions or in any subgroup of the population in general.

We are going to introduce the statistical problem underlying disease mapping studies with the help of the following example, where the underlying problem is clearly evidenced.

Example 4.2

We turn back again to the municipal oral cancer mortality data set used in the previous example. There, we already calculated the SMRs corresponding to each municipality in the Valencian Region. Those SMRs have been plotted at the left-hand side of Figure 4.1 by means of a choropleth map. In a first attempt to make sense of this map of SMRs, we have also plotted (right-hand side of Figure 4.1) a choropleth map with the population of each municipality in the Valencian Region. The first striking issue in both plots is that a high proportion of the municipalities in the highest risk group corresponds to municipalities with low population. Indeed, the median number of men living in the municipalities in the highest risk group (472 per municipality) is

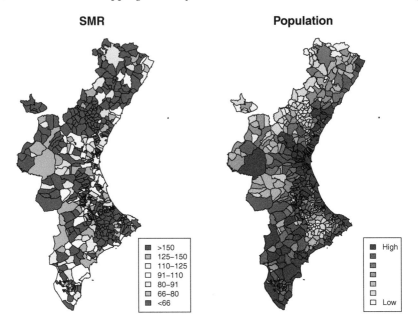

Figure 4.1
Left: SMRs for the municipalities in the Valencian Region. Right: Population in the municipalities of the Valencian Region (cuts correspond to septiles of the municipal populations).

lower than that median value for the whole Valencian Region (692 per municipality). This difference is much higher, for instance, for municipalities with SMRs higher than 500 (54 men per municipality). This result invites us to conclude that oral cancer shows higher mortality in the rural areas of the Valencian Region. Paradoxically, if we repeat the same exercise with the municipalities in the lowest risk group, we find something similar. The median number of men in the municipalities of that group is 197. Consequently, the rural (less populated) areas basically contain those municipalities with more extreme SMRs, regardless of whether they are particularly high or low.

In order to discover what can be happening here, we can take a closer look at the data. The municipality with the highest SMR (3977.0) is Castell de Cabres. This municipality, besides having the highest SMR, is also the least populated in the whole Valencian Region with 10.2 men, on average, living there during the period of study. This municipality has had the "bad luck" of registering one death of oral cancer among their men during the follow-up period. Although oral cancer is not a rare cause of death, it is neither among the most frequent ones, which makes the expected number of deaths for this cause and municipality very low (0.025 deaths). Therefore, the presence of a single observed case in this municipality (jointly with its low population) makes its SMR so extreme. On the contrary, if no oral cancer death had occurred in Castell de Cabres during the period of study, the corresponding SMR would have taken 0 as value, the lowest possible value. As a result, Castell de Cabres (and all those municipalities with a similar population) is always forced to show extreme SMRs just as a consequence of its size, regardless of whether there is a genuine risk excess there (caused by a factor modifying its mortality) or not.

The effect just evidenced in Castell de Cabres in the previous example is a general fact in all units of low population. This may also be seen as a consequence of Expression (4.3), which states that the variance of the SMRs grows as long as the number of expected cases of a unit decreases. Consequently, choropleth maps of SMRs do not achieve the original goal that they intended to, depicting the geographical distribution of risks or, at least, they do not achieve it in a satisfactory way. SMRs show some specific problems, such as higher volatility in low populated areas, which make the choropleth map show some artifacts as, for example, the geographical distribution of the population as just shown. This makes SMRs valuable statistical indicators for disease mapping but with obvious drawbacks that disease mapping practitioners would clearly want to solve.

The statistical problems of SMRs, when used on units with low population, can be summarized as follows:

- As just pointed out, the least populated units, will always show extreme SMRs whether their true risks are high or low, so choropleth maps of these indicators will show particular 'noise' at the rural, less populated, areas. As a consequence, units with the highest and lowest risks will systematically be placed at the less populated areas, whether or not there is a genuine risk factor underneath increasing the mortality in those units.

- When assessing the SMR significance, we would find that only those units that are more populated show SMRs significantly different from 100 (even if their SMRs are not so different from 100). This is a consequence of the higher variance of the SMRs in the least populated units. Therefore, significance maps will just point towards well-populated areas although the disease could be mostly typical of rural areas.

- SMRs of units with no observed deaths are always equal to 0, regardless of the expected observations of the corresponding units. This makes SMRs unsensible to the statistical evidence corresponding to those observations, when it is obviously very different to have 0 observed cases when having 0.1 or 10 expected cases.

- SMRs are maximum likelihood estimates of model (4.2). This is a saturated model which contains a parameter for fitting each observed data in our data set. This makes SMRs not be parsimonious at all and, consequently, SMRs are extremely sensible to changes in the observed data.

- Low-populated units tend to cluster together in rural areas. This makes extreme observations (sometimes of opposite sense) to also cluster. Consequently, SMR choropleth maps tend to represent neighbouring units with extreme opposite risks. This fact goes against the usual existence in real settings of risk factors covering several neighbouring units that make them have similar risk estimates and therefore be spatially dependent in general. Thus, SMR choropleth maps tend to draw noisy geographical patterns that go against the typical spatial dependence of risks in real settings.

All these problems related to the use of naive SMRs advise against its use for dealing with units of low population.

The statistical inference problem just described, which is the basis of disease mapping as a research area, is not an exclusive problem of epidemiology. This inference problem related to the size of the units of study is also present in many other contexts, such as official statistics in general and is usually known even beyond disease mapping applications as *small area estimation* problems. The small area concept is also very popular in the disease mapping literature, although there is not a clear definition of this term used by this set of professionals. Sometimes epidemiologists ask us about the concept of small areas: is a municipality a small area? and a census tract? and etc.? Epidemiologists, in general, seek geographical criteria to guide their definition of a small area, since they are aware that dealing with these kinds of units requires more sophisticated methods for estimating their statistical indicators. In our opinion, the better and less ambiguous way to define small areas is according to statistical criteria. Thus, Rao (2003) defines small areas as those 'for which direct estimates of adequate precision cannot be produced'. This definition can be used in a strict way, setting a desired precision and therefore determining the small areas that correspond to that threshold. Nevertheless, we consider the small area definition more useful when read in a more general manner. Thus, we will consider that we have a small area estimation problem when the size of the geographical areas used poses a statistical problem for the statistical indicators that we want to estimate. Consequently, and coming back to the epidemiologic context, we could work at a census tract level (lower than the municipality level) without having any specific small area estimation problem, for example when studying the hospitalization rate for all causes, a health event of very high frequency. On the contrary, we can work at the country level in worldwide studies and have a small area estimation problem, such as when monitoring the monthly incidence of Ebola disease. Therefore, geographical units can be either small or not depending on the specific problem and not just on its dimension. In any case, at this stage we must be aware that when dealing with a small area estimation problem, either in epidemiology or any other context, we must resort to more elaborate statistical estimators instead of using naive statistical proposals.

At this stage of the book, one could easily presume the important role that statistics is going to play in all this mess. Anyway, we would like to recall that *SMR*s can be considered, from a statistical point of view, as (the maximum likelihood) risk estimates corresponding to the model in (4.2). That model is quite simple and maybe that is why it leads to such naive risk estimates, which is perfectly worth it when working with not-so-small areas. Our task, from here on, will be to explore alternative risk estimates, usually corresponding to more elaborate models that may lead to new estimates with better statistical properties and better performance when dealing with small areas.

4.2   Non-spatial smoothing

The use of *SMR*s in disease mapping small area studies has historically been an exception. Few statistical analyses of such an amount of data (sometimes hundreds or even thousands of spatial units) would consider saturated models with fully independent estimates for analyzing the data. *SMR*s are exactly that, statistical risk estimates of saturated models considering exclusively information on the corresponding geographical unit for estimating each *SMR*. This would be equivalent to as if, in a scatter plot of two variables, we estimated the expected value of the y component of any observation as exactly that component on the corresponding observed value, ignoring the information of the rest of the data. Leaving aside parsimony issues, this could have some sense if the amount of variability in the observations is low, but we cannot pretend to hold this premise when dealing with small areas. Consequently, *SMR*s definitely would not be the risk estimators that we would wish for, although the model leading to them (Expression (4.2)) will be a good starting point for deriving improved risk estimates.

Most statistical analyses, in general, resort to parametric proposals (deterministic transformations of one or several covariates) for modeling the relationship between two, or more, variables. In disease mapping problems, we would have at least two obvious covariates for modeling the risk of the disease under study: longitude and latitude of each spatial unit. Therefore, there is room in principle for parametric models also in these kinds of studies. In more detail, parametric models usually assume the data to follow Expression (4.2) and define the logarithm of the risks (the logarithm is the canonical link function for Poisson regression models) as

$$\log(\theta_i) = f(x_i, y_i, \ldots)$$

for a parametric function f. An obvious choice would be to define f as a linear combination of the covariates and their interaction, thus if x_i and y_i respectively denote the longitude and latitude of the centroid of the i-th unit, that parametric risk function could be defined as

$$f(x_i, y_i) = \beta_0 + \beta_1 x_i + \beta_2 y_i + \beta_3 x_i y_i \qquad (4.4)$$

This function fits the log-risks to a plane, yielding much more parsimonious risk estimates than their own $SMRs$. Risk estimates, as any other statistical estimator, should be a tradeoff between parsimony and fit and obviously the linear fit above will be often too restrictive to properly describe the geographical risk variations in a large number of settings. Therefore, it will be convenient to use more flexible processes for modeling the geographical variability of risks. An obvious proposal here would be to incorporate higher-order polynomial terms (on both x_i and y_i) in Expression (4.4). This will enable the fitted surface to reproduce, if needed, local maxima and minima at some specific locations, more maxima and minima as long as the degree of the polynomial function used increases. However, the bad news on the use of polynomial functions is that reproducing, for example, a local maxima at some place may impose strange (and often unwanted) performances of the parametric function $f()$ in very distant places. Thus polynomial functions do not have a local scope, which is what makes them unsuitable tools to be used in disease mapping studies.

The use of spline, or methods based in bases of functions in general, is a straightforward alternative to polynomial parametric functions (Lee and Durban, 2009; Goicoa et al., 2012). These models consider the $f()$ function above to be a linear combination of a basis of functions, whose elements are linked to a fixed set of knots scattered along the region of study. Several bases of functions have been proposed for fitting spatial areal data, and since each of their elements is linked to any of the knots considered, they usually have a more local scope than raw polynomial functions, which makes them particularly suited for disease mapping studies. These models usually consider a high number of knots and consequently the fit of a high number of parameters. Nevertheless, that number is lower than the number of units in the study; therefore, these models perform a kind of low-dimensional fit of the geographical distribution of risks, as parametric models in general.

Example 4.3

We are going to illustrate now the use of basis of functions in disease mapping models by applying them to the municipal oral cancer data set. We have built a set of knots in the following way. We have considered a set of equidistant values $\{x_i : i = 1, \ldots, 11\}$, with x_{i+1} placed 20 kilometers to the east of x_i, covering the longitudes of the municipalities of the Valencian Region. We have repeated this process for their latitudes, yielding the set $\{y_j : j = 1, \ldots, 19\}$ where y_{j+1} is placed 20 kilometers to the north of y_j. The set of knots finally used corresponds to those points $\{(x_i, y_j) : i = 1, \ldots, 11, j = 1, \ldots, 19\}$ which are placed closer than 20 kilometers of any of the municipalities of the Valencian Region (we further explain below the reason for trimming the original set arising from the cartesian product of $\{x_i : i = 1, \ldots, 11\}$ and $\{y_j : j = 1, \ldots, 19\}$). This yields a total of 95 knots for building the model that we pursue. The basis used is composed of bidimensional Gaussian functions centered at each one of the previous knots, with standard deviation of 20 kilometers along both axes. Alternative basis could also be used (possibly with better properties), but for illustrative purposes we have chosen the mentioned Gaussian functions. Our modeling proposal sets $f(x_i, y_i) = \mu + \boldsymbol{B}\boldsymbol{\gamma}$ where $\boldsymbol{B}$ is a 540×95 matrix with B_{ij} being the evaluation of the j-th Gaussian basis function considered on the centroid of the i-th municipality.

We have made two different proposals for the $f(x_i, y_i)$ function. The first considers the coefficients of the basis of Gaussian functions ($\boldsymbol{\gamma}$) as fixed effects, i.e., they have independent vague prior distributions. In contrast, the second model considers those parameters as Gaussian random effects with a common, although unknown, standard deviation that should be estimated. We expect this second model to yield a more parsimonious fit since the common distribution of the γ_is will avoid them to take whatever value according just to data. The random effects model will also require all the γ_i values to be in agreement, since all of them can be considered elements of a common population determining the variability of the risk surface.

Both models have been fitted in `WinBUGS`. The syntax used for fitting the fixed effects model is the following

```
model{
 for(i in 1:n){
  O[i]~dpois(lambda[i])
  log(lambda[i])<-log(E[i])+log.theta[i]
  log.theta[i]<-mu+inprod(basis[i,],gamma[])
  sSMR[i]<-100*exp(log.theta[i])
  P.sSMR[i]<-step(sSMR[i]-100)
 }
 #Prior distributions
 for(j in 1:nbasis){gamma[j]~dflat()}
 mu~dflat()
}
```

This model assumes the observed deaths in the i-th municipality, o_i, to follow a Poisson distribution of mean

$$e_i \cdot exp(\mu + \sum_{j=1}^{95} B_{ij}\gamma_j).$$

The terms multiplying the expected deaths e_i, θ_is in Expression (4.2), were previously identified as the risk estimates that we want to derive. Therefore, this new model implicitly defines those risks as the exponential of a linear combination of the terms in the basis (`sSMR[i]<-100*exp(log.theta[i])`), in contrast to traditional SMRs which are independent estimates for each municipality. We refer to these new risk estimates (multiplied by 100), and any other model-based risk estimates henceforth, as *smoothed SMRs* or simply ($sSMR$), in order to distinguish them from conventional SMRs. The above `WinBUGS` syntax also contains a line `P.sSMR[i]<-step(sSMR[i]-100)` for evaluating the probability of each $sSMR$ to be higher than 100, i.e., the probability of observing a risk excess for any municipality. These probabilities are usually of great interest for epidemiologists (Bernardinelli et al., 1995a) since they can be understood as a kind of 'significance' measure of any potential risk excess that we could find.

Regarding the prior distributions used, the fixed effects model considers both μ and γ as coefficients in a Poisson regression model and therefore they are assigned improper flat prior distributions. The alternative random effects model changes the prior distributions for the components of γ to:

```
for(j in 1:nbasis){gamma[j]~dnorm(0,tau)}
tau<-pow(sd.g,-2)
sd.g~dunif(0,10)
```

Therefore, the components of γ now are supposed to share a common Normal distribution with standard deviation `sd.g`. A uniform prior distribution is chosen for this parameter with 10 as the upper limit. Bearing in mind that the components of γ are coefficients modeling the log-risks, i.e., in a logarithmic scale, that value indeed yields a vague prior distribution for `sd.g`. Example 2.3 already showed evidences of the convenience of using random effects for the parameters in those models in order to obtain more parsimonious fits.

Both models were run by means of two calls to the `pbugs` function in R. For the random effects model, 5,500 iterations, with the first 500 iterations used as burn-in, sufficed for obtaining satisfactory convergence statistics for all the variables saved. Remember that we considered good convergence if the `R-hat` statistic is lower than 1.1 and the `n.eff` statistic is higher than 100 for all the parameters saved. These statistics are routinely calculated and shown by the `pbugs` function. The fixed effects model showed far more convergence problems, indeed we had to run 55,000 iterations, whose initial 5,000 iterations were used as burn-in, which took about 4.6 hours to compute on a laptop. The main convergence problems were observed in those nodes placed at the boundaries (or even outside) of the Valencian Region. The likelihood function for these variables provides very little information, as well as their vague prior distributions; this is the reason of these convergence problems and the reason why we trimmed the original candidate points to be used as knots in the model.

Figure 4.2 shows the posterior means for the $sSMR$s for the above-described models. The left plot corresponds to the $sSMR$s estimated from the fixed effects model, while that on the right corresponds to the results of the random effects model. The less populated municipalities in these two plots do not show now a particular performance and they seem as variable as the rest of the geographical units, in contrast to the SMRs map (see Figure 4.1). Although

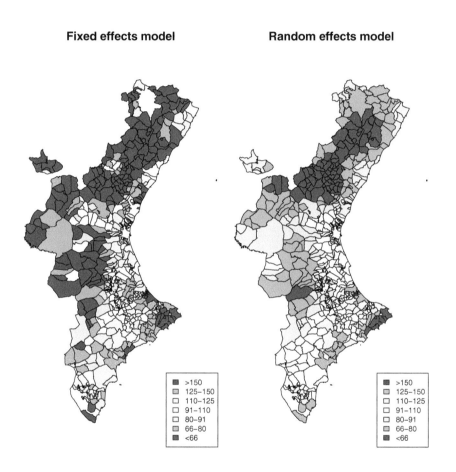

Figure 4.2
Left: *sSMR*s for the fixed effects Gaussian basis model. Right: *sSMR*s for the random effects Gaussian basis model.

both plots show far more parsimonious geographical patterns than the original
SMRs choropleth map, differences between both are evident. The random
effects model shows a much more parsimonious performance. We already saw
this feature in Example 2.3, which can be more dramatic when considering
a higher number of knots. The parsimony of the fixed effects model greatly
depends on that number, while the random effects model is less sensible to
that factor.

Regarding which of these two models is more adequate, the fixed effects model
has a DIC of 1844.6 with 98.0 effective parameters (very close to the real
number of parameters in the model). On the other hand, the random effects
model has a DIC of 1790.4 with 29.1 effective parameters, far less than the
real number of parameters since they share information through their prior
distribution. Therefore, the more parsimonious pattern of the random effects
model seems to yield a better depiction of the geographical pattern that we
want to estimate. This result discourages the use of SMRs as risk estimates
since these are even less parsimonious than the $sSMR$s for the fixed effects
model above.

The random effects model took 27.4 minutes to run the $3 \cdot 5500$ iterations
corresponding to all three chains, using three different processors and the
pbugs function. We have alternatively implemented this same model in INLA
by executing the following syntax

```
> form= O ~ f(id.node,model="z",Z=basis,
              hyper=list(prec=list(prior=sdunif)))
> result.INLA=inla(form,family="poisson",data=data,E=E,
                  control.compute=list(dic=TRUE))
```

where data is a data.frame with columns O, E (as used in the WinBUGS model)
and id.node=1:540, a variable indexing the municipalities composing the Valencian Region. The argument basis is once again the 540×95 matrix used in
WinBUGS and sdunif is the uniform prior on the standard deviation as defined
in Section 3.2. You will have to define the sd.unif prior before executing the
inla call above (see the annex online material for this example). We have also
run INLA with the safest option control.inla=list(strategy="laplace")
in order to assess its computing time. INLA took 4.0 seconds to fit the model
with the regular fitting options, 18.3 seconds with the safer options; therefore,
the change in computing time in comparison to WinBUGS for this data set is
huge for both options, making evident the supposed computational advantage
of INLA vs. WinBUGS.

This first disease mapping example shows that the use of traditional SMRs,
when dealing with small areas, should be completely dismissed. The models
implemented in this example are quite simple and their fit could be easily improved by introducing some slight modifications to them. Nevertheless, Example 4.3 makes clear that simple models, describing the geographical variability

of risks as linear combinations of a basis of functions clearly outperform the original *SMR*s risk estimates by just introducing a bit of statistical modeling.

Example 4.3 has additionally shown that random effects may be a useful device for estimating risks, yielding smoother estimates. On the other hand, as mentioned in the previous section *SMR*s can be considered Bayesian fixed effects estimates (posterior modes) of risks under a naive Poisson model, therefore there is room for a random effects-based alternative to traditional *SMR*s. Our goal will be now to model directly the municipal risk estimates as random effects, instead of using them as a device for modeling the parameters of some given function. Therefore, we will avoid the use of intermediate parametric functions to model the risks and the effect that they could have on the final estimates. As we will check during the rest of the book, the direct modeling of risks as random effects is, by far, the most frequent device in the literature for improving naive *SMR*s when dealing with small areas.

We turn back again to Expression (4.2), the starting point for identifying the *SMR*s as risk estimates. In order to model the risks $\boldsymbol{\theta}$ as random effects, it will be necessary to propose a common prior distribution for all its components depending on some parameters to be fitted. Bearing in mind that all components of $\boldsymbol{\theta}$ are Real positive values, an obvious choice would be to assume a gamma prior distribution for them. Therefore, we may assume a $Gamma(\alpha, \beta)$ prior distribution for $\boldsymbol{\theta}$, i.e., a gamma distribution with mean and variance:

$$\mu = \alpha/\beta, \ \sigma^2 = \alpha/\beta^2 \tag{4.5}$$

The gamma prior distribution for the risks has historically been a very popular choice, leading to what is known in the literature as the *Poisson-gamma model* (Clayton and Kaldor, 1987; Tsutakawa, 1988). This prior distribution has the particularity of, given α and β, producing known posterior distributions without resorting to MCMC or any other numerical device. Thus, the posterior distribution for θ_i is simply a $Gamma(o_i + \alpha, e_i + \beta)$ distribution, i.e., once again a gamma distribution. This is what Bayesians call a *conjugate prior distribution*, a prior distribution (in this case for the θ_i's) leading to a posterior distribution of the same family. As a consequence, the posterior mean of θ_i for the Poisson-gamma model is just

$$E(\theta_i | \boldsymbol{o}, \alpha, \beta) = \frac{o_i + \alpha}{e_i + \beta}.$$

We could easily derive the following expressions $\alpha = \mu^2/\sigma^2$ and $\beta = \mu/\sigma^2$ from Expression (4.5), therefore we would have

$$E(\theta_i | \boldsymbol{o}, \alpha, \beta) = \frac{o_i + \frac{\mu}{\sigma^2}\mu}{e_i + \frac{\mu}{\sigma^2}} = \frac{e_i}{e_i + \frac{\mu}{\sigma^2}}\frac{o_i}{e_i} + \frac{\frac{\mu}{\sigma^2}}{e_i + \frac{\mu}{\sigma^2}}\mu = w_i SMR_i + (1 - w_i)\mu \tag{4.6}$$

where $w_i = e_i/(e_i + \mu/\sigma^2)$. This expression clearly shows the tradeoff between data and prior distribution on the posterior distribution of θ_i. The posterior mean above is a weighted mean of the risk estimate arising from the data, SMR_i, and its prior mean μ. Moreover, the weights of these two components (w_i) depend on the number of expected values of each spatial unit and a second parameter μ/σ^2 which becomes lower as the prior distribution is vaguer. Therefore, θ_i's posterior mean will be closer to SMR_i, i.e., will be more influenced by the data, whether the prior distribution is vaguer or the corresponding municipality is larger (having therefore a higher number of expected deaths). Consequently, the $sSMRs$ arising from the Poisson-gamma model weight, for each municipality, the reliability of its data and whenever it is lower, the common prior mean plays a more active role on the final $sSMR$. In this sense, Equation (4.6) evidences that for two municipalities having the same SMR, specifically for two municipalities with no observed deaths, their posterior means of the $sSMR$ for the Poisson-gamma model are not necessarily the same since they also depend on the size of the municipality. Lack of sensitivity to the size of spatial units was highlighted above as a drawback of the $SMRs$ that would be solved for this (and the following) model(s).

The non-MCMC-dependence of the Poisson-gamma model made it very popular at the dawn of Bayesian disease mapping, when MCMC inference was not completely developed. Nevertheless, the popularization of MCMC has made this model to be replaced by other alternative proposals. Inference in Poisson-gamma models is usually made by means of *empirical Bayes methods* (Carlin and Louis, 2000). As mentioned, the risks in the Poisson-gamma model are completely determined given the parameters of their prior distribution, α and β. Empirical methods estimate both values as a function of the data $\hat{\alpha}(\boldsymbol{o})$ and $\hat{\beta}(\boldsymbol{o})$ and use both values to derive the corresponding $sSMRs$. This is not a fully Bayesian analysis since it would require us to derive the posterior distribution of both α and β and therefore deriving the corresponding $sSMRs$, accounting for the uncertainty of both parameters. In this sense, empirical Bayes methods, after the generalization of MCMC methods, are considered a kind of approximate Bayesian inference methods. There is specific software implementing empirical Bayes inference on the Poisson-gamma model, indeed the **Dcluster** package (Gómez-Rubio et al., 2005) of **R** has the function **empbaysmooth** for this specific purpose.

A restrictive feature of the Poisson distribution is that it depends on just one parameter and all the statistics of the corresponding variable are a function of just that variable. As a consequence, the mean and variance of any variable following a Poisson distribution should be necessarily equal, since this is a particular feature of this distribution. Regretfully, spatial variability and other processes usually make the variance of the observed counts to be substantially larger than their mean, which is usually known as *overdispersion* and which invalidates the Poisson distributed data assumption. When overdispersion is noticed in a data set, a frequently used and more flexible alternative to the Poisson distribution is the *negative binomial* distribution, which may be interpreted as the distribution of the number of observed successes in an independent series of Bernoulli trials (of probability p) before observing a fixed number (r) of failures. The negative binomial distribution is a biparametric function, depending on both p and r so in this sense it is a more flexible alternative to the Poisson distribution. The Poisson-gamma model above, once integrated out the risks $\boldsymbol{\theta}$, is equivalent to assuming a negative binomial distribution of parameters $r = \alpha$ and $p = \beta/(\beta + e_i)$ on the observed counts corresponding to each municipality (see Bivand et al. (2008), page 315). In this sense the underlying gamma distribution on the risks in the Poisson-gamma model can be considered as a generalization of the Poisson distribution of a common mean for all the observations, leading to a more flexible and known distribution for the observed counts.

A second random effects-based proposal for estimating smoothed SMRs consists of modeling the logarithms of the relative risks, $\log(\boldsymbol{\theta})$, as independent Normal variables of common and unknown variance that will be estimated within the model. Specifically, the likelihood of this model follows the usual Poisson assumption (4.2) and the rest of the model assumes

$$log(\theta_i) \sim N(\mu, \sigma_\gamma)$$

$$\mu \sim U(-\infty, \infty)$$

$$\sigma_\gamma \sim Uniform(0, a)$$

for a a high enough value so that is does not constrain the posterior distribution of σ_γ. This model is usually known as the *Poisson-lognormal model*. This proposal would be equivalent to model the relative risks as variables following a lognormal distribution, a biparametric distribution for positive Real variables, like the gamma distribution. Both the lognormal and the gamma distribution are similar prior choices for the relative risks, leading to similar estimates so the $sSMR$s of both models will be similar in general. Nevertheless, there are some advantages that make the lognormal alternative particularly interesting. First, we are used to assigning prior distributions to parameters of Normal distributions so we can make that choice 'safely'. On the contrary, the assignment of prior distributions to the parameters of the gamma distribution in a Poisson-gamma model (for inference without empirical Bayes methods) is a less standard task, requiring considerable care and attention. Second, Normal distributions are more prone to modeling than gamma distributions, which makes it possible to induce dependence between the relative risks in the lognormal case an affordable task. Instead of modeling the $\log(\theta_i)$'s as independent Normal variables, we could jointly model $\log(\boldsymbol{\theta})$ as a multivariate Normal distribution whose covariance matrix could induce a convenient dependence structure. Dealing with geographically referenced data as we usually do, it is not hard to anticipate that this feature makes the Normal assumption on the log-relative risks a very attractive choice for further modeling in disease mapping problems.

Example 4.4

We are going to apply now the Poisson-gamma and Poisson-lognormal random effects models to the municipal oral cancer example. For the empirical Bayes fitting of the Poisson-gamma model, we have made use of the `empbaysmooth` function of the `DCluster` package in R. This function has a very simple syntax and we can fit this model by simply typing in R

```
> library(DCluster)
> PoisGamma=empbaysmooth(Obs=Obs.muni,Exp=Exp.muni,maxiter=100)
> PoisGamma.sSMR=100*PoisGamma$smthrr
```

where `maxiter` controls the maximum number of iterations allowed in the empirical Bayes estimation of the $sSMRs$. On the other hand, fully Bayesian inference can be made on the Poisson-lognormal model, either with MCMC simulation (that can be performed in `WinBUGS`) or alternatively with INLA. The syntax used to run this model in `WinBUGS` has been the following

```
model{
 for(i in 1:n){
  O[i]~dpois(lambda[i])
  log(lambda[i])<-log(E[i])+log.theta[i]
  log.theta[i]<-mu+het[i]
  het[i]~dnorm(0,tau)
  sSMR[i]<-100*exp(log.theta[i])
  P.sSMR[i]<-step(sSMR[i]-100)
 }
 mu~dflat()
 tau<-pow(sd.het,-2)
 sd.het~dunif(0,10)
}
```

The mean of the log-relative risks, μ, can either be placed outside of the heterogeneous random effects `het` or inside as their mean. Obviously, in this latter case it should be removed of the linear term defining the log-risks. That is, the fifth and sixth lines in the previous model should be changed to

```
  log.theta[i]<-het[i]
  het[i]~dnorm(mu,tau)
```

both models are equivalent in terms of the estimation of the $sSMRs$ although, as we will see in the next section, slight modifications of this kind can have sometimes a substantial effect on models convergence. We run three chains with 2200 iterations per chain, whose first 200 iterations were used as burn-in. The R-hat statistic was lower than 1.1 and the effective sample size higher than 100 for each parameter in the model.

For comparison purposes, we have also implemented this model in INLA by executing the following syntax

```
> form = 0 ~ f(id.node,model="iid",hyper=list(prec=list(prior=sdunif)))
> result = inla(form,family="poisson",data=data,E=E,
                control.compute=list(dic=TRUE))
```

for `sdunif` as defined in Section 3.2 and `0`, `E` and `id.node=1:540` being columns of the data.frame `data`. The posterior means of the *sSMR*s of both implementations showed a correlation of 0.997, pointing out the close similarity of these results (except maybe some Monte Carlo or other numerical approximation errors). `WinBUGS` took 13.5 seconds to run the $3 \cdot 2{,}200$ simulations sampled (using three processors and the `pbugs` function), while `INLA` took just 2.7 seconds to run with its default options. With the safest settings `control.inla=list(strategy="laplace")`, `INLA` took 9.2 seconds to run, still less than for `WinBUGS`. In any case, the differences in computing times for this example are not as large as for Example 4.3. From now on, we will focus on the `WinBUGS` results since they are in general identical to those derived from `INLA`.

Regarding the parameters controlling the geographical pattern of the risks, we have the following posterior summaries

```
          mean   sd 2.5%   25%   50%   75% 97.5% Rhat n.eff
mu        -0.1  0.0 -0.2  -0.1  -0.1  -0.1  -0.1    1  1000
sd.het     0.2  0.0  0.2   0.2   0.2   0.3   0.3    1  1000
```

The intercept of the model, `mu`, takes values close to zero. This is something that could be expected at a first glance since the expected values used were calculated using the Valencian Region as reference population (internal standardization). Therefore, the sum of total observed deaths coincides with the sum of expected deaths in our data set, which would make the quotient of observed and expected deaths on every municipality to be around 1 and thus its logarithm to be around 0. Nevertheless, the posterior mean and in general the posterior distribution of `mu` is below zero. This is something typical of Poisson-lognormal mixed regression models. In these models the expected counts follow a lognormal distribution of parameters μ and σ^2, where μ corresponds to the intercept in our model and σ^2 to the variance of the random effects. This makes the mean of the risks to be $\exp(\mu + \sigma^2/2)$, the mean of the mentioned lognormal distribution. Therefore, in contrast to Normal models, the mean of the risks does not depend on just the intercept of the model, but also on the variability of the random effects. Thus, any increase in the variance of the random effects should be compensated with a decrease in μ since; otherwise, that increase will modify the expected counts of the Poisson distribution. As a consequence, it is very usual to find posterior distributions of the intercept in Poisson-lognormal models with substantial mass below zero in order "to make room" to the variability of the random effects.

On the other hand, the posterior distribution of `sd.ind` is concentrated well above zero. This suggests the need of the random effect into the model and, as a consequence, the need of geographical variability for explaining the spatial variation in the risk of oral cancer mortality in the Valencian Region.

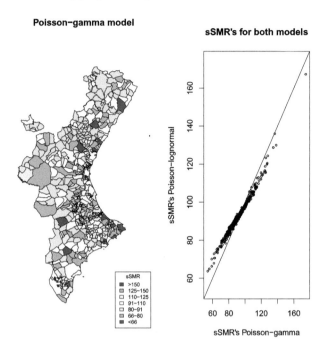

Figure 4.3
Left: $sSMR$s choropleth map for the Poisson-gamma model. Right: $sSMR$s
for the Poisson-gamma and Poisson-lognormal models.

Figure 4.3 (left) shows the map of the smoothed SMRs for the Poisson-gamma
model. This map has filtered much of the noise in the map of the raw SMRs
(Figure 4.1), pointing out only a few municipalities with high risk. Castell
de Cabres, the tiny municipality with the highest SMR in the Valencian
Region (3977) and just 1 observed death, now has an $sSMR$ of 100.4. On the
contrary, Oliva, a municipality with a population of around 11,000 men during
the period of study and 47 oral cancer deaths, has an $sSMR$ of 174.5, while it
had a SMR of 214.7. Therefore, it is evident that the Poisson-gamma model
has smoothed the SMRs mostly wherever they are unreliable risk indicators
based in few observed cases.

Figure 4.3 (right) shows the relationship between the $sSMR$s derived from the
Poisson-gamma and the Poisson-lognormal models. Both sets of $sSMR$s show
a correlation of 0.99 that summarises a clear linear relationship among them.
Nevertheless, the standard deviation of the Poisson-gamma $sSMR$s (12.89)
is higher than that of the Poisson-lognormal $sSMR$s (9.64). This makes the
scatter plot in the right side of Figure 4.3 deviate from the line $y = x$. As a
consequence the Poisson-lognormal $sSMR$s are smoothed more (shrunk towards 100) than those from the Poisson-gamma model. That is, although both

choropleth maps for both models would point out the same municipalities as of high risk, the scales of the corresponding $sSMR$s are different, making both estimates differ for each municipality.

In order to decide which of these $sSMR$s could make more sense, we have calculated the corresponding DIC for every model. The DIC for the Poisson-gamma model is not straightforward to be calculated since it is not based in an MCMC sample. Since for this model we do not have such a sample, but we have the analytical expression of the posterior distribution for each risk, we have drawn for each municipality a sample from that posterior distribution. Thus the DIC for the Poisson-lognormal model has been 1815.1, meanwhile for the Poisson-gamma model is 1804.2. Therefore, the differences between both models are remarkable, being the Poisson-gamma $sSMR$s more appropriate in terms of this criterion. Thus, although smoothing is good in general, this example shows that an excessive smoothing may not be so good.

A comparison with the Gaussian basis models of Example 4.3 is worth also a comment. The random effects model in that example attains a DIC lower than the models in this example. The main difference between the Gaussian basis models and those in this example is that the first makes a local smoothing, where every element in the basis feeds off the municipalities around the corresponding node. This is not the case of the models in this example where the new source of information that we have incorporated, the common prior distribution of the random effects, does not take at all into account the geographical arrangement of the municipalities. On the contrary, when estimating a specific $sSMR$, this distribution weighs equally the information of the neighbouring municipalities and that coming from municipalities placed much farther. This may explain the particular good performance of the Gaussian basis models in comparison to the non-spatial random effects models just shown.

4.3 Spatial smoothing

The previous section has led us to two important conclusions regarding disease mapping. First, smoothing risks by means of a model may improve the estimated geographical pattern when dealing with small areas. Nevertheless, oversmoothing is a potential problem when smoothing risks that should be kept in mind. On one hand, we have the SMRs, which are completely unsmoothed risk estimates being the result of a saturated model. On the other hand, we could assign a single common value to every $sSMR$, which would be the most extreme case of smoothing. Obviously, these two extreme cases are useless. Attaining an appropriate degree of smoothing between those two extreme settings is one of the key goals in disease mapping studies.

The second important conclusion from the previous section concerns taking advantage of local dependence. The modeling of temporal data is a related field to disease mapping where dependence among observations is frequently considered. Since the temporal evolution of time series could be very intricate, the parametric modeling of this kind of data is often avoided. Instead, data dependence is the main tool used for explaining and forecasting the available time series. With spatial areal data, something similar happens. It is hard to find a parametric proposal flexible enough to appropriately fit the wide variety of spatial patterns that could be observed throughout a region of study. This is why (low-dimensional) parametric models have not been so popular in the disease mapping literature. As shown, independent random effects are very flexible devices able to fit very different geographical patterns. Nevertheless, the random effects models introduced above do not consider dependence on data, in contrast to time series models. This makes non-spatial models not appropriately account for spatial dependence when it is present in the data, a very frequent situation in disease mapping studies. As a consequence, residuals in these models generally show the spatial auto-correlation that has not been properly absorbed by the random effects (Lawson et al., 2000). This makes the fit of non-spatial models poor and shows the typical problems arising when data dependence is ignored (bias, inaccurate uncertainty estimates, etc.).

As we showed for the Poisson-gamma model, smoothed risk estimates are basically the original SMRs shrunk towards the global mean risk for the whole region of study. This is the consequence of considering a common prior distribution for all the risks, regardless of the geographical location that they are placed in. Nevertheless, it would be much more convenient to shrink the $sSMR$s towards their local mean instead of the common global mean. The existence of risk factors influencing more than one contiguous municipalities would make the risks of neighbouring municipalities similar, and therefore the $sSMR$s would clearly benefit of shrinkage towards a local mean. This makes the incorporation of the spatial arrangement of the risks a clear way of improvement of non-spatial methods. This is going to be our specific goal from now on.

4.3.1   Spatial distributions

We are going to introduce now the family of *Conditional Auto-Regressive (CAR) distributions*, which is by far the most common tool for inducing spatial dependence in areal referenced vectors of random variables. CAR distributions were first introduced by Besag (1974). For a random vector $\varphi = (\varphi_1, \ldots, \varphi_I)$, a (Gaussian) CAR model is defined as the following set of conditional distributions

$$\varphi_i | \varphi_{-i}, \mu, \sigma \sim N\left(\mu_i + \sum_{j \neq i} b_{ij}(\varphi_j - \mu_j), \sigma_i^2\right), \quad i = 1, \ldots, I, \qquad (4.7)$$

where the term φ_{-i} refers to all the elements in φ leaving its i-th component out. We will just focus now on the Gaussian version of CAR distributions, although we will introduce later an alternative Laplace (or double-exponential) version of this distribution too. Nevertheless, it is interesting mentioning that analogous CAR distributions have been also proposed for binary (auto-logistic models) or count (auto-Poisson models) data (Besag, 1974), for example. We will not pay any attention to these non-Gaussian models, since they have focussed very scarce consideration in the disease mapping literature.

Expression (4.7) makes it clear why this model is known as auto-regressive; the mean for each φ_i is regressed against the rest of the components in that vector. Obviously, the estimation of all the regression coefficients b_{ij} in the expression above cannot be done as there would be much more quantities to estimate than available data. Hence, those elements are either fixed, as for the ICAR distribution that we will introduce below, or modeled as a function of one (or at most a few) variable(s), as for the proper CAR distribution also introduced below.

A notable difference between temporal and spatial auto-regressive processes is that, for the first, each component φ_i depends only on previous observations $\varphi_1, \ldots, \varphi_{i-1}$ in the time series. However, for the spatial case, there is no similar ordering to be used in the definition of the conditional distributions in (4.7), therefore, φ_i's distribution depends on the rest of elements in φ_{-i}. This makes, for any two components i and j with $i \neq j$, φ_i's conditional distribution to depend on φ_j, whereas φ_j's conditional distribution also depends on φ_i. These settings with crossed dependence relationships do not necessarily yield valid joint multivariate distributions for φ so this requires particular care. Specifically, Besag (1974, 1975) shows that the set of conditional distributions in (4.7) yields the following joint multivariate distribution for φ

$$\varphi | \boldsymbol{\mu}, \boldsymbol{\sigma} \sim N_I(\boldsymbol{\mu}, (\boldsymbol{I}_I - \boldsymbol{B})^{-1} diag(\boldsymbol{\sigma}^2)), \tag{4.8}$$

where $\boldsymbol{B}$ is the $I \times I$ matrix with $B_{ij} = b_{ij}$, $B_{ii} = 0$ and $diag(\boldsymbol{\sigma}^2)$ a diagonal matrix with diagonal terms $(\sigma_1^2, ..., \sigma_I^2)$. Nevertheless, this expression does not necessarily correspond to a well-defined multivariate Normal distribution for any value of $\boldsymbol{B}$ and $\boldsymbol{\sigma}$. So, care should be taken in order to guarantee that the conditional distributions in Expression (4.7) conduce to a valid multivariate joint distribution in (4.8).

In order to guarantee that Expression (4.7) leads to a valid distribution, we should check that its associated joint distribution (4.8) has also a valid (symmetric and positive definite) covariance matrix. The symmetry condition can be either checked on the covariance or precision matrix. That is, a valid CAR process should fulfill $(\boldsymbol{I} - \boldsymbol{B})diag(\boldsymbol{\sigma}^{-1}) = ((\boldsymbol{I} - \boldsymbol{B})diag(\boldsymbol{\sigma}^{-1}))'$ or, alternatively,

$$b_{ij}\sigma_j^2 = b_{ji}\sigma_i^2 \tag{4.9}$$

for any $i \neq j$. Therefore, if $\boldsymbol{\varphi} = (\varphi_1, \varphi_2)$, the stochastic processes

$$\varphi_1 | \varphi_2, \sigma \sim N(\varphi_2, \sigma^2), \quad \varphi_2 | \varphi_1, \sigma \sim N(\varphi_1, 2\sigma^2),$$

or

$$\varphi_1 | \varphi_2, \sigma \sim N(\varphi_2/2, \sigma^2), \quad \varphi_2 | \varphi_1, \sigma \sim N(\varphi_1, \sigma^2),$$

for example, would not yield valid CAR distributions, since they do not fulfill the symmetry condition above. In the first of these cases, the symmetry condition could be fixed by setting the variance of $\varphi_2 | \varphi_1, \sigma$ equal to σ^2. In that case φ_1 would be centered in φ_2 and vice versa but, additionally, both conditional distributions would share the same variance, balancing the expected distance of φ_2 with respect φ_1, and vice versa. That coherence of both conditional distributions makes the corresponding process well defined. That is the kind of requirements needed for CAR distributions to be valid. Note that condition (4.9) is just necessary but is not sufficient to guarantee the validity of the CAR process. Additionally, the positive definiteness of $(\boldsymbol{I}_I - \boldsymbol{B})^{-1} diag(\boldsymbol{\sigma}^2)$ should be further fulfilled so that the corresponding CAR distribution was well defined.

So, if CAR models do not necessarily yield well-defined processes, why are they so popular modeling devices? The main advantage of CAR models is that they make it easily possible to model local dependence between each observation and those corresponding to nearby geographical units, as typically done in time series modeling. Thus, conditional independence can be set between two distant units i and j by just setting $b_{ij} = 0$ in (4.7). In that case, the conditional dependence of $\varphi_i | \boldsymbol{\varphi}_{-i}$ would not depend on φ_j. Thus, inducing conditional independence in CAR distributions is an easy task, which makes it possible to relate each component of $\boldsymbol{\varphi}$ to just a very few components of that vector, in principle a local set of neighbouring spatial units. For large irregular regions, like those arising in disease mapping problems, this way of defining local dependence between observations by means of local relationships seems an intuitive and sensible alternative to defining a global covariance structure on those complex regions, as usually done in geostatistical models. Therefore, dependence could be induced in disease mapping models either locally, throughout conditional distributions of the elements in $\boldsymbol{\varphi}$, or globally, throughout the modeling of the joint distribution of $\boldsymbol{\varphi}$. The first of these options can be done by means of CAR models, which provide a formal framework guaranteeing the validity of the corresponding joint distribution and setting the theoretical properties of these locally dependent spatial models. Additionally, the conditional formulation of CAR models has considerable computational benefits. In fact many spatial proposals which directly model the joint distribution of all the available observations rely on CAR conditional models for its inference (Lindgren et al., 2011). Therefore, at least for these reasons, CAR models should be kept in mind for modeling disease mapping problems and they are indeed the main modeling tool used for those kind of studies.

As b_{ij} is intended to be 0 for all pairs of units which are considered to be distant, the concept of *neighbour* units will be useful for delimiting those distant units in a CAR model. Thus, we will say two spatial units i and j to be neighbours if the conditional distribution of φ_i in (4.7) depends on φ_j, i.e., if $b_{ij} \neq 0$. In other words, we say two regions i and j to be neighbours if, given $\varphi_{-(i,j)}$, they are in some sense close enough so that φ_i and φ_j are still dependent. Since each spatial unit will typically have just a few neighbours, then matrix $\boldsymbol{B}$ will be sparse with just some non-zero cells per row. Obviously, if i and j are said to be neighbours, j and i will be also as a consequence of the symmetry condition (4.9). It is common to denote as $i \sim j$ if municipalities i and j are neighbours, although some other authors also denote the set of neighbours of the i-th municipality as ∂_i. We will henceforth use these two useful notations indistinctly. The sparse matrix $\boldsymbol{B}$ defines a graph where the vertices are the spatial units of the region of study and edges defined by the pairs of neighbouring units (non-zero elements in $\boldsymbol{B}$). This (optionally edge-weighted) undirected graph is known as the *graph* of the corresponding CAR distribution, which is a convenient way to summarize the neighbouring structure assumed for a region of study. Note that any weighted graph on the units of study unequivocally defines the matrix $\boldsymbol{B}$ used in the definition of CAR distributions, and vice versa.

Spatial units can be defined as neighbours according to a wide variety of criteria, for example, we can consider two units to be neighbours if they share common boundaries, if their centroids are located closer than a fixed distance, if there is a direct road joining them without visiting another intermediate municipality, etc. (Earnest et al., 2007). For any pair of neighbouring units i and j, the strength of their dependence can be modulated with the value b_{ij}, provided that the corresponding CAR model for the corresponding $\boldsymbol{B}$ and $\boldsymbol{\sigma}$ yields a valid model. The most common criterion for setting neighbour relationships on a graph is to set $b_{ij} = 1/m_i$, where m_i is the number of neighbours of unit i, for all those units i and j which share common boundaries and 0 otherwise. This criterion is usually known as *adjacency* between units and weighs equally all the neighbours of any spatial unit. Nevertheless, this is not at all the only criterion for summarizing the geographical structure of the region of study (Best et al., 1999; Earnest et al., 2007).

Neighbouring-based CAR models are said to be *Markovian*, this means that, given $\{\varphi_j : j \in \partial_i\}$, φ_i is conditionally independent of φ_k for any other $k \notin \partial_i$. Markovian (Gaussian) CAR models, for appropriate choices of $\boldsymbol{B}$ and $\boldsymbol{\sigma}$, are also known as *Gaussian Markov random fields*, or simply GMRF (Rue and Held, 2005). A GMRF, with respect to a given graph, is defined on a vector $\boldsymbol{\varphi}$ by simply assuming $\boldsymbol{\varphi} \sim N_I(\boldsymbol{\mu}, \boldsymbol{\Sigma})$ where $\boldsymbol{\Sigma}^{-1}$ is a sparse matrix corresponding to a (weighted) graph of some region of study. Both definitions of CAR distributions and GMRFs are equivalent, that is any CAR distribution can be expressed as a GMRF, or vice versa. Nevertheless, CAR distributions put particular emphasis on the conditional distribution of each of its elements and GMRF puts more emphasis on its joint distribution, which has a sparse precision matrix. We will use both concepts indistinctly knowing that they are equivalent. That is, we will equivalently say henceforth that φ is a GMRF or that it follows a CAR distribution. Rue and Held (2005) is an excellent and comprehensive reference if you are interested in the use of spatial dependent models under that approach.

4.3.1.1 The Intrinsic CAR distribution

As defined, CAR distributions are a huge family so, in practice, some subfamilies of particular interest should be defined. The Intrinsic CAR distribution is one of those particular cases of CAR distributions of particular interest. Let us consider $\boldsymbol{W}$, an $I \times I$ sparse weights matrix summarizing the neighbouring structure of the units of study. That is, $\boldsymbol{W}$ takes into account conditional dependence of the spatial units and the strength of conditional dependence in the corresponding graph. Given $\boldsymbol{W}$, the *intrinsic conditional auto-regressive distribution* (also called simply intrinsic CAR or ICAR) is usually defined as the following set of conditional distributions (Kunsch, 1987; Besag and Kooperberg, 1995):

$$\varphi_i | \{\varphi_j : j \in \partial_i\}, \sigma \sim N\left(\sum_{j \in \partial_i} \frac{w_{ij}}{w_{i+}} \varphi_j, \frac{\sigma^2}{w_{i+}}\right), \quad i = 1, \ldots, I, \qquad (4.10)$$

where $w_{i+} = \sum_{k \in \partial_i} w_{ik}$ is the i-th row sum of $\boldsymbol{W}$. The conditional expectation of φ_i, for any i, in an ICAR distribution is a weighted mean of φ for unit i's neighbouring regions. Those municipalities with a higher weight in $\boldsymbol{W}$, i.e., those being "closer" in some sense to unit i, will have a higher contribution to that mean. Moreover, the conditional variance of φ_i also depends on $\boldsymbol{W}$ in such a way that those municipalities that are more connected (those with more neighbours or with neighbours with higher weights) will show lower variability. Therefore, the information contributed by unit i's neighbours reduces the uncertainty on φ_i as a result of their spatial dependence. Note that for the quite common case of adopting adjacency as neighbouring criteria, all the non-zero elements of $\boldsymbol{W}$ should be equal to 1, and then Expression (4.10) would reduce to the simpler expression

$$\varphi_i | \{\varphi_j : j \in \partial_i\}, \sigma \sim N\left(m_i^{-1} \sum_{j \in \partial_i} \varphi_j, \frac{\sigma^2}{m_i}\right), \quad i = 1, \ldots, I \qquad (4.11)$$

where m_i is just $|\partial_i|$, i.e., the number of neighbours of the i-th geographical unit, yielding a simplified unweighted formulation of the original definition.

The Intrinsic CAR distribution is a particular case of CAR model with $\boldsymbol{B} = diag(w_{1+}^{-1}, \ldots, w_{I+}^{-1})\boldsymbol{W}$ and $\boldsymbol{\sigma}^2 = \sigma^2(w_{1+}^{-1}, \ldots, w_{I+}^{-1})$. Note that w_{ii} will necessarily be 0 for any i, since otherwise φ_i's mean would depend on itself. Moreover, if $w_{ii} \neq 0$ for some i, Expression (4.10) would not fulfill the definition of CAR model, where the sums involved in the conditional means were done for $i \neq j$. This will be achieved if any unit i is not a neighbour of itself, which will be assumed by convention. As formulated, the ICAR distribution also defines a Gaussian Markov random field since φ_i's conditional distribution depends only on those φ_j so that $j \in \partial_i$.

The ICAR distribution, as defined in (4.10), yields the following joint distribution (Brook, 1964; Besag, 1974)

$$P(\boldsymbol{\varphi}|\sigma) \propto \exp\left(\frac{-\boldsymbol{\varphi}^t(\boldsymbol{D} - \boldsymbol{W})\boldsymbol{\varphi}}{2\sigma^2}\right) \qquad (4.12)$$

with $\boldsymbol{D} = diag(w_{1+}, \ldots, w_{I+})$ and $\boldsymbol{W}$ the weights matrix defined above. This also can be seen as a consequence of the CAR formulation of ICAR distributions, which would yield the joint distribution in Expression (4.12), as can be easily derived from (4.8). Bearing in mind that $\boldsymbol{D}$ is diagonal, matrix $\boldsymbol{W}$ will have to be symmetric in order to guarantee the symmetry of the variance-covariance matrix of $\boldsymbol{\varphi}$.

Expression (4.12) has a particularity, namely, its precision matrix always fulfills

$$\sigma^{-2}(\boldsymbol{D} - \boldsymbol{W})\mathbf{1}_I = \sigma^{-2}((w_{1+}, \ldots, w_{I+}) - (\sum_{j\neq 1} w_{1j}, \ldots, \sum_{j\neq I} w_{Ij})) = \mathbf{0}_I.$$

As a consequence, that precision matrix is not positive definite (just positive semidefinite), which makes the ICAR distribution ill defined in principle (Besag and Kooperberg, 1995). The latter expression implies also that the columns of $(\boldsymbol{D} - \boldsymbol{W})$ are linearly dependent and, therefore, that precision matrix among other things is neither of full rank nor invertible. This makes Expression (4.12) a peculiar multivariate Normal distribution that requires some care to work with it.

At this stage of the book, we would rather avoid technical details on the ICAR distribution that will be further discussed in Chapter 6. Nevertheless, by now, we anticipate that for fixing the rank-deficiency of $(\boldsymbol{D} - \boldsymbol{W})$, the vectors following an ICAR distribution are usually restricted in some way. Thus, for the common case of having a fully connected region of study, $\boldsymbol{\varphi}$ is usually restricted so that $\boldsymbol{\varphi}' \cdot \mathbf{1}_I = 0$, i.e., a sum-to-zero restriction is imposed to their components. That is, we require $\boldsymbol{\varphi}$ to be orthogonal to the vector $\mathbf{1}_I$, the vector which makes the precision matrix $(\boldsymbol{D} - \boldsymbol{W})$ rank-deficient. This restriction makes the number of independent variables of $\boldsymbol{\varphi}$ to be lower than its number of components and to match the rank of $(\boldsymbol{D} - \boldsymbol{W})$. So, in this sense ICAR distributions can be considered legitimate low-dimensional multivariate

Normal distributions on a hyperplane of a higher dimensional space. For any vector $\varphi \neq 0$ in this subspace, the precision matrix of the ICAR distribution accomplishes: $\varphi(\boldsymbol{D} - \boldsymbol{W})\varphi \neq 0$, thus $(\boldsymbol{D} - \boldsymbol{W})$ is positive definite for the elements of that subspace. Thus the sum-to-zero restriction on φ makes the precision matrix of the ICAR positive definite for all the vectors having that distribution, so the positivity condition of the precision matrix is solved in this manner.

If the rank-deficiency of $(\boldsymbol{D} - \boldsymbol{W})$ was higher than 1, further restrictions corresponding to the linear combinations that make $(\boldsymbol{D} - \boldsymbol{W})$ rank-deficient should be imposed so that the ICAR distribution was well defined. It can be shown that the number of connected components ("islands") composing the region of study coincides with the rank-deficiency of $(\boldsymbol{D} - \boldsymbol{W})$ (Hodges et al., 2003). Therefore, we should impose as many restrictions on the ICAR distributions as islands compose the region of study. Therefore the matrix $(\boldsymbol{D} - \boldsymbol{W})$ will be positive definite for any vector in that hyperplane and, as a consequence, the ICAR distribution will be well defined therein. Specifically, in that case, it will be convenient to impose a particular sum-to-zero restriction for any of the islands composing the region of study.

Note that Expression (4.12) is just proportional to the kernel of a multivariate Normal distribution and we have not fixed any proportionality constant there. That proportionality constant should be proportional to $\sigma^{-(I-k)/2}$ (Hodges et al., 2003) where k corresponds to the number of connected components forming the region of study. The term k in the exponent of the proportionality constant is set to reflect the lower dimensionality of the subspace arising from the sum-to-zero restriction(s) imposed, one per connected component. In case of putting the typical proportionality constant for I-dimensional multivariate Normal distributions $(\sigma^{-I/2})$, Expression (4.12) would yield an improper prior distribution. Paradoxically, if sum-to-zero restriction(s) were not imposed on the ICAR distribution, alternative (and distinct) expressions of the proportionality constant could be derived, which would yield valid (and different) expressions of this distribution (Lavine and Hodges, 2012).

A consequence of the global sum-to-zero restriction of ICAR distributions is that, as you may have noticed in Expression (4.10), in contrast to general CAR distributions, ICARs do not depend on a mean argument $\boldsymbol{\mu}$. Under the sum-to-zero restriction, it makes no sense to try to estimate the mean of any ICAR-distributed vector since that mean is itself fixed. Thus, the definition made of the ICAR distribution implicitly assumes $\boldsymbol{\mu} = \boldsymbol{0}_I$. Therefore, if we used an ICAR random effect to model the variability of a vector and wanted the mean of this vector to take whatever value, we should put that mean as a separate intercept term to the ICAR component, given the inability of the ICAR distribution to model that mean. A second consequence of sum-to-zero restrictions preclude the use of ICAR distributions as a tool to directly model the data, i.e., as a probability density function for the data likelihood. The only case where this use would be suitable would be when the observed (random) data accomplished the restrictions imposed on φ, but this has in general probability 0. Therefore, ICAR distributions are used just as devices for modeling the spatial dependence of random effects and this is the typical use that we will have for this distribution.

The ICAR distribution depends on a single parameter, its variance σ^2. This parameter controls the variability of the whole distribution. Nevertheless σ^2 should be interpreted with care since it cannot be considered the typical marginal variance of Normal distributions. Each element φ_i in an ICAR distribution will have a different marginal variance equal to $\sigma^2((\boldsymbol{D} - \boldsymbol{W})^-)ii$, where $(\boldsymbol{D} - \boldsymbol{W})^-$ denotes the Moore-Penrose generalized inverse of $\boldsymbol{D} - \boldsymbol{W}$. We will justify the use of this generalized inverse in Chapter 6. The variance parameter σ^2 models the conditional variability of any observation around its neighbours' mean; therefore, it is better understood as a conditional variance. Expression (4.12) makes evident that σ^2 does not have any effect on φ's correlation, which depends just on the matrix $(\boldsymbol{D} - \boldsymbol{W})$. It seems paradoxical that the ICAR distribution, which is conceived to induce spatial dependence on vectors of variables, does not have any specific parameter allowing to tune the spatial correlation of φ. In this sense the ICAR distribution can be considered as somewhat restrictive although, on the contrary, it may be also considered an appealing tool due to its particular simplicity. Additionally, the ICAR distribution can be considered as a spatial parallel of random walks processes for time series, which do not have any parameter controlling the strength of temporal dependence.

WinBUGS has a specific sentence for setting intrinsic CAR distributions up. This sentence, the `car.normal` function, avoids explicitly coding the set of conditional distributions defining an ICAR process. The function used to define intrinsic CAR distributions has the following syntax

```
> sp[1:n]~car.normal(adj[],weights[],num[],tau)
```

This sentence is somewhat particular, since it does not have to be run separately for all the components of `sp` within a `for` loop, as customarily done in the BUGS language. Since `car.normal` defines a multivariate distribution, instead of a set of independent univariate distributions, it is defined as a single function. This rule applies also to all the multivariate distributions in BUGS such as the multivariate Normal (`dmnorm`) or the proper CAR distribution that we will introduce below. Regarding the left-hand side of the WinBUGS sentence above, it is compulsory to put within the brackets the set of indexes which correspond to the ICAR distribution; otherwise, WinBUGS returns the error 'empty slot not allowed in variable name'.

The `car.normal` function has 4 arguments, the first three are vectors of fixed values, i.e., these values are not allowed to be variables in the model. The fourth argument corresponds to the precision of the ICAR distribution, which will be typically one more variable in the model that we will be interested to learn about, and therefore we will have to assign it a prior distribution. The `adj[]` argument is a vector concatenating, as an ordered sequence, the neighbours of all units in the region of study, i.e., adj=(first unit's neighbours, second unit's neighbours, etc.). The argument weights[] is a vector of the same length as adj with the weights corresponding to every one of these neighbours. Thus weights contains the values of w_{ij} in Expression (4.10), which are also the non-zero elements of matrix W. The order of the elements in weights will be the same as the order used for introducing the vector adj. For the case of using adjacency as criteria for defining neighbours, all the w_{ij}s would be equal to 1, which can be coded even within the model syntax as

```
for(i in 1:nadj){
 weights[i]<-1
}
```

where nadj stands for the length of the vector of adjacencies adj. Finally, num[] is a vector of length equal to the number of units in the region of study whose i-th component contains the number of neighbours of the corresponding areal unit. Therefore, sum(num[]) will have to be equal to nadj. The first three arguments of the car.normal function for an adjacency matrix will be typically obtained from a call to the nb2WB function of the spdep package of R (already introduced in Chapter 3), with the boundary file of the region of study as the main argument. The precision argument of the car.normal distribution will be typically modeled as any other precision of random effects in any other hierarchical Bayesian model. In general we propose to use a uniform prior distribution on this parameter by making

```
tau<-pow(std.dev,-2)
std.dev ~ dunif(0,a)
```

for some large value for a. Typically, setting a to some moderate value, such as 5 or 10, should be vague enough since we are talking about random effects modeling a quantity corresponding to a logarithmic scale, although this could change for some models. A more thorough discussion of this and other prior choices for modeling the variability of random effects in disease mapping models will be developed at Subsection 4.3.2.1 of this chapter.

The car.normal function automatically implements the sum-to-zero restriction usually assumed for intrinsic CAR distributions, so we will not have to take specific care of this issue. This restriction is incorporated into the posterior sample of φ by just subtracting its mean from the sampled random effects at every step of the MCMC, as suggested by Besag et al. (1995). Moreover, it is not necessary to take specific care of fulfilling this restriction when initializing the sp vector above, since WinBUGS does not require those initial values to fulfill it. In case of having a region of study composed of several connected components, several sum-to-zero restrictions should be imposed; to do this, it would be convenient to consider a different ICAR distribution for each connected component. This will induce a different sum-to-zero restriction for each connected component in the region of study. In that case it will be convenient to include a separate intercept in the model for each "island" of the region of study, since otherwise all of them will be forced to take a common overall risk which seems to be a hard and unrealistic constraint.

Regarding the implementation of the `car.normal` function in `WinBUGS`, we have repeatedly noticed that the calculation of the DIC statistic is inefficiently implemented for those models containing this distribution. Namely, these models, when executed with the option `DIC=TRUE` of the `pbugs` function of R, suddenly slow down at the moment that the DIC starts to be computed (just after the burn-in period). Moreover, computing the deviance (the statistic in which DIC is based) for each iteration of the MCMC, regardless of the thinning of the Markov chains is inefficient since most of the calculated deviances are ignored. These inefficiencies invite us to calculate the DIC on our own, for example in R, instead of doing it in `WinBUGS` during the MCMC run. At the accompanying online material of the next example, you will find R code suitable for calculating the DIC in Poisson-based disease mapping models in general. Convenient adaptations of that R code at the spatio-temporal or multivariate settings will be also provided in the corresponding online material when required. The use of this code speeds up in a significant manner `WinBUGS` in comparison to runs that calculate the DIC therein and contain the `car.normal` distribution.

`WinBUGS` has a second sentence implementing a non-Gaussian version of the ICAR distribution, the `car.l1` function. This function implements, for every observation, a conditional process of the kind of Expression (4.10) but based on a Laplace (or double exponential) distribution instead of on conditional Normal distributions (Besag et al., 1991). The Laplace distribution is a robust alternative to the Normal distribution with expression

$$P(y|\mu, \lambda) = \frac{1}{2\lambda} \exp\left(-\frac{|y - \mu|}{\lambda}\right). \tag{4.13}$$

The mean and variance of this distribution are, respectively, μ and $2\lambda^2$. The Laplace distribution has heavier tails than the Normal distribution, making it more prone to reproduce subtle jumps between contiguous areal units; thus it is more prone to reproduce discontinuities in spatial patterns (Best et al., 1999). The syntax for the `car.l1` function is exactly the same as that in the Normal-based ICAR distribution, i.e.,

```
> sp[1:n]~car.l1(adj[], weights[], num[], tau)
```

where `adj`, `weights`, `num` and `tau` have the same meaning as for the `car.normal` distribution.

Alternatively, `INLA` has also implemented the intrinsic CAR distribution. As mentioned, this distribution cannot be used as data likelihood; therefore, it will have to be necessarily used as latent model. For setting an intrinsic CAR distribution in `INLA` as prior distribution of a set of random effects, we should use the `f(...)` function with the `model="besag"` option. On the contrary to `WinBUGS`, `INLA`'s implementation of the ICAR distribution does not allow us to use different weights for the different neighbours of any geographical unit. Thus, in this software the ICAR model necessarily assumes the expected value of any observation to be the mean of that variable in the corresponding neighbours instead of a more general weighted mean.

The main options of the intrinsic CAR distribution in `INLA` are `hyper` and `graph`. The first has the usual meaning for any random effect; it is used to set up the prior distribution of the log-precision of the random effects. We will typically set the option `hyper=sdunif` as defined in Section 3.2, which assumes a uniform prior distribution on the positive real line for the corresponding standard deviation. The `graph` argument is used to introduce the geographical structure of the region of study into `INLA`. Specifically, this argument should contain the path to the `.graph` file created by the `nb2INLA` function of the `spdep` package, as described in Section 3.4. `INLA` assumes by default the usual sum-to-zero restriction for the whole region of study. Nevertheless, on the contrary to `WinBUGS`, if the region of study was composed of several islands, the intrinsic CAR distribution constrains by default the random effects of each island with an additional sum-to-zero restriction. Therefore, in that case, it will be convenient for the models to include a different intercept term for each island in order to allow them to have different overall means.

4.3.1.2   Some proper CAR distributions

The intrinsic CAR distribution is just one member in the family of CAR distributions, as it is defined in Expression (4.7). Nevertheless, for any valid choice of B and σ, we would have a different member of the family of CAR distributions. A CAR alternative to the ICAR distribution is the *Proper Conditional Auto-Regressive distribution*, known as proper CAR or PCAR. We want to stress that there are far more CAR processes which define proper CAR distributions. Nevertheless, the popularity of the proposal introduced just below has made it to be coined as "the" proper CAR distribution for many authors.

Given a graph on a vector of variables, the PCAR distribution is defined by means of the following set of conditional distributions (see the rejoinder of Besag et al. (1991) or Cressie (1993))

$$\varphi_i | \{\varphi_j : j \in \partial_i\}, \boldsymbol{\mu}, \sigma, \rho \sim N\left(\mu_i + \rho\left(\sum_{j \in \partial_i} \frac{w_{ij}}{w_{i+}}(\varphi_j - \mu_j)\right), \frac{\sigma^2}{w_{i+}}\right), \quad (4.14)$$

for $i = 1, \ldots, I$. As a consequence of Expression (4.8), this set of conditional distributions yields the following multivariate Normal distribution for $\boldsymbol{\varphi}$

$$\boldsymbol{\varphi} | \boldsymbol{\mu}, \sigma, \rho \sim N_I\left(\boldsymbol{\mu}, \sigma^2(\boldsymbol{D} - \rho \boldsymbol{W})^{-1}\right), \quad (4.15)$$

with $\boldsymbol{D} = diag(w_{1+}, \ldots, w_{I+})$ and $W_{ij} = w_{ij}$ if $i \sim j$, and 0 otherwise. Note that for $\rho = 1$ the PCAR's precision matrix coincides with that of the ICAR distribution; therefore, the intrinsic case can be considered as a limit case of

PCAR with additional sum-to-zero restrictions. Specifically, for the PCAR distribution, the conditional expected value of each $\boldsymbol{\varphi}$ component no longer coincides with its neighbours' (weighted) mean; on the contrary, that value is regressed against that mean. In this sense, the proper CAR distribution may be seen as a generalization of the 1st-order auto-regressive model of time series to the spatial case; meanwhile the intrinsic CAR distribution makes a similar generalization of the 1st-order random walk process (Botella-Rocamora et al., 2012). Thus, although related, both ICAR and PCAR distributions are qualitatively different, yielding processes with very different properties.

In contrast to the ICAR distribution, the latter two expressions depend on a vector $\boldsymbol{\mu}$, the marginal mean of $\boldsymbol{\varphi}$. Nevertheless, the effect of that vector can be separately modeled by considering $\boldsymbol{\varphi} = \boldsymbol{\mu} + \boldsymbol{\psi}$, for $\boldsymbol{\psi}$ a vector following a PCAR distribution of mean $\boldsymbol{0}_I$. Therefore, for simplicity, from now on we will consider in general $\boldsymbol{\mu}$ to be equal to $\boldsymbol{0}_I$ in Expression (4.14), which yields a simplified zero-centered version of the PCAR distribution. As for ICAR, adjacency is the most widely used graph building criterion for PCAR distributions, in which case (and for $\boldsymbol{\mu} = \boldsymbol{0}_I$), the proper CAR distribution arises as the following simplified set of conditional distributions

$$\varphi_i | \{\varphi_j : j \in \partial_i\}, \sigma, \rho \sim N \left(\rho \left(m_i^{-1} \sum_{j \in \partial_i} \varphi_j \right), \frac{\sigma^2}{m_i} \right), \ i = 1, \ldots, I \quad (4.16)$$

where m_i stands for the number of neighbours of unit i.

In contrast to ICAR, PCAR distributions are biparametric since they depend on its standard deviation σ and a second parameter, ρ, controlling the strength of the spatial dependence. Thus, for higher values of ρ, the PCAR distribution shows stronger spatial dependence than for $\rho \approx 0$, for which $\boldsymbol{\varphi}$'s components are independent given σ. Nevertheless, that independence is somewhat strange since the variance of any of $\boldsymbol{\varphi}$'s elements depends also on the number of neighbours of the corresponding unit. That is, the conditional variances in the PCAR distribution depend on the shape of the region of study, when one would typically want them to have equal variances in order to reflect full spatial independence.

For $\boldsymbol{W}$ being a symmetric matrix, $\boldsymbol{D} - \rho \boldsymbol{W}$ is obviously also symmetric. Thus, if $\boldsymbol{D} - \rho \boldsymbol{W}$ was a positive definite matrix, the PCAR distribution defined above would yield a valid (proper) distribution. Provided the non-zero elements of $\boldsymbol{W}$ were positive, for $|\rho| < 1$ the matrix $\boldsymbol{D} - \rho \boldsymbol{W}$ is diagonally dominant and therefore positive definite. Thus, sufficient conditions for the validity of the PCAR distribution will be $\boldsymbol{W}$ being symmetric, with positive non-zero values and $-1 < \rho < 1$.

Since ρ could take also negative values, the PCAR distribution admits the expected value for any site to go in the opposite direction than the consensus of its neighbours showing, therefore, negative spatial dependence. Nevertheless, for $\rho < 0$ the PCAR distribution shows some non-intuitive performances, such as, pairs of neighbouring units having, a priori, positive correlation when it was expected to be negative (Wall, 2004). However, for the case of a Gaussian likelihood, these problems are shown to be alleviated in the posterior distribution (Assunçao and Krainski, 2009). Moreover, it has also been adduced that the PCAR distribution induces high correlations among neighbours only if ρ takes values very close to 1. As a consequence, this distribution could find some difficulties for fitting strongly dependent spatial patterns (Besag, 1974). This kind of problem has made the PCAR distribution to be criticized for modeling spatial areal data (Wall, 2004). Nevertheless, the ability of the PCAR distribution to adapt itself to the strength of the spatial pattern at hand is an unquestionable advantage over, for example, the ICAR distribution. Finally, the fact that the PCAR distribution is proper makes dealing with it easier than with the ICAR distribution from both theoretical and practical points of view, avoiding some technical issues. Namely, the PCAR distribution does not require adding any particular restriction and avoids other technical and controversial issues such as setting an appropriate proportionality constant on the corresponding joint multivariate Normal distribution (Lavine and Hodges, 2012). Therefore, we find the PCAR distribution to be a competitive alternative to the intrinsic case which would also deserve attention.

WinBUGS has a specific function available that implements a wide family of proper CAR distributions, the `car.proper` function. This function could be used for fitting PCAR random effects. Namely, the `car.proper` function in WinBUGS fits random effects of the form

$$\boldsymbol{\varphi}|\boldsymbol{\mu}, \sigma, \rho \sim N_I(\boldsymbol{\mu}, \sigma^2(\boldsymbol{I}_I - \rho\boldsymbol{C})^{-1}\boldsymbol{M}). \qquad (4.17)$$

which coincides with the general expression of CAR distributions (Expression (4.8)) with $\boldsymbol{B} = \rho\boldsymbol{C}$ and $\sigma^2\boldsymbol{M} = diag(\boldsymbol{\sigma}^2)$. Thus, $\boldsymbol{M}$ in this expression is expected to be a diagonal matrix with the different weights for the specific conditional variances for each component in $\boldsymbol{\varphi}$. On the other hand, matrix $\boldsymbol{C}$ will be typically a sparse matrix. This function allows implementing CAR models with $\boldsymbol{B}$ known up to a multiplicative constant ρ. Obviously, $(\boldsymbol{I}_I - \rho\boldsymbol{C})^{-1}\boldsymbol{M}$ should be symmetric and positive definite so that the corresponding distribution is well defined.

PCAR distributions could be implemented with the `car.proper` function by making $\boldsymbol{M} = diag(w_{1+}^{-1}, ... w_{I+}^{-1})$ and $\boldsymbol{C}_{ij} = w_{ij}/w_{i+}$ for $i \sim j$, and 0 otherwise, which would reproduce the multivariate expression of PCAR distributions in (4.15). Nevertheless, the general expression (4.17) in terms of $\boldsymbol{C}$ and $\boldsymbol{M}$ allows the `car.proper` function to fit more CAR models besides "the" PCAR distribution. Thus, an alternative to PCAR is what Cressie and Kapat (2008) name as *Autocorrelation CAR (ACAR) model* , which is defined by setting $C_{ij} = A_{ij}(w_{j+}/w_{i+})^{1/2}$ for $i \sim j$, or 0 otherwise, and $\boldsymbol{M} = diag(w_{1+}^{-1}, ..., w_{I+}^{-1})$ for a graph $\boldsymbol{W}$. Cressie and Kapat (2008) set an adjacency graph $\boldsymbol{W}$ with $W_{ij} = 1$ if $i \sim j$ and 0 otherwise and $A_{ij} = 1$ for all i and j. Nevertheless, A_{ij} could be alternatively used to weigh the contribution of the adjacent neighbours as a function of, for example, the Euclidean distance between units

(Cressie and Chan, 1989). Matrix C could be also defined as a function of the expected values in each unit as $C_{ij} = (e_j/e_i)^{1/2}$ if $i \sim j$ and 0 otherwise (Stern and Cressie, 1999), making those units with higher expected values more influential instead of those 'more connected' in the graph. In this case M should be set to $diag(e_1^{-1}, ..., e_I^{-1})$ so that the model defines an appropriate variance-covariance matrix. Nevertheless, care should be taken with the use of these distributions since some of them have been criticized for the weird conditional means that they could be implicitly proposing (Wakefield et al., 2000). Finally, setting it out $C_{ij} = 1$ if $i \sim j$, or 0 otherwise, and $M = diag(1, ..., 1)$ we would also define an additional valid proper CAR distribution, the *homogeneous CAR (HCAR) distribution* of Cressie (1993) and Cressie and Kapat (2008). The `car.proper` function allows us to fit all these CAR models, among others, in `WinBUGS`.

For the parameterization used in (4.17), and therefore for the models above, that expression defines a proper distribution if and only if $\rho \in]\lambda_{(1)}^{-1}, \lambda_{(I)}^{-1}[$, where $\lambda_{(1)}, \ldots, \lambda_{(I)}$ are the increasingly ordered eigenvalues of $M^{-1/2}CM^{1/2}(=D^{-1/2}WD^{-1/2}$ for a PCAR distribution). Sun et al. (1999) show a proof of the sufficiency of this condition, although its necessity can also be derived from that proof. This precludes ρ to be considered as a traditional correlation parameter. Note that the condition above is both necessary and sufficient in contrast to the $-1 < \rho < 1$ condition on the PCAR distribution which was only sufficient. This means that for the PCAR distribution $] - 1, 1[\subseteq]\lambda_{(1)}^{-1}, \lambda_{(I)}^{-1}[$. Moreover, since for $\rho = 1$ the covariance matrix of the PCAR distribution is singular, then $\lambda_{(I)}^{-1}$ for the PCAR distribution is exactly 1. Thus, for the particular case of PCAR distributions, the range of valid values is $]\lambda_{(1)}^{-1}, 1[$ with $\lambda_{(1)}^{-1} < -1$.

The syntax of the `car.proper` distribution of `WinBUGS` is the following

```
sp[1:n]~car.proper(mu[], C[], adj[], num[], M[], tau, rho)
```

Four of these seven arguments: C, `adj`, `num` and M (those setting the values of C and M in (4.17)) are necessarily non-stochastic, i.e., the matrices C and M should be completely known. On the other hand, the other three arguments in this function may be either fixed to specific values or inference could be made on them. The arguments C, `adj` and `num` define the C matrix in `WinBUGS` in a similar way to that made by `weights`, `adj` and `num` for matrix W in the `car.normal` function. Thus, `num` will contain the number of neighbours of each geographical unit and `adj` an ordered sequence of those neighbours which will be typically obtained from the `nb2WB` function in R (`spdep` package). The argument C will be a vector with the (row-wise) ordered sequence of non-zero elements in C, which is equal to $D^{-1}W$ for the PCAR distribution. Note that C is a row-standardized transformation of the weights matrix W so, in contrast to the `car.normal` function, where the non-zero elements of matrix W were all usually fixed to 1, the non-zero elements of C will be in general different. Thus, if we wanted to define an adjacency-based C matrix for the

PCAR distribution, where $C_{ij} = 1/m_i$ for $i \sim j$ and 0 otherwise, we could simply do in R

```
> Cmat=rep(1/num,num)
```

where `num` is the vector containing the number of neighbours for each unit. The vector M (of the same length as `sp`) will contain the diagonal elements of the matrix M. For the proper CAR distribution, this vector will be the diagonal elements of D^{-1}, that is, $(w_{1+}^{-1}, ..., w_{I+}^{-1})$ and in case of defining the graph for `sp` in terms of adjacency, this would be simply $(m_1^{-1}, ..., m_I^{-1})$, what can be done within WinBUGS by typing

```
for(i in 1:n){M[i]<-1/num[i]}
```

into the corresponding model.

Regarding the arguments of `car.proper` that could be stochastic, `mu` will be a vector of the same length as `sp` with the marginal expected values of this vector. As mentioned, frequently `mu` will be separately modeled outside of the vector `sp` in which case `mu` should be set to 0_I. This can be made within WinBUGS by including the sentence

```
for(i in 1:n){mu[i]<-0}
```

into the corresponding model. In this case, an intercept (or whatever appropriate expression) should be included in that model to substitute `mu`'s effect in `sp`. Argument `tau` stands for the precision of the PCAR distribution, which is usually unknown, so it will be typically assigned a uniform prior distribution on the corresponding standard deviation, as for the ICAR distribution.

The last argument in the `car.proper` function, `rho`, corresponds with the parameter ρ controlling the spatial dependence in (4.17). As mentioned, this parameter produces valid distributions when ranging in the interval $]\lambda_{(1)}^{-1}, \lambda_{(I)}^{-1}[$, where $\lambda_{(1)}$ and $\lambda_{(I)}$ are, respectively, the lowest and largest eigenvalue of $M^{-1/2}CM^{1/2}$, $D^{-1/2}WD^{-1/2}$ for the PCAR distribution. WinBUGS has specific functions for calculating these two eigenvalues, these are

```
min.bound(C[], adj[], num[], M[])
```

and

```
max.bound(C[], adj[], num[], M[])
```

whose arguments should be filled with the same arguments used for calling to the `car.proper` function. As previously mentioned, for the PCAR distribution `max.bound` will always return 1; nevertheless, this function will be useful for more general proper CAR distributions (Cressie and Chan, 1989; Stern and Cressie, 1999; Cressie and Kapat, 2008). The output of these two functions will typically define the lower and upper limits of a uniform distribution to be used as prior distribution for `rho`. However, other alternatives are also possible, such as a uniform distribution on $]0, \lambda_{(I)}^{-1}[$ considering only 'positive spatial correlations', or a beta distribution overweighing `rho` values close to $\lambda_{(I)}^{-1}$, since these are the only values producing geographical patterns with substantial spatial dependence (Besag et al., 1991; Carlin and Banerjee, 2003). Obviously these latter options would be informative choices for ρ's prior distribution.

INLA allows implementing several different proper CAR distributions, although it does not have any function implementing specifically the same models reproduced with the `car.proper` function in WinBUGS. As a consequence, the PCAR distribution, for example, cannot be reproduced in INLA. The first option for implementing proper CAR distributions in `inla` is called by putting the `model="besagproper"` argument on a corresponding `f()` function. This defines a proper CAR model corresponding to the following set of conditional distributions

$$\varphi_i | \{\varphi_j : j \in \partial_i\}, \sigma, \delta \sim N \left((\delta + m_i)^{-1} \sum_{j \in \partial_i} \varphi_j, \frac{\sigma^2}{\delta + m_i} \right), \ i = 1, \ldots, I$$

or, equivalently,

$$\varphi | \sigma, \delta \sim N_I \left(\mathbf{0}, \sigma^2 (\delta \mathbf{I}_I + \mathbf{D} - \mathbf{W})^{-1} \right)$$

for $\mathbf{W}$ being a symmetric adjacency matrix with $W_{ij} = 1$ if $i \sim j$, or 0 otherwise, and $\mathbf{D} = diag(m_1, \ldots, m_I)$ (see page 285 of Blangiardo and Cameletti (2015)). Note that, in contrast to the `car.proper` function in WinBUGS, the `besagproper` family in INLA neither includes a marginal mean for φ (it is assumed to be equal to $\mathbf{0}_I$) nor allows us to introduce different weights in $\mathbf{W}$. In contrast to the PCAR distribution, which makes its precision matrix diagonally dominant by including ρ into the model, this new alternative achieves the same goal by adding δ to the diagonal elements of $\mathbf{D} - \mathbf{W}$, which makes its precision matrix positive definite. This model behaves as if each geographical unit had δ imaginary neighbours with their corresponding values in φ being equal to 0. This shrinks φ's components towards 0 as a function of δ. Moreover, that shrinkage will be higher for those units with fewer neighbours since the information provided by the imaginary neighbours will be proportionally higher in that case. This could induce some differences in comparison to the PCAR distribution which would not show this effect on the conditional means.

For $\delta = 0$ and φ constrained to sum zero, this distribution coincides with the ICAR distribution. For $\delta > 0$ this distribution is proper as a consequence of the diagonal dominance of its precision matrix. For high values of δ this distribution tends to the multivariate Normal distribution

$$\varphi | \sigma, \delta \sim N_I \left(\mathbf{0}, \sigma^2 \delta^{-1} \mathbf{I}_I \right).$$

Thus, for high enough values of δ, this distribution mostly reproduces independence and homoscedasticity, which seems a nice feature. Hence, δ is in charge of quantifying the strength of the spatial dependence in this distribution. By default, INLA puts a $Gamma(1, 1)$ prior distribution on this parameter, which seems to be an informative choice precluding δ to take moderately high values, so when using this prior, we advise making sensitivity analyses in order to assess the effect of this prior assumption. The syntax used for putting this distribution in inla is the same as for the ICAR distribution, so it will be compulsory to add a graph argument to the statement f(...,model="besagproper") in order to make it work.

The second option available in INLA for fitting proper CAR distributions is the generic1 latent model. This model implements the multivariate Normal distribution

$$\boldsymbol{\varphi}|\sigma, \beta \sim N_I(\mathbf{0}, \sigma^2(\mathbf{I} - \frac{\beta}{\lambda_{(I)}}\mathbf{C})^{-1}) \tag{4.18}$$

for $\mathbf{C}$ a (typically sparse) fixed symmetric matrix accounting for the geographical structure of the region of study and $\lambda_{(I)}$ the maximum eigenvalue of $\mathbf{C}$. This joint distribution can also be seen as the following set of conditional distributions

$$\varphi_i|\{\varphi_j : j \in \partial_i\}, \sigma, \beta \sim N(\frac{\beta}{\lambda_{(I)}}\sum_{j \in \partial_i} C_{ij}\varphi_j, \sigma^2), \ i = 1, ..., I.$$

Choosing $\mathbf{C}$ as a typical adjacency matrix could be a sensible choice where the mean of every observation would be proportional to the corresponding neighbours' sum. This choice would reproduce the previously mentioned Homogeneous CAR (HCAR) distribution of Cressie and Kapat (2008). In this case, those units with more neighbours will have a more volatile expected value in contrast to ICAR and PCAR distributions. This assumption seems questionable for many causes of death and contrary to the hypothesis of (positive) spatial dependence, which should make neighbours reduce the uncertainty on any geographical unit. On the other hand, the conditional variances in the HCAR distribution are equal for all the values of $\boldsymbol{\varphi}$. This seems appropriate for $\beta \approx 0$ since in that case this distribution reproduces independent and identically distributed Normal observations, regardless of the number of neighbours of each unit. On the contrary, for higher values of β, all the values of $\boldsymbol{\varphi}$ are, in average, equally distant to their mean, whether these are more or less reliable, i.e., whether the corresponding geographical unit has more or less neighbours, respectively. This second property of HCAR distributions does not seem so appealing.

The HCAR distribution can be invoked in inla by means of the syntax f(...,model="generic1") with the Cmatrix argument ($\mathbf{C}$ matrix in Expression (4.18)) being the adjacency matrix of the region of study. The inclusion of $\lambda_{(I)}$ in the parameterization of the expressions above makes the upper limit of the distribution of β exactly 1; otherwise, the corresponding covariance matrix would not be positive definite. Although β could take values lower than 0, INLA assumes it to be necessarily within the interval $[0, 1[$, i.e., INLA's implementation implicitly assumes that the `generic1` function will always be used for modeling spatial patterns with positive correlations. This should not be a serious limitation since, as mentioned, some authors also advocate for constraining PCAR distributions so that they only take positive spatial auto-correlations (Carlin and Banerjee, 2003). By default, `INLA` assumes a vague Normal prior distribution ($N(0, 10)$) on $logit(\beta)$, which puts substantial mass on the extremes of the [0,1] interval for β. Once again we advise `INLA` users to carry sensitivity analyses out on this prior distribution.

The `generic1` latent model can also be used for implementing another common proper CAR distribution in `INLA`, the Leroux et al. CAR process (Leroux et al., 1999; MacNab, 2003), also known as *LCAR distribution* or process for some authors. Leroux et al.'s process defines a proper CAR distribution resembling Besag et al.'s proposal (Besag et al., 1991) that is introduced in the next subsection, but using a single random effect, which may be more convenient in several senses. Indeed some works, such as Lee (2011), show their preference of LCAR based models in terms of robustness for a variety of settings over different alternatives as for example the Besag et al. proposal. The LCAR distribution may be defined as the following set of conditional distributions

$$\varphi_i | \boldsymbol{\varphi}_{-i}, \sigma, \lambda \sim N\left(\frac{\lambda}{1 - \lambda + \lambda m_i} \sum_{j \sim i} \varphi_i, \frac{\sigma^2}{1 - \lambda + \lambda m_i}\right) \quad i = 1, ..., I. \quad (4.19)$$

For $\lambda = 0$ this process reproduces independence between geographical units and homoscedasticity, while for $\lambda = 1$ this is equivalent to the ICAR distribution, except for the sum-to-zero restriction(s) that usually accompany that distribution. Therefore, the parameter λ in the LCAR distribution, which is supposed to vary in the interval [0,1], controls the amount of spatial dependence reproduced by the model.

The LCAR distribution could be also equivalently formulated as a joint multivariate Normal distribution as

$$\boldsymbol{\varphi} | \sigma, \lambda \sim N_I \left(\boldsymbol{0}_I, \sigma^2((1 - \lambda)\boldsymbol{I}_I + \lambda(\boldsymbol{D} - \boldsymbol{W}))^{-1}\right)$$

where $\boldsymbol{W}$ is a binary adjacency matrix of the corresponding graph and $\boldsymbol{D}$ a diagonal matrix with elements given by the number of neighbours of each geographical unit. This distribution solves the impropriety problems in the ICAR distribution by means of λ, which makes a mixture of the covariance matrices of the ICAR and independent processes, which is no longer a singular matrix for λ in [0,1[. Moreover, this distribution solves also the heteroscedasticity problems shown by the PCAR distribution when reproducing independent patterns.

Leroux et al.'s distribution, as described in Ugarte et al. (2014), can be implemented in `INLA` by making use of the `generic1` latent model, in a similar manner to the HCAR distribution above. For implementing the Leroux et al.

distribution, we should change the $\boldsymbol{C}$ matrix used for the HCAR distribution by the following

$$\boldsymbol{C} = \boldsymbol{I}_I - (\boldsymbol{D} - \boldsymbol{W}) = \begin{cases} -m_i + 1, & i = j \\ 1, & i \sim j \\ 0, & \text{otherwise} \end{cases}$$

The covariance matrix of the Leroux et al. proposal can be expressed as

$$\sigma^2((1 - \lambda)\boldsymbol{I}_I + \lambda(\boldsymbol{D} - \boldsymbol{W}))^{-1} = \sigma^2(\boldsymbol{I}_I - \lambda(\boldsymbol{I}_I - (\boldsymbol{D} - \boldsymbol{W})))^{-1} \quad (4.20)$$

which is equal to $\sigma^2(\boldsymbol{I}_I - \lambda\boldsymbol{C})^{-1}$ for the definition of $\boldsymbol{C}$ just proposed. This is the format of the covariance matrix required for the `generic1` latent model in INLA, therefore. Moreover, it can be shown (Ugarte et al., 2014) that the highest eigenvalue of $\boldsymbol{C}$, as it is defined just above, is equal to 1; therefore, the λ parameter of the Leroux et al. model coincides with the β parameter of the `generic1` latent model. Thus, we can resort to that latent model for fitting the LCAR distribution. Ugarte et al. (2014) suggest to put a `logitbeta` prior on logit(β), the parameter used by INLA to parameterize the `generic1` latent model. This is equivalent to putting a beta distribution on β, which seems a reasonable choice for this parameter varying in the [0,1] interval. A uniform prior on β would be achieved by putting `param=c(1,1)` as hyperparameters of the `logitbeta` prior distribution, which seems also a sensible prior choice.

Note that all the CAR implementations available in INLA, and many more, can be also implemented in WinBUGS despite the fact that there is no prebuilt function programmed for them. This can be done by coding in WinBUGS the set of conditional distributions corresponding to each of the CAR distributions just introduced. For example, the LCAR distribution could be programmed in WinBUGS by coding all the conditional distributions in Expression (4.19) using a `for` loop as

```
for(i in 1:n){
  ler[i]~dnorm(mean.ler[i],prec.ler[i])
  prec.ler[i]<-(1-lambda+lambda*num[i])/(sd.ler*sd.ler)
  mean.ler[i]<-sum(ler.adj[(index[i]+1):index[i+1]])*
               lambda/(1-lambda+lambda*num[i])
}
for(j in 1:n.adj)){
  ler.adj[i]<-ler[adj[i]]
}
```

where `ler` would be the LCAR vector of random effects, `lambda` the parameter controlling the spatial dependence, `ler.adj` is the value of `ler` for each adjacent neighbour to each spatial unit and `index` is a vector delimiting the neighbours of each spatial unit. Specifically, `index` should have length $I + 1$ and their elements would be equal to $(0, m_1, m_1 + m_2, ...)$ for m_i being the number of neighbours of unit i. The vector `index` can be easily computed in R by doing `c(0,cumsum(num))`, where `num` is a vector with the number of neighbours of each spatial, typically calculated by means of the `nb2WB` function.

4.3.2 Spatial hierarchical models

Section 4.2 showed random effects to be a powerful tool for modeling the spatial variation of risks in small areas. Random effects shrink risk estimates towards their overall mean, avoiding the overfitting of the fixed effects saturated model that yielded the SMRs as (usually naive) risk estimates. We also saw that models based in bases of functions show a convenient performance because they could profit from local features affecting several neighbouring sites. Thus, merging the information of nearby units, which would provide regional risk estimates in random effects models, seems a promising modification of this kind of models. The CAR distributions introduced above are clear candidates for performing this task.

The non-spatial lognormal random effects model in Section 4.2 assumed, given μ and σ^2, the log-risks to be distributed as $N(\mu, \sigma^2)$ independent variables. A straightforward way for including spatial dependence on this model would be to assume the log-risks to follow a proper CAR distribution. In this case the log-risks would follow a multivariate Normal distribution with a spatially structured covariance matrix, instead of considering them to be independent Normal variables. The stochastic variable ρ of the proper CAR distribution would be in charge of putting more or less dependence into the model as a function of the amount of dependence shown by the data. Inference on ρ would be performed into the model and this would determine the degree of smoothness of the fitted spatial pattern. This slight modification of the independent random effects proposal is enough to incorporate dependence in $sSMR$s, while also illustrating the modularity of hierarchical models. It is enough to change the 'piece' of the model (recall the Lego analogy in Chapter 2) which assumed independence between risks, by a new 'piece' assuming the data to be spatially dependent, in order to fix that inappropriate feature of the lognormal model.

We could also resort to the ICAR distribution for inducing spatial dependence. This could solve some of the already mentioned problems associated with the proper CAR (PCAR) distribution. However, the ICAR distribution has also its particular problems. We pointed out that the spatial pattern defined by the ICAR distribution is not able to adapt itself to the amount of spatial dependence shown by the data. Thus, the ICAR distribution would not be able to reproduce, for example, independence between sites in case that the observed values showed that particular behaviour (Leroux et al., 1999; Lee, 2011). Consequently, the ICAR distribution is rarely used alone for smoothing risks. On the contrary, it usually complements the independent Normal random effects introduced in the previous section, usually referred to as the heterogeneous term. That is, the log-risks, when modeled with an ICAR distribution are usually defined as

$$\log(\theta_i) = \mu + \psi_i + \varphi_i$$
$$\psi_i \sim N(0, \sigma_\psi^2)$$
$$\varphi \sim ICAR(\sigma_\varphi^2)$$
$$\dots$$

This proposal, assuming the log-risks as the sum of ICAR and independent Gaussian random effects, was originally proposed by Besag et al. (1991) and, since then, has been the most popular modeling choice for smoothing risks when dealing with small areas. Several works in the literature refer to this proposal as the *BYM* (*Besag, York and Mollié*) model; we will also henceforth use this acronym. The BYM model is nowadays an indubitable benchmark in the disease mapping literature, being the basis of lots of proposals that extend this kind of studies to more complex settings (spatio-temporal, multivariate, etc.).

Note that in the formulation above of the BYM model, we have a third term used to model the log-risks, the intercept. The sum-to-zero constraint(s) imposed on the ICAR distribution makes it necessary to include this term into the model to account for the constrained dimension(s) that cannot be fitted by the ICAR term (Besag and Kooperberg, 1995). Moreover, the mean of the heterogeneous term is set to 0; therefore, a specific term is needed to model the mean of the log-relative risks which cannot be modeled by any of the two random effects in this model. The intercept μ will typically be modeled as a fixed effect with a vague prior distribution such as an improper uniform or a vague Normal distribution of large variance.

The BYM proposal models the log-risks as the sum of two random effects of different covariance matrices. These matrices depend, and hence the covariance structure of the log-risks, on two parameters: σ_ψ^2 and σ_φ^2. Thus, in case that the data were mostly independent, the corresponding random effects term would take higher variance. Therefore, this term would explain a high proportion of the whole variance in the data and the covariance matrix of the log-risks would mostly resemble a diagonal covariance matrix corresponding to an independent process. On the contrary, if the data showed substantial spatial dependence, the ICAR random effect would take higher variance so that most of the variance in the model would be fitted by the spatially structured term. Therefore, under the BYM proposal, the final fit consists of a tradeoff between these two random effects, which is achieved by means of the balance of their variances. These variances are in charge of giving higher or lower weight to the random effects in the model as if they were the weights in a mixture model mixing these two random effects.

The epidemiological justification for including two random effects in the BYM model would be the following. Risk factors modifying the mortality of a site can be of two different kinds. On one hand, risk factors can have an effect on a large area including several neighbouring sites. Risk factors as dietary habits, lifestyles, weather, etc. would be expected to vary with a geographically smooth pattern, so causes of mortality depending on them should show similar performances on nearby sites. Therefore, the ICAR distribution would be suitable for modeling these kinds of risks. On the other hand, risk factors may instead have a local scope affecting just a single site. The effect of mobile phone antennas or parks, for example, is expected to be very local and, in the case of dealing with not too small sites (in a geographical sense) such as counties, they should not have an effect beyond the geographical unit that contains them. The modeling of these effects would be more suitable by means of heterogeneous random effects. This effect makes it possible for nearby sites to take very different risks if it was necessary; otherwise, the ICAR random effect would smooth out the corresponding geographical jump giving similar risk estimates to all the units in that area.

The implementation of the BYM model in `WinBUGS` does not require any particular comment. We will just have to code in this software the inclusion of both heterogeneous and spatial random effects for modeling the log-risks. Regarding `INLA`, it allows us to implement the BYM model by putting a single `f()` term into the corresponding formula. In order to do it, we should include into the formula a term of the kind `f(...,model="bym")`. In the case that the region of study was composed of n geographical units, the `bym` option of `INLA` fits $2n$ random effects. The first n of these are the sum of the spatial and heterogeneous random effects for each geographical unit, while the last n contain just the fit of the spatial random effects. The benefit of using the `bym` option instead of putting separate `besag` and `iid` random effects into the model is that the first turns back the marginal distribution of the sum of both effects in the model, which may be of more interest than the separate marginal distributions of both effects. `INLA` assumes by default a $Gamma(1, 5e - 4)$ prior distribution on the precisions of both random effects involved in the `bym` model. In order to change this prior distribution in both parameters of the BYM model, we would have to modify the `hyper` argument of the corresponding call to the `f(...,model="bym")` function with the argument `hyper=list(prec.spatial=list(prior=<whatever>)`, `prec.unstruct=list(prior=<whatever>))`. We will typically put a uniform prior distribution on the positive real line for the standard deviations of both random effects by setting `sdunif` for both `prior` arguments in the previous expression.

Example 4.5

We follow with the analysis of the municipal oral cancer mortality data set in the Valencian Region. We assess now if modeling the log-risks with the spatially correlated random effects just introduced produces any improvement in the *sSMR*s. We have implemented two models: first, we have modeled the log-risks by means of a proper CAR distribution, and second, we have modeled them by means of the BYM proposal. The BUGS syntax implementing the proper CAR model proceeds as follows

```
model{
 for(i in 1:n){
  O[i]~dpois(lambda[i])
  log(lambda[i])<-log(E[i])+log.theta[i]
  log.theta[i]<-sp[i]
  sSMR[i]<-100*exp(log.theta[i])
  P.sSMR[i]<-step(sSMR[i]-100)
 }


 #The proper CAR "piece"
 sp[1:n]~car.proper(mu.sp[], C[], adj[], num[], M[], tau, rho)
 for(i in 1:n){mu.sp[i]<-mu}


 #Prior distributions
 rho~dunif(rho.low,rho.up)
 rho.low<-min.bound(C[], adj[], num[], M[])
 rho.up<-max.bound(C[], adj[], num[], M[])
 tau<-pow(sd.sp,-2)
 sd.sp~dunif(0,10)
 mu~dflat()
}
```

We have used adjacency as a criterion for defining the spatial structure in the `car.proper` distribution in the model above. The posterior distribution of the parameters defining the geographical pattern just fitted can be summarized as follows

	mean	sd	2.5%	25%	50%	75%	97.5%	Rhat	n.eff
mu	-0.1	0.1	-0.3	-0.2	-0.1	-0.1	0.1	1	1000
sd.sp	0.5	0.1	0.4	0.4	0.5	0.5	0.6	1	1000
rho	1.0	0.0	0.9	1.0	1.0	1.0	1.0	1	1000
...									

We have run the model for 3 chains with 150,000 iterations per chain, whose first 20,000 iterations have been discarded as burn-in. Such a long number of iterations were required to achieve convergence; however, we will see at the next example several tricks to solve this issue. The model was fitted by calling WinBUGS from R with the pbugs function. The R-hat and n.eff statistics for mu, sd.sp and rho and the rest of the variables in the model are, respectively, below 1.1 and above 100 which suggests a correct convergence of the model.

The intercept mu takes values slightly lower than 0. This was stated in Example 4.4 as a common fact in Poisson-based disease mapping models. Note that μ could be included also in the linear term as a separate intercept centring, additionally, sp in 0. Both models would yield identical *sSMR*s. Regarding rho and sd.sp, the parameters ruling the variance structure of the random effects, we find that the random effects have a substantial contribution to the fit. The standard deviation of the random effect has a 95% credible interval of [0.4,0.6], well above 0, which points out the necessity of the random effects in order to introduce spatial variability into the model. Moreover, the parameter controlling the correlation structure of the random effects, rho, has its posterior mean and most of its posterior mass close to 1. Since the car.proper distribution has been used for implementing a PCAR distribution, rho.up will be equal to 1. Therefore, rho takes values as high as possible, suggesting a geographical pattern of considerable spatial dependence. When introducing the PCAR distribution, we pointed out that it needed very high values of the correlation parameter to reproduce spatial patterns of substantial dependence. The model seems to capture a strong spatial pattern in the data and, therefore, rho takes very high values in order to be able to reproduce a pattern of that kind.

As a second spatial alternative proposal, the BYM model could also be implemented by substituting the PCAR term in the model above by the sum of ICAR and independent random effects. This could be done by reproducing the following WinBUGS code

```
model{
 for(i in 1:n){
  O[i]~dpois(lambda[i])
  log(lambda[i])<-log(E[i])+log.theta[i]
  log.theta[i]<-mu+sp[i]+het[i]
  het[i]~dnorm(0,tau.het)
  sSMR[i]<-100*exp(log.theta[i])
  P.sSMR[i]<-step(sSMR[i]-100)
 }

 #The intrinsic CAR "piece"
 sp[1:n]~car.normal(adj[], weights[], num[], tau.sp)
 for(i in 1:nadj){weights[i]<-1}

 #Prior distributions
 tau.het<-pow(sd.het,-2)
 sd.het~dunif(0,10)
 tau.sp<-pow(sd.sp,-2)
 sd.sp~dunif(0,10)
 mu~dflat()
}
```

In this case, the posterior summaries of the main parameters in the model yield

```
        mean   sd 2.5%   25%  50%   75% 97.5% Rhat n.eff
mu      -0.2  0.0 -0.2 -0.2 -0.2 -0.1  -0.1    1  1000
sd.het  0.1  0.1  0.0  0.0  0.1  0.1   0.2    1   180
sd.sp   0.4  0.1  0.3  0.4  0.4  0.4   0.5    1   390
...
```

These two standard deviations are not directly comparable since that corresponding to the spatial term is a conditional standard deviation (the variability of each random effect given those in the surrounding units), whereas that of the heterogeneous term corresponds to a marginal standard deviation. Nevertheless, the heterogeneous term has a standard deviation with considerable mass, and mode (result not shown), close to 0 in contrast to the spatial term which has most of its mass well above this value. As a consequence, we expect the spatial term to have a higher contribution to the geographical pattern fitted than the heterogeneous random effect.

Both models in this example show quite similar DIC statistics: 1786.5 for the BYM model vs. 1788.2 for the proper CAR model. This difference in the DICs is not conclusive at all, so none of these models can be claimed to have a better fit. Nevertheless, with regard to the models introduced in previous examples, differences in terms of DIC are however quite conclusive. The lognormal model showed a DIC of 1815.1, while the Gaussian basis model showed a DIC of 1790.4, 4 units above the DICs of the models in this example. The effective number of parameters of each of these models is also illustrative: 83.3 for BYM, 83.7 for the proper CAR based model, 88.1 for the lognormal model and 29.1 for the random effects Gaussian basis model. Thus, the random effects spatial models are less complex than their non-spatial alternative. The spatial term makes information to be shared among geographical units, which reduces the number of parameters needed to explain the spatial variability in mortality. Nevertheless, Gaussian basis models are much less complex than CAR-based models. Consequently, their fits are markedly different. Fit in terms of DIC is a balance between parsimony and flexibility, according to this criterion the CAR models achieve the best balance among those models considered up to now.

Figure 4.4 shows the geographical distribution of the $sSMR$s (left) and their probability of being higher than 100 (right). The $sSMR$s map shows a completely different pattern than that of the original SMRs (Figure 4.1), which hardly provided any information of interest. The BYM $sSMR$s map shows two regions at the south-eastern side of the map with higher risk than the rest of the Valencian Region. The higher $sSMR$ achieves a value of 170.2, that is, nearly a 70% risk excess in comparison to the risk of the whole Valencian Region, which corresponds to one of the municipalities placed at the most northern of these two regions. These high risk regions did not show up or, at least, they did not attract any particular attention among the amount of municipalities in the highest risk group in the original SMRs map. These two regions concentrate a high proportion of the risk excesses in the Valencian Region since, excluding them and a few more municipalities, the rest of the sites in the map show risk values below the Valencian Region as a whole.

Figure 4.4 (right) also shows the probability of risk excess for each municipality in the Valencian Region. According to this map, we have substantial evidence of risk excess in some of the municipalities belonging to the two south-eastern 'clusters' mentioned above. Moreover, we find some evidence of risk excess

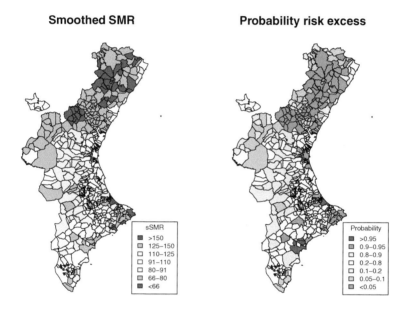

Figure 4.4
Left: *sSMR*s posterior means for the municipalities in the Valencian Region
according to the BYM model. Right: Probability of risk excess ($sSMR_i > 100$)
for the municipalities in the Valencian Region according to the BYM model.

in Valencia, the city in the middle of the north-eastern gulf in the Valencian Region, and Alcoy, the city at the inner-south side of the Valencian Region. These two cities did not show particularly high $sSMR$s at the left-hand side plot of Figure 4.4, they just have $sSMR$s above 100 (slightly above in the case of Valencia). These $sSMR$s combined with the particularly high population of these two municipalities make them show moderate evidence of risk excess, although their $sSMR$s are not so high. That is, for the assessment of the evidence of risk excess for each spatial unit it does not only matter the value of the corresponding $sSMR$ estimate, but also the population of that unit.

Correlations between $sSMR$s posterior means corresponding to the lognormal (non-spatial) and the BYM models is 0.633 and that between the proper CAR and BYM model is 0.989. Therefore, introducing spatial dependence into the model substantially modifies the estimates of the risks. Neighbours' information changes risk estimates, making them more accurate since they are based on a much higher amount of information. On the contrary, the PCAR and BYM proposals yield quite similar estimates; in fact we do not plot the PCAR based estimates since they are quite similar to those shown in Figure 4.4. For this data set, the specific way of inducing spatial dependence does not have particular relevance, at least it is much less important than the fact of introducing it into the model. We will see in Chapter 6 some settings where this does not necessarily hold.

The $sSMR$s standard deviation ($sd(\overline{\boldsymbol{\theta}})$, where $\overline{\boldsymbol{\theta}}$ stands for the vector of posterior means of the $sSMR$s) for the lognormal model is 9.6, meanwhile it is 17.1 for the proper CAR and 18.5 for the BYM model. Thus these standard deviations are substantially higher for the spatial models. This lower variability in the lognormal model means more smoothing as compared to its spatial alternatives. According to DIC, that extra smoothing in the lognormal model can be considered as simply oversmoothing, since it does not yield any improvement on the final fit. Spatial models shrink risk estimates towards their local mean, which also show geographical variability, instead of shrinking them to a common mean for the whole region. This gives the spatial $sSMR$s an extra source of variability (the local variability), reducing the oversmoothing of the lognormal non-spatial model.

The BYM model shown in this example can also be implemented with INLA. The syntax used to do it with the safest INLA computing options would be the following

```
> form= O ~ f(id.node,model="bym",graph="/Data/VR.graph",
            hyper=list(prec.spatial=list(prior=sdunif),
            prec.unstruct=list(prior=sdunif))
> BYM.inla=inla(form,family="poisson",data=data,E=E,
            control.inla=list(strategy="laplace")))
```

Likewise, some proper models could also be fit with INLA. For example, the following formula would correspond to the fit of the INLA version of the PCAR distribution introduced above

```
> formProper= 0 ~ f(id.node,model="besagproper",
                    graph="/Data/VR.graph",
                    hyper=list(prec=list(prior=sdunif)))
```

or the following one would fit an HCAR distribution for smoothing the original *SMRs*

```
> formGeneric= 0 ~ f(id.node,model="generic1",
                     Cmatrix="Data/Cmat.inla",
                     hyper=list(prec=list(prior=sdunif)))
```

with an appropriate `Cmatrix` argument (see the annex online material). These formulas should be called from `inla` with the same syntax as that used for the BYM model, but obviously changing its formula argument by that corresponding to each one of these alternative models.

The output below shows the correlation of the estimated *sSMRs* (posterior means) for the different spatial models and implementations considered in this example.

	BYM.inla	PCAR.inla	HCAR.inla	BYM.WB	PCAR.WB
BYM.inla	1.0000	0.9881	0.8072	0.9995	0.9893
PCAR.inla	0.9881	1.0000	0.8516	0.9877	0.9993
HCAR.inla	0.8072	0.8516	1.0000	0.8077	0.8432
BYM.WB	0.9995	0.9877	0.8077	1.0000	0.9891
PCAR.WB	0.9893	0.9993	0.8432	0.9891	1.0000

As shown, correlations between *sSMRs* for the different spatial alternatives considered are in general rather high. It is very rewarding to check that the highest among these correlations is that corresponding to both implementations of the BYM model (`INLA` and `WinBUGS` implementations) since they too should report virtually the same *sSMRs*, leaving aside the numerical errors arising from the different implementations. As a consequence, those errors do not seem to be very high. All models and implementations yield correlations higher than 0.98, except for those corresponding to the *sSMRs* of the HCAR model. So, in general all these models, except those depending on the HCAR distribution, are flexible enough as to reproduce the same geographical pattern, despite their dependence structures being somewhat different. The posterior distribution of the β parameter in the HCAR distribution is 0.906. This points out a high spatial dependence for the *sSMRs*. Maybe this can explain the different results yielded by this model since its main feature was that it was able to define completely independent observations if required, but at the cost of putting the same conditional variance to all *sSMRs* regardless of its spatial dependence. In this case, with high spatial dependence, this makes a difference since it does not take into account that municipalities with more neighbours should have less variability as a consequence of the information gained from those neighbours.

Finally, the following output shows the standard deviation of the *sSMRs* for each one of the models run.

	BYM.inla	PCAR.inla	HCAR.inla	BYM.WB	PCAR.WB
sd	18.6	17.3	11.7	18.6	17.3

Once again, it is very rewarding to check the concordance between the results of the BYM model for both implementations. These standard deviations show also that the model performing a lower smoothing is BYM, followed by PCAR and finally by the HCAR model, which makes substantially more smoothing than the rest of the models, removing far more variability in the $sSMR$s than the rest of the alternatives. According to the worse fit of this model in terms of DIC, this lower variability would be producing a kind of oversmoothing on the $sSMR$s estimates.

Identifiability is an important issue in the BYM model. The log-risks in this model are defined as the sum of two random effects of different covariance structures. Whilst the data provide us information on the sum of these two terms, which is perfectly identifiable, data do not yield separate information on each of these two components, which have to be inferred from their own (noisy) risk estimates instead of from the data. This makes these two random effects weakly identifiable, and specific inference on each one of them is even discouraged (Eberly and Carlin, 2000). Some proposals have been done trying to fix this issue such as Leroux (2000) or MacNab (2011) that will be introduced in more detail in Chapter 6.

4.3.2.1   Prior choices in disease mapping models

Choosing prior distributions for the variables in a model is surely the most controversial and sensitive issue in Bayesian statistics in general. We are not going to get into deep theoretical discussions on the convenience of some specific prior distributions on the parameters of the models already introduced. Nevertheless, the importance and sensitivity of these priors is worth some consideration that we cannot circumvent in a book with so many Bayesian models.

Prior choices in the disease mapping literature have not focussed much attention from a theoretical point of view, although extensive sensitivity analyses have been carried out (see Natario and Knorr-Held (2003); Ferrándiz et al. (2003); Tzala and Best (2008); Lee (2011); MacNab (2011); Schrödle and Held (2011a); Botella-Rocamora et al. (2012); Ugarte et al. (2014), to cite just some). The common procedure in the disease mapping literature has been guided by tradition due to the lack of more sound theoretical arguments. Authors often choose prior distributions in their models according to the prior choices proposed by other colleagues in previous publications, with the hope that those choices should not be bad for the new model and with the endorsement that they have undergone scrutiny of supposedly expert referees. This is surely a convenient or justifiable procedure since when you lack other arguments, making something similar to what other colleagues have found reasonable is often a good idea. Moreover – being now a bit ironic – you could always blame other researchers in case your prior choices were shown to not be so good, which may be even more important in practical terms. Nevertheless, this procedure has two major flaws. First, the criteria of other authors or reviewers are not a guarantee of anything. This makes possible that a wrong proposal in the literature becomes, by contagion, a bad habit followed in lots of papers or, even worse, in an unfounded dogma for the prac- titioners of a research area. Second, prior choices that could be appropriate for some models are not necessarily good for similar models. So mimicking the procedures followed in similar situations may be a dangerous procedure, sometimes prone to making wrong prior choices. Regretfully, as long as no more theoretical research is developed on this issue, we are forced to rely on the common knowledge (or beliefs) of the people working, and using exten- sively the models in a research area. In this sense, and trying to be a bit more optimistic, we hope that the maturity of a research field will lead, or has led, to a solid common knowledge and the vast experience of their researchers will make them more unlikely to make big common mistakes.

We are going to focus on the prior choices of two specific parameters in disease mapping models. First, we will focus on the parameters modeling the fixed effects in the linear predictor of the models introduced above and afterwards we will focus on the prior distribution of the parameters controlling the variability of the random effects. Regarding the fixed effects, note first that up to now we have used a single parameter of this kind in the models already introduced, the intercept of the linear predictor (μ). Nevertheless, it is quite common to include additional fixed effects into disease mapping models putting, for example, a term of the form $\sum_{j=1}^{J} \beta_j x_j$ into the linear predictor, where $\{x_j : j = 1, ..., J\}$ are J covariates. We will talk much more in depth about this possibility in the following chapter.

Traditionally, fixed effects parameters in linear Normal models have been given improper uniform priors on the whole real line. Indeed, this prior can be shown to be the Jeffreys prior (a recognized and theoretically supported non-informative prior choice) for these parameters (Ibrahim and Laud, 1991). Moreover, this uniform prior on these parameters makes their posterior mode coincide with the frequentist Maximum Likelihood Estimate, which seems a convenient feature. These properties, jointly with the computational conve- nience of this choice, have made it to be nearly omnipresent in linear Normal models. An exception to the use of improper uniform priors for these parame- ters is the objective variable selection setting, where inference is also made on which of the considered covariates should be included into the linear Gaussian model. Improper or arbitrarily vague prior distributions are not admissible in this setting since they make Bayes factors, the model selection criterion usually applied in this area, to be also arbitrary. In this case alternative non-arbitrarily vague prior distributions are used for these variables. Typical choices in this setting (Zellner, 1986; Bayarri et al., 2012) are usually of the kind

$$\beta|\sigma \sim N_J(\mathbf{0}, \sigma^2(\mathbf{X}'\mathbf{X})^{-1}) \qquad (4.21)$$

where σ is an additional hyperparameter to be fitted within the model and $\mathbf{X}$ is the design matrix whose columns contain the covariates considered. The correlation structure of this prior distribution mimics that of β Maximum Likelihood Estimate arising so that the information within this non-vague prior distribution does not have a large impact on β's posterior distribution. Therefore, in Normal linear models, improper uniform and Normal prior distributions seem to be the single prior distributions with widespread acceptance and use in the literature.

Nevertheless, as disease mapping models have typically Poisson or binomial likelihood functions (and typically include some random effects), they are not traditional Normal linear models. Therefore, the optimal properties mentioned of the improper uniform prior on β do not necessarily hold for these models. Namely, Jeffreys priors for the fixed effects in generalized linear models have their own expressions, which are not in general improper uniform prior distributions (Ibrahim and Laud, 1991). Nevertheless, although objective prior distributions have been developed for generalized linear models, the improper uniform and vague Normal prior distributions are also omnipresent in the disease mapping literature, without a sound justification up to our knowledge beyond its appropriateness for the Normal case. In principle, the use of improper uniform priors for fixed effects in generalized linear models does not necessarily lead to proper posterior distributions (Ibrahim and Laud, 1991). Although some conditions have been set guaranteeing the propriety of posterior distributions (Sun et al., 1999, 2001). Nevertheless, the checking of posterior propriety in disease mapping models has generally focussed hardly any attention on applications.

In practical terms, and we will do this for the rest of this book, we will use improper uniform distributions for fixed effects, in accordance to the rest of the disease mapping literature. Although we do not have a sound reason for this choice, beyond the statistical tradition in the disease mapping literature, we do not have a better sensible option in practical terms. We prefer to use improper uniform instead of vague Normal prior distributions for β in our models since the first is a vaguer limit case of the second, so in this sense it would be a preferable choice. Moreover, although Normal vague prior distributions could avoid posterior impropriety problems, they could be just masking those problems. In that case, posterior inferences would be very sensitive to the (arbitrary) vagueness of the Normal prior distributions (Berger, 2006). So, in general, we prefer to use improper uniform priors for β since they can make us aware of posterior impropriety problems by means of the strange behaviours that the Markov chains could show. In that case, extreme care and attention should be put on specifying alternative prior distributions for those potentially dangerous parameters or on the proposal of alternative models fixing the problems found.

However, we find Normal prior distributions adequate in at least three settings in the disease mapping context. On one hand, if objective variable selection was to be made, arbitrarily vague or improper priors are not an option for $\boldsymbol{\beta}$, as previously mentioned. In that case, Equation (4.21) should be adapted in order to apply it to generalized linear models. For a Poisson regression model with an intercept μ and expected deaths $\boldsymbol{e}$, the adaptation of Equation (4.21) would yield the following expression (Ibrahim and Laud, 1991; Martinez-Beneito et al., 2011)

$$\boldsymbol{\beta} \sim N_J(\mathbf{0}, (\boldsymbol{X}' diag(\boldsymbol{e} \exp(\mu)) \boldsymbol{X})^{-1}) \tag{4.22}$$

So this expression could be used as a non-arbitrarily vague alternative to the previous prior distributions. The dependence structure of this prior distribution once again reproduces the dependence of the variables in the model, which makes both $\boldsymbol{\beta}$'s prior distribution and the corresponding covariates to be in agreement.

Second, in the case of having a large number of covariates (let's say hundreds), we would want to shrink $\boldsymbol{\beta}$'s estimates towards 0 in order to control the effect of covariates without a real association with the outcome. In that case, ridge regression or lasso (O'Hara and Sillanpää, 2009; Kyung et al., 2010) could be used to get that shrinkage. Ridge regression could be carried out by defining $\boldsymbol{\beta}$ as a vector of Normal random effects

$$\beta_j \sim N(0, \sigma^2), \ j = 1, ..., J$$

for an unknown σ, which will be estimated within the model. On the other hand, Bayesian lasso could be carried out by simply defining $\boldsymbol{\beta}$ as a vector of Laplace (or double exponential) random effects

$$\beta_j \sim Laplace(0, \sigma^2), \ j = 1, ..., J.$$

Recall that the Laplace distribution was introduced in Section 4.3 as a robust alternative to the Normal distribution. This distribution (which is referred to in `WinBUGS` as the `ddexp` distribution) has a sharper peak around its mean than the Normal distribution. This will make several of the components of $\boldsymbol{\beta}$ to be shrunk towards 0 and just a few of their components to take values substantially different to 0.

Finally, a third setting where Normal prior distributions could be advisable is when the available covariates are highly dependent. The reasons for using a Normal prior in this case are computational (`WinBUGS` specific to be more precise) instead of theoretical. In this case, dependence between covariates could make the univariate Gibbs sampling steps in the MCMC to be highly dependent, which could make the chains to converge very slowly. Putting a multivariate Normal prior distribution on $\boldsymbol{\beta}$, instead of independent univariate distributions, would allow the elements of that vector to be updated in a joint multivariate step of the Gibbs sampling algorithm. Moreover, this multivariate step would take into account the covariance of the variables which will yield an improved updating algorithm with substantial benefits in terms of convergence. Thus, in this case, setting this prior distribution for β in a `WinBUGS` model

```
beta[1:J]~dmnorm(zeros[],prec.beta[,])
for(j in 1:J){
  zeros[j]<-0
  for(i in 1:I){
    prec.beta[i,j]<-0.0001*equals(i,j)
  }
}
```

instead of

```
for(j in 1:J){
  beta[j]~dnorm(0,0.0001)
}
```

or

```
for(j in 1:J){
  beta[j]~dflat()
}
```

although mathematically equivalent for the univariate Normal priors, can make a huge difference in terms of convergence of the MCMC.

The variability parameters of random effects are the second kind of variables that will typically have to be assigned prior distributions in disease mapping models. Prior distributions can be assigned on either the precision, variance or standard deviation of the random effects since this automatically entails an associated prior distribution on the rest of parameters. Setting prior distributions on these parameters is a sensitive issue in Bayesian mixed effects models and much attention should be put on this task, surely more attention than previously paid in the literature. For example, Berger (1985) shows that the reference prior (an objective prior optimal in many senses) for the standard deviation of a Normal likelihood is an improper prior proportional to σ^{-1}. Nevertheless, this same prior on the standard deviation of a vector of Normal random effects (also in a Normal model) would yield an improper posterior distribution. This is just an example, without exiting of Normal models, of the sensitivity of models to the priors of variability parameters in Normal distributions, which invites us to take extreme care when selecting them.

In the case of disease mapping models with Poisson or binomial likelihoods, there is not a consensus at all on the selection of prior distributions for these random effects parameters. Prior choices in this case depend on 'personal preferences', which vary mainly for different authors and the year of publication of the corresponding work. One of the most common prior choices for these parameters is setting a gamma prior distribution on the precision parameter of random effects. Historically, this prior distribution was the most common choice for the first Bayesian disease mapping models. The reason for this is that the gamma prior is the conjugate distribution for the precision of Normal random effects and this made computations much easier for the first MCMC algorithms, or even before the proposal of MCMC. Nowadays, with the maturity of MCMC and other Bayesian inference tools, conjugacy is an almost irrelevant property in practical terms, but the common use of these prior distributions has been kept alive in the literature. Indeed, even nowadays setting gamma distributions on precision parameters is possibly the most common choice in Bayesian disease mapping models, even the default choice in INLA.

For the BYM model, a common vague gamma prior distribution is set usually for the precisions of both random effects. Nevertheless, some works use different parameters for those gamma distributions according to different criteria. Thus, Best et al. (1999) adduce convergence criteria for putting a gamma prior of lower variability to the spatial precision parameter than for the heterogeneous precision. On the other hand, Bernardinelli et al. (1995a) propose the use of informative gamma priors for those precisions. For example, if only a heterogeneous random effect of variance σ_h^2 was included into the model they would expect that

$$\log(z_{SMR,.95}) - \log(z_{SMR,.05}) = 2 \cdot 1.64\sigma_h$$

where $z_{SMR,\alpha}$ stands for the α-th percentile of the set of raw SMRs and 1.64 is the 95th percentile of a standard Normal distribution. This assumes that 90% of the raw log-SMRs should fall within the interval $[-1.64\sigma_h, 1.64\sigma_h]$, which corresponds to a 90% central interval of a $N(0, \sigma_h^2)$ distribution. Similar arguments could be followed for the ICAR distribution although, in that case, σ_s^2 does not stand for the marginal variance of the random effect but for the conditional variance of that distribution (Bernardinelli et al., 1995a; Wakefield, 2007; Lee and Durban, 2009; MacNab, 2011). Bernardinelli et al. determine that the relationship between the marginal variance of the ICAR distribution $\tilde{\sigma}_s^2$ and the conditional variance is $\tilde{\sigma}_s^2 \approx 0.7\sigma_s^2$ in their particular case study on an irregular lattice division of Sardinia. Thus, the former relationship for the spatial term would be

$$\log(z_{SMR,.95}) - \log(z_{SMR,.05}) = 2 \cdot 1.64\tilde{\sigma}_s = 2 \cdot 1.64 \cdot 0.7\sigma_s.$$

Note that the 0.7 term in this last expression is specific of the Sardinian lattice and should be recalculated for other different lattices (Schrödle and Held, 2011a). For the BYM model, containing both heterogeneous and spatial terms, the former two relationships would yield

$$\log(z_{SMR,.95}) - \log(z_{SMR,.05}) = 2 \cdot 1.64 \cdot \sqrt{\sigma_h^2 + 0.49\sigma_s^2}.$$

Bernardinelli et al. propose to choose gamma prior distributions for the heterogeneous and spatial terms so that the former equation is mostly preserved. According to the conclusions of that paper, when this is done, the posterior results are hardly sensitive to changes in the priors preserving that equation.

Given the different nature of the standard deviations in a BYM model (marginal for σ_h and conditional for σ_s), putting them in the same prior distribution with common parameters, could give the corresponding random effects, a priori, very different weights. As a consequence, the prior marginal variances of these two random effects could be very different, which does not seem to be a sensible assumption. In this sense, some authors (see for example Mollié (1996), Ferrándiz et al. (2003) or Section 6.4.3.2 of Banerjee et al. (2014)) advise to choose gamma prior distributions for the precisions of these two random effects so that their marginal variabilities are equal. That is, they advise to set gamma prior distributions which make σ_h and $\tilde{\sigma}_s$ share similar distributions. In this manner, they implicitly assume the same prior contribution (in terms of the marginal prior variability) of the two random effects in the BYM model. In other context, the use of Penalized complexity priors for spatial models, Riebler et al. (2016) propose to rescale the weights matrix $\boldsymbol{W}^* = w^* \cdot \boldsymbol{W}$ of the ICAR distribution so that the overall marginal variability in that distribution is comparable to that of the heterogeneous term. The rescaling of the weights matrix makes the precision parameter of the ICAR random effect to be interpretable also in marginal terms. As a consequence, a similar prior gamma distribution could be put on the precision parameters of the heterogeneous and spatial random effects. Anyway, as mentioned, once that rescaling is made, Penalized complexity priors are set on the hyperparameters in the model instead of putting gamma prior distributions on the precisions. Interestingly, `INLA` has a function implemented `inla.scale.model` that could be used in general, not just for Penalized complexity priors, for making the marginal scales of the heterogeneous and spatial terms in BYM models comparable.

Despite the efforts for balancing the prior distribution for both precision parameters in BYM models, the use of common independent vague gamma priors for both parameters has been the most frequent choice in the literature. The most typical prior distribution for the precision parameters in BYM models has been a $Gamma(\epsilon, \epsilon)$ distribution, with ϵ taking a low value. These prior distributions assume a prior mean of 1 for the corresponding precisions and a large variance equal to ϵ^{-1}. That large variance should allow in principle those precisions to take any reasonable value. Nevertheless, a brief look at the literature shows how the election of the ϵ parameter in the works published is basically arbitrary. We can find papers assuming ϵ equal to 1 (Lawson and Clark, 2002), 0.01 (Reich et al., 2006, 2007), 0.001 (Marí-Dell'Olmo et al., 2014; Assunção et al., 2001) or 0.0001 (Assunçao, 2003; MacNab, 2014; MacNab and Gustafson, 2007), for example. The main purpose for all of these choices is the same, trying to set non-informative prior distributions, although this is done with lower or higher prior variance. The specific value of ϵ chosen for the previous prior would be expected to have a negligible role.

Surprisingly, putting prior distributions with a large variance on precisions of random effects could be less innocuous than it seems at a first glance. Hence, that procedure entails weird assumptions in the model in terms of the corresponding standard deviations (Lambert et al., 2005). Thus, assuming a $Gamma(\epsilon, \epsilon)$ prior on a precision means putting most of the mass of the standard deviation on very large values of this parameter. For example, for $\epsilon = 0.001$ the corresponding standard deviation has its 1st percentile at 6.4 and accumulates most of its mass at disproportionately large values of this parameter (Kelsall and Wakefield, 1999). You can easily check this fact, and related similar facts of other gamma distributions on precisions, by generating large samples $\{x_1, x_2, ...\}$ of those gamma distributions and transforming them as $\{x_1^{-1/2}, x_2^{-1/2}, ...\}$. The summaries of this transformed sample will approximate the main statistics of the prior distribution of the corresponding standard deviation. Thus, you can easily check that the prior distribution of the standard deviation of the random effects will be even more awkward for lower values of ϵ. As a consequence these priors will always tend to induce spatial and heterogeneous variability into the BYM model, regardless of whether they are really present in the data, or not. For fixing this performance, Kelsall and Wakefield (1999) propose the use of a Gamma(0.5, 0.005) prior distribution for precisions. This choice yields a prior distribution on the standard deviation with median 0.047 and 2.5th and 97.5th percentiles equal to 0.014 and 1.024, respectively, which seem like much more reasonable values. This prior choice has been also very popular in the literature (see, for example, Wakefield and Morris (2002); Wakefield (2003); Haining et al. (2010); Nathoo and Ghosh (2013); and Neyens et al. (2017)). Moreover, similar related priors for precisions have also been proposed in the literature with substantial popularity such as the $Gamma(1, 0.0005)$ (Natario and Knorr-Held, 2003; Gschlößl and Czado, 2008; Blangiardo et al., 2013), which is the default prior for precisions in INLA; the $Gamma(1, 0.01)$ prior (Rue et al., 2009; Schrödle et al., 2011; Ugarte et al., 2014; Gerber and Furrer, 2015). All these prior proposals would share the same philosophy as the $Gamma(0.5, 0.0005)$ prior of Kelsall and Wakefield (1999). In summary, this arbitrariness in this key aspect of Bayesian hierarchical models does not seem to be good news for a supposed well-established research area and makes it advisable that more theoretical research be done in this respect.

A reassuring consequence of using vague proper prior distributions in general is that they lead to proper posterior distributions. Thus, the use of vague proper gamma prior distributions for precisions in disease mapping models has been supported by many authors according to the posterior propriety of the corresponding model (Maiti, 1998; Sun et al., 1999, 2001). Nevertheless, in our point of view, the use of these borderline proper gamma distributions is much more troublesome than acknowledged and they may just give a false and unfounded sense of safety which, at the end, is the cause for the posterior sensitivity evidenced by lots of authors (see Best et al. (1999) or MacNab et al. (2006) for a couple of examples). In the words of Berger (2006): 'when an improper prior produces an improper posterior, using a vague proper prior can only hide – not solve – the problem' or 'the common perception that using a vague proper prior is safer than using improper priors, or conveys some type of guarantee of good performance, is simply wrong'. Berger (2006) also adds that the 'use of vague proper priors will work well only when the vague proper prior is a good approximation to a good objective prior' and this is not the case of gamma prior distributions for precisions in disease mapping models. In this sense, Theorem 1 in Appendix 1 provides some theoretical explanation for this conclusion. Specifically, we show how a $Gamma(\alpha, 0)$ prior distribution for the precision of independent Normal random effects in a typical disease mapping model yields an improper posterior distribution for any $\alpha \geq 0$. Similarly, this could also be proved for more general (spatial) random effects, although that proof would be more elaborated. Therefore, all the gamma prior distributions for precisions in the previous paragraphs are proper approximations of an improper prior distribution which yields an improper posterior, the $Gamma(\alpha, 0)$. This flat prior leads to a misleading point so we should try to avoid that performance with proper priors that mimic this inadvisable improper prior.

In some sense, approaching an improper prior distribution leading to an improper posterior by an alternative vague prior distribution is like trying to approximate an improper integral, such as $\int_0^1 \sigma^{-1} d\sigma$ by $\int_\epsilon^1 \sigma^{-1} d\sigma$ for a small $\epsilon > 0$. Regardless of the value of ϵ, the value of the second integral will be always infinitely far from the first. Moreover, the value of that second integral will vary to a larger extent as ϵ gets closer to 0. Thus, the results derived will be more sensitive as we try to get closer to the value that we would like to approach. The problem of vague gamma distributions on precision parameters is that ϵ, the hyperparameter of the gamma distribution small values, is the only ones responsible for avoiding the posterior distribution to integrate infinitely. Getting closer or farther away from the improper posterior distribution corresponding to the $Gamma(\alpha, 0)$ prior, which will be always infinitely far, depends just on the arbitrary value chosen for ϵ. Therefore, the posterior distribution corresponding to a $Gamma(\alpha, \epsilon)$ prior will vary wildly as ϵ approaches 0. This will make the posterior distribution for those gamma priors necessarily very sensitive to the choice of ϵ (Gelman, 2005b). Thus, in that case we have guaranteed that the posterior distribution that we get will always depend on the arbitrary value chosen of ϵ Kelsall and Wakefield (1999). Therefore, in this sense the posterior distribution obtained will be somewhat arbitrary. In our opinion, this reason would be enough for discarding the use of vague gamma prior distributions for precisions in disease mapping models.

Several alternatives have been proposed to the use of vague gamma priors on the precision of random effects. Spiegelhalter et al. (2004) or Lambert et al. (2005) show interesting disquisitions on the choice of prior distributions for these, or other related, parameters. One important issue for choosing an alternative prior distribution for the variability of random effects is that a uniform prior on the precision or variance or standard deviation does not entail a uniform prior distribution on the alternative parameterizations. Thus, what could seem as a non-informative flat distribution on one parameter would not be so flat on the grounds of the other transformations of the parameters. As a consequence, we should have a clear idea on what parameter, if there is one, we would want to be non-informative. In our opinion, assessing the effect of any prior distribution in terms of the standard deviation of the random effects is a good idea since that parameter is measured in the same scale as the data, in contrast to the variance and the precision. This makes us have some intuition on the assumptions, and the scale, underlying that probability distribution. For example, Spiegelhalter (2001); Gelman et al. (2003) and Lambert et al. (2005) propose uniform prior distributions on the positive real line, or a related subset, for the variance of random effects. As shown in Spiegelhalter et al. (2004) and Lambert et al. (2005), this prior distribution would be equivalent to the improper prior $P(\sigma) \propto \sigma$, which favours high standard deviations and therefore will make random effects tend to have a meaningful contribution regardless of whether they should do it, or not. Moreover, the prior density function at $\sigma = 0$ is 0, so in general this prior distribution will be prone to overfit the data (Simpson et al., 2017).

A popular group of prior distributions for the standard deviation of the random effects σ are the half-Normal or half-t distribution centered at zero (Thompson et al., 1997; Gelman, 2005b). That is, these prior distributions consider the right positive tail of those distributions as priors for σ. Those distributions have their mode at 0 so they are intended as parsimonious choices, favouring the random effects to be disregarded if they really had no an important contribution to the model. Although both half-Normal and half-t distributions achieve the former goal, the half-t distribution has a heavier tail, making it a more robust alternative to the half-Normal distribution. In fact, Gelman (2005b) advocates for a half-Cauchy distribution (i.e., a t distribution with 1 degree of freedom) according to its robustness. One issue for these prior distributions is the choice of a scale parameter for them. If the scale of the half-Normal or half-t was fixed to a large value, the decreasing right tail of the prior distribution, argued to be positive, would lose its effect, making that prior distribution mostly locally flat. Therefore, the scale of these prior distributions is usually fixed according, and in agreement, to the data. In this sense, these prior distributions are informative, although the choice of their scale is intended to be as uninformative as possible.

A second prior on σ which has become very popular is an improper uniform distribution on the positive real line ($U(0, \infty)$), or a uniform distribution between 0 and an upper limit A, intended to be non-informative. Setting a uniform prior distribution on a standard deviation – a scale parameter that we have intuition of – seems a much safer option than putting a degenerate gamma distribution on a precision, a parameter that we lack any intuition. The improper uniform distribution could be seen as a limit case of the half-Normal of half-t priors when their standard deviations tend to infinite, as these two distributions become infinitely flat as that standard deviation increases. Thus, in this sense, they are related prior choices. One advantage of the uniform prior distribution is that it does not depend on any parameter that we should choose, possibly in agreement to the data, as for the half-Normal or half-t distributions. The parameter A, instead of fixed, should be simply high relative to the scale of the data. Gelman (2005b) reports a small overestimation in the distribution of σ when a uniform prior is used, that is why he supports the half-Cauchy prior. Nevertheless, he reports that overestimation for the case of having a very low number of levels for the random effects, less than 10 levels, which is never the case in disease mapping models. In our experience, the posterior distributions in disease mapping studies when half-Normal, half-t or uniform distributions are used are hardly sensitive to which of these prior distributions is used. For lattices having, let's say, more than 100 spatial units we have not found sensitivity to the prior distribution chosen among these three options.

Proper versions of the uniform improper prior distribution, $U(0, A)$, with A being 'high', are often used because WinBUGS does not admit an improper uniform distribution on the positive real line. Thus the $U(0, A)$ prior is just a proper approximation to that distribution, just for practical purposes. Regarding the choice of A, any high enough value would be good. Note that if $\sigma \sim U(0, A)$, then the posterior distribution would be proportional to $f(\boldsymbol{\omega}; \boldsymbol{o}, \boldsymbol{e}) 1_{[0,A]}(\sigma)$, where $\boldsymbol{o}$ and $\boldsymbol{e}$ are the vectors of observed and expected cases, respectively, $f()$ the likelihood function, $\boldsymbol{\omega}$ is the set of parameters in the model and $1_{[0,A]}(\sigma)$ is equal to 1 if $\sigma \in [0, A]$ and 0 otherwise. In case of assuming a $U(0, A')$ prior distribution, with $A' > A$, the posterior distribution would change accordingly by substituting $1_{[0,A]}(\sigma)$ by $1_{[0,A']}(\sigma)$. If, for the first case, the marginal posterior distribution of σ had most of its mass below A, the posterior distribution under the second choice would be completely equivalent in practical terms. Thus, the choice of the upper limit of the uniform prior for σ becomes irrelevant for high enough values of that parameter (Lee, 2011). The limit where that value becomes irrelevant is given by any value for which most of the mass of the posterior distribution of σ keeps to its left. Although it would be tempting to set A to a very high value, such as 1,000 or even higher, this is a dangerous procedure as for disease mapping models random effects are modeling the risks but in a logarithmic scale. If a logarithm takes values around the thousands, we could be at a serious risk of a numeric overflow if that value is later exponentiated, so it is safer in practical terms to fix A to a more moderate value. Bearing this in mind it would be safer to fix A to 5, 10 or a quantity of this order, which will be for sure wide enough for modeling risks in a logarithmic scale. Anyway, it will be convenient to check always that the upper percentiles of the posterior distribution of σ are far below from the value set for A, otherwise that value should be increased as it could be influential. In some sense, this is another good property of the uniform prior distribution on σ, we can check if the values of its hyperparameter are influencing the posterior distribution as compared to other alternative choices of A. This is not a very straightforward task for the vague gamma prior distributions on precisions.

In general, for the rest of the book, we will use the uniform prior distribution on the positive real line as prior distribution for σ as default choice for the variability of random effects. This choice is also becoming very popular in the literature (see Lee (2011); Song et al. (2011); Marí-Dell'Olmo and Martínez-Beneito (2015); MacNab (2016a), for just a few examples). According to the previous comments, we will use a uniform proper distribution $U(0, A)$, with A having a moderate value (let's say 5 or 10) when using WinBUGS for fitting our models. When using INLA, we will not have any practical limitation that forced us to use a proper prior so we will use the improper uniform distribution on the positive real line. The implementation of the improper uniform prior in the positive real line is described in Section 3.2 and has already been used in several examples of this book.

Finally, we find it also convenient to mention Penalized Complexity Priors (Simpson et al., 2017), a proposal for assigning priors in Bayesian hierarchical models, which is becoming very popular. Penalized Complexity Priors (PC priors) have been also used for proposing prior distributions in disease mapping models (Simpson et al., 2017). PC priors are defined as priors fulfilling a series of criteria which in principle should yield reasonable priors distributions. Anyway, these priors are subjective since they are defined as a function of the modeler's opinion on the admissible range of values of some of their parameters. The BYM model has to be previously reparameterized in order to derive sensible PC priors for its hyperparameters. Thus, the linear predictor in the reparameterized model becomes $\mu + \tau^{-1/2}(\sqrt{1 - \phi}\boldsymbol{\psi} + \sqrt{\phi}\boldsymbol{\varphi})$, where τ is the overall precision of the set of random effects and ϕ models the proportion of variance corresponding to either the spatial or the heterogeneous random effect. The PC prior for τ in this model is a type-2 Gumbel prior. The PC prior for ϕ, which depends on the specific lattice used for the analysis, does not belong to any known or popular family of distributions. In summary, the use of PC priors for the BYM model is far more complex than the use of uniform prior distributions on standard deviations, our default proposal, and the advantages of PC priors over the uniform priors in this context are still unclear. Therefore we maintain the uniform distribution on standard deviations as the default prior choice for the variability of random effects in disease mapping models for the rest of this book.

4.3.2.2   Some computational issues on the BYM model

As introduced in Chapter 2, MCMC inference should be iterated until convergence is achieved and sufficiently long chains, and of enough quality, are generated. This process may be time consuming, mainly for those proposals extending the BYM model to more complex settings, such as spatio-temporal or multivariate models. Therefore, computational tricks that could speed up the inference process in disease mapping problems could be very useful, mainly when this inference process has to be repeated for a series of diseases, such as when developing mortality atlases. This is the goal that we are now going to discuss.

The first tool to be used to speed the inference up for the BYM model is INLA. As mentioned in Chapter 3, INLA avoids MCMC for making inference in Bayesian hierarchical models, which can yield substantial savings in computing times for a large collection of models. INLA is particularly suited for fitting lots of disease mapping models; indeed it was originally devised as a tool for fitting Gaussian Markov random fields. As a consequence, the number of tools developed in the INLA package for spatial modeling is very high in comparison, for example, to the tools implemented for fitting temporal data. The previous examples have already illustrated the computational advantages of fitting models within this software as compared to MCMC-based tools such as WinBUGS.

The second tool suitable for speeding up the inference in spatial models is the **pbugs** function of the **pbugs** package of R. This package, already introduced in Chapter 3, parallelizes the MCMC inference in WinBUGS by using a different core of the available processor(s) for simulating each chain. WinBUGS, by default, computes all the MCMC chains with a single core and **pbugs** makes it possible to use the computing power of several cores instead of just one of them. Ideally, if J chains were run for making inference on a model, the **pbugs** function should reduce the computing time of the MCMC in a factor close to $1/J$ as compared to the corresponding call to **bugs**. Nevertheless, since some of the tasks performed by **pbugs** are not parallelized (preparing the data to be sent to WinBUGS, retrieving the results from WinBUGS, etc.) the time saved is generally higher than that factor. Luckily, the procedures of the MCMC that are parallelized are precisely those consuming more time in computational demanding problems. Therefore, the benefit achieved by parallelizing is higher (and so the computing time closer to the $1/J$ factor) precisely when it is really required.

As mentioned, the amount of time saved by the **pbugs** function is (ideally) inversely proportional to the number of chains simulated. Thus, further computing time may be saved with the **pbugs** function if the number of chains run is increased. For example, let us assume that we run 3 chains with a burn-in period of 1,000 iterations followed by 10,000 additional iterations per chain. Let us also assume that we used a thinning value of 1 out of 10 simulations per chain, yielding a sample size of 1,000 iterations saved per chain. In this case the **pbugs** function would reduce the computing time by about one third of the time spent by the **bugs** function of the R2WinBUGS package. Alternatively, if we run 6 chains instead of 3, we would run the same 1,000 iterations needed as burn-in period followed by 5,000 additional iterations per chain, with a thinning value of 10, in order to obtain comparable samples. In this case, we would obtain 6 random samples of size 500 and of similar autocorrelations than in the 3-chain simulation. The time spent by the 6-chain simulation with the **pbugs** function would be the time needed by one core to sample 6,000 simulations. On the contrary, the **bugs** function of the package R2WinBUGS would spend the time needed by the same core to sample 33,000 simulations. Therefore, the time needed by **pbugs** to run would be $6/33 \approx 19\%$ of the time spent by the corresponding call to `bugs` for simulating 3 chains. So, the more chains are sampled, the higher reduction of time will be achieved by `pbugs`.

Nevertheless, the time saved by `pbugs` will be limited by two factors. First, the number of cores available to perform computations. Obviously, drawing several chains may speed up the process, provided that each chain is simulated in a different core. If our machine had, let's say, 4 cores the benefit of the `pbugs` function will be limited to sampling, at most, 4 chains. If more chains were sampled, they should share the cores available and therefore no more benefit would be achieved by sampling more chains. Second, the time saved with `pbugs` is also constrained by the burn-in period. All chains have to simulate their own burn-in period, which cannot be reduced by simulating further chains. So, the burn-in period sets an additional lower limit for the amount of time that can be reduced by using `pbugs`.

DIC computation will also affect the computing time needed to make inference on the BYM model in `WinBUGS`. For some reason, the computation of this criterion for the BYM model, and in general for any model containing the ICAR distribution, slows down `WinBUGS` in an unjustifiable amount. We suspect that the coding of the calculation of DIC in `WinBUGS` is inefficient for models containing the ICAR distribution since we have not noticed such a delay when the simulated model does not contain this distribution. As an illustrative example, we simulated the BYM model for the municipal oral cancer data set for 3 chains and 1,000 iterations of burn-in followed by another 10,000 iterations. We used the `bugs` function of `R2WinBUGS` for this purpose. This took 238 seconds with the option `DIC=FALSE`, meanwhile it took 334 seconds when executed with the option `DIC=TRUE`. The complexity of the calculation of DIC does not justify this difference. Therefore, we advise in general to avoid the calculation of DIC in `WinBUGS` at least for the BYM model. If the $sSMR$s are saved, which will typically be done for any disease mapping study, it will be possible to calculate the DIC of the model afterwards in `R` in a much more efficient way. The annex online material for Example 4.5, between others, contains an `R` function for calculating the DIC for the BYM model, which is also valid for disease mapping models in general with Poisson data likelihoods. These functions will save you substantial computing time if, hereafter, you decide to avoid the calculation of DIC in `WinBUGS`.

The computation of DIC in `R` for `WinBUGS` models has also a second advantage. Thus, the DICs reported by `WinBUGS` and `INLA` are not directly comparable. That is, those DICs are comparable except for a constant that will depend on the data set at hand. Hence, if the DICs for two models run in `WinBUGS` differ in d units, that same difference will also be equal to d for the same models if they were run in `INLA`. Nevertheless, for each of these two models, the `WinBUGS` and `INLA` DICs would not be equal but they will differ, surprisingly, by an unknown quantity c. Thus, if one model was run in `WinBUGS` and a second model was run in `INLA`, the DICs reported by these tools would not be comparable. By calculating the DIC of `WinBUGS` models in

R, in exactly the same manner as `INLA`, we could solve the non-comparability of the DICs of these two tools. In this manner, we will be able to compare any two models regardless if they are run in either `WinBUGS` or `INLA`. The code used in Example 4.5 for computing the DIC implements the same DIC expression than that used by `INLA`, so by using that function you will make DICs comparable whether they are run in `INLA` or `WinBUGS`.

A second related issue to the DIC inefficiency just mentioned would be the following. `WinBUGS` models are frequently run with a thinning parameter of T, where $T > 1$. This makes only 1 out of every T iterations to be saved, and the rest of them to be discarded from the posterior sample. In the case of DIC, which is inefficiently programmed in `WinBUGS`, this means that the deviance (the statistic being the base of DIC) is calculated for every iteration of the MCMC, whether that iteration is saved or not. This makes the calculation of DIC in `WinBUGS` even more inefficient, whether the ICAR distribution is contained or not in the corresponding model. This issue is solved once again by calculating the DIC in R since it is calculated directly on the thinned sample instead of on every iteration of the MCMC, which is a much more efficient alternative. Bearing this in mind, we can make `WinBUGS` slightly more efficient by avoiding to calculate direct transformations of any other variable in the model that was intended to be returned as an outcome. This will allow us to calculate the corresponding transformation in R instead, but only for the thinned sample that will make the calculation of this variable more efficient. A clear example of this kind of variables is the probability of the $sSMRs$ to be above 100 (`P.sSMR` in the models in the examples above). This is just a deterministic transformation of the $sSMRs$ which can be perfectly calculated in R by means of the sentence

```
> apply(ResulBYM$sims.list$sSMR,2,function(x){mean(x>100)})
```

where `ResulBYM` is the R object containing the results of the corresponding BYM model. The calculation of these probabilities in R will not produce a substantial acceleration of `WinBUGS` since it corresponds to a quite simple transformation. Nevertheless, in other settings, such as the spatial prediction in Bayesian geostatistical models (which may be known to many of the readers of this book), its calculation on the thinned sample in R may produce substantial savings in the time spent by `WinBUGS`. In any case, the calculation of the above probabilities in R will avoid the corresponding **bugs** objects to be larger than really needed. This issue may be of considerable importance when the region of study is very large (thousands of units) or in spatio-temporal or multivariate models where several $sSMRs$ are saved for every site.

There is a final tool making it possible to speed the inference up of the BYM model in `WinBUGS`. This is the reparameterization of this model in an alternative way so that the resulting chains have better convergence properties. It is acknowledged that reparameterizing may substantially change the converged properties of a model (Gelfand et al., 1995a,b) so this is the goal that we pursue now. The reparameterization that we are going to propose is based on the following: For any random variable θ and any fixed scalar σ, the variance of $\sigma\theta$ satisfies $Var(\sigma\theta) = \sigma^2 Var(\theta)$. This result entails that, if $\boldsymbol{y}$ is a random I-vector with distribution $\boldsymbol{y} \sim N_I(\boldsymbol{0}, \sigma^2\boldsymbol{C})$, then $\boldsymbol{y}$ may be alternatively expressed as $\boldsymbol{y} = \sigma\boldsymbol{x}$ where $\boldsymbol{x} \sim N_I(\boldsymbol{0}, \boldsymbol{C})$. That is, a model containing $\boldsymbol{y}$ or an alternative model reparameterized in terms of $\sigma\boldsymbol{x}$ instead of $\boldsymbol{y}$ would yield equivalent fits, although the convergence of the corresponding MCMC algorithms may be very different. Namely, according to this new parameterization, the BYM model could be alternatively formulated as

$$o_i \sim Pois(e_i\theta_i)$$
$$\log(\theta_i) = \mu + \sigma_\varphi \cdot \varphi_i + \sigma_\psi \cdot \psi_i$$
$$\psi_i \sim N(0,1)$$
$$\varphi \sim ICAR(1)$$
$$\dots$$

In our experience, this reparameterization of the BYM model in `WinBUGS` may yield considerable benefits in terms of the convergence of σ_φ and σ_ψ, usually the variables with a more problematic convergence in the BYM model. As a consequence, the number of iterations needed to fulfill the convergence criteria of an MCMC simulation may be considerably reduced in case of using the reparameterized model just proposed instead of the original BYM model formulation.

Finally, to end with the computational considerations, we would like to point out that the considerations made in this section on speeding up the MCMC are cumulative. That is, we could call to `WinBUGS` by means of `pbugs` to simulate from the reparameterized BYM model, leaving the DIC calculation and the probability of risk excess for every unit for a posterior computation in `R`. This implementation of the BYM model would be much more efficient than other more conventional implementations of this model without the computational 'tricks' that we have just mentioned. For small data sets, the difference in computing times between both implementations can be insignificant; nevertheless for larger data sets, or for some extensions of the BYM model to more complex settings, this advice can really make a large difference so we advise you to bear it in mind.

Example 4.6

We are going to turn back to the analysis of the oral cancer data set. We have fitted now several different implementations of the BYM model in that data set in order to assess, in practical terms, the impact of the computational tricks introduced. Specifically, we have fitted those models in `WinBUGS` implementing different combinations of the computational tricks that we have just introduced. Thus, the model runs are:

- **BYM.naive:** A naive version of the BYM model has been run with the `bugs` function of the library `R2WinBUGS`. This naive version also calculates the DIC of the model within `WinBUGS` and puts the standard deviation of the random effects as a parameter of the corresponding distributions.

- **BYM.DIC:** This is a modified version of the BYM.naive implementation but without calculating DIC within `WinBUGS`. DIC can be later calculated in R with hardly any computational cost.

- **BYM.DIC.pbugs:** This is a modified version of the BYM.DIC implementation but run with the `pbugs` function of the library of that same name.

- **BYM.Reparam**: This is a modified version of the BYM.DIC.pbugs implementation. In this case, the standard deviations of the random effects are placed in the linear predictor multiplying the corresponding random effects, whose standard deviations are fixed to 1. This is supposed to improve the convergence summaries of the variables in the model.

We have run all 4 versions of the BYM model in `WinBUGS` 10 times for 5,000, 10,000 and 25,000 iterations for each of the 3 chains. The burn-in period for all these runs is set to a 10% of the number of iterations per chain. The mean computing times for all 4 versions and 3 different numbers of iterations are shown in Table 4.1. We can see how the differences in computing time for the different versions of the BYM model run are substantial. Thus, we see how the computing of the DIC within `WinBUGS` takes about 30 seconds on average, regardless of the number of iterations run. Thus, the DIC computation in `WinBUGS` for the BYM model is particularly expensive when a lower number of iterations are going to be run. Moreover, calling `WinBUGS` with `pbugs`, instead of calling it with `bugs`, speeds up the computation by factors between 2 and 3. These factors are closer to 2 when the number of iterations is lower, and closer to 3 when they are higher. However, in contrast to calculating the DIC in `WinBUGS`, the advantage of using `pbugs` is not constant for the different number of iterations. On the contrary the reduction of computing time for `pbugs` is mostly proportional to the time taken for the model without parallelization. Finally, the reparameterization proposed of the BYM model does not seem to bring any advantage in computing time, as compared to the BYM.DIC.pbugs version. In contrast, it takes about 20% more seconds to run than BYM.DIC.pbugs regardless of the number of iterations run.

Tables 4.2 and 4.3, respectively, show the median Brooks-Gelman-Rubin statistics (R-hat) and effective sample sizes (n.eff) for the standard deviations of the random effects for each setting run. We only explore the convergence for these two parameters since they are by far the most problematic variables for all the runs of the BYM model. For these two tables, we can see how the BYM.Reparam model has achieved convergence easily even for 5,000 iterations, i.e., the R-hat statistics are lower than 1.1 and n.effs are higher than 100 for both monitorized variables. On the contrary, the rest of the versions

Version	5,000 iterations	10,000 iterations	25,000 iterations
BYM.naive	92.0	147.7	318.7
BYM.DIC	59.6	118.7	289.3
BYM.DIC.pbugs	27.1	51.2	121.3
BYM.Reparam	32.1	61.4	149.6

Table 4.1
Mean computing time (in seconds) for all 10 runs, 4 implementations and 3 different numbers of iterations of the MCMC.

Iterations	σ_φ			σ_ψ		
	5,000	10,000	25,000	5,000	10,000	25,000
BYM.naive	1.17	1.17	1.15	1.04	1.02	1.00
BYM.DIC	1.15	1.32	1.17	1.05	1.03	1.01
BYM.DIC.pbugs	1.35	1.17	1.08	1.05	1.03	1.01
BYM.Reparam	1.01	1.00	1.00	1.00	1.00	1.00

Table 4.2
Median value of the Brooks-Gelman-Rubin statistic for all 10 runs and 3 different numbers of iterations of the MCMC.

of runs of the BYM model find serious problems to achieve convergence even for 25,000 iterations, mainly for the standard deviation of the heterogeneous term (σ_φ). Note that the convergence statistics for BYM.naive, BYM.DIC and BYM.DIC.pbugs should be equal except for Monte Carlo error, thus the convergence statistics for those three settings could be read jointly. Regarding the R-hat, we see that the spatial standard deviation does not show any problem in general; on the contrary the heterogeneous part shows problems (R-hat>1.1) even for the longest simulation. Moreover, strikingly, the improvement in the R-hat statistic for the non-reparameterized models when the number of simulations increases is quite low. This suggests that at least 100,000 simulations would be needed to achieve the convergence criteria that we have set for the non-reparameterized models.

Very similar conclusions, although more clear, could be drawn from Table 4.3. Interpreting this table, note that the maximum suitable value for n.eff would be 1,000 since that is the number of samples saved from the simulations. The reparameterized model achieves frequently n.effs of 1,000 for both variance parameters, mainly when the numbers of iterations are higher. In contrast, for the non-reparameterized model, the heterogeneous standard deviation never achieves (median) n.effs higher than 100 and the spatial component is in general higher than that value, although just slightly for 5,000 iterations. Moreover, once again, the improvement in the n.effs as a function of the number of simulations is very mild so, for the non-parameterized model, the number

	σ^2_φ			σ^2_ψ		
Iterations	5,000	10,000	25,000	5,000	10,000	25,000
BYM.naive	18.0	17.5	23.5	105	140	210
BYM.DIC	20.5	11.5	49.5	64	104	325
BYM.DIC.pbugs	10.0	22.5	48.5	54	105	315
BYM.Reparam	440.0	1000	1000	345	1000	1000

Table 4.3
Median effective sample size for all 10 runs and 3 different numbers of iterations of the MCMC.

of simulations required to achieve convergence should be much higher than 25,000.

Therefore, as a summary, for the reparameterized model we would achieve satisfactory convergence with just 5,000 iterations (or even surely less). That setting would take 32.1 seconds to be fitted if the DIC was later calculated in R and the **pbugs** function was used to run the model. In contrast, the naive version of the BYM model would take far more than 318.7 seconds to run with acceptable convergence statistics. Therefore, the difference between a naive or an 'advanced' version of the BYM model could be huge in practical terms. Thus, the amount of time needed for a naive implementation of the BYM is more than 10 times higher (easily 30 or 50 times higher according to our results) than an advanced implementation of the BYM model.

Additionally, we have run the BYM model with **INLA** also with different approximation strategies in order to compare the computational performance of this tool versus **WinBUGS**. The **int.strategy** for all these runs was fixed to **auto**, the default option of **INLA**. We have found that **INLA** takes 6.2 seconds to run with the Gaussian approximation, 6.7 seconds with the simplified Laplace approximation and 64.3 with the full Laplace approximation. We can see how the computing options in **INLA** may also increase computing times substantially, up to 9 times in multiplicative terms. Interestingly, the summaries for the precisions of the random effects for all these different runs in **INLA** coincided completely up to 6 decimal digits (those shown by **INLA**). So there is no apparent difference between the results of the most and least accurate options, in theory, for the oral cancer data set.

4.3.2.3   Some illustrative results on real data

We are going to conclude this chapter with some results of the BYM model on two real studies. First, we show some results corresponding to the *Mortality Atlas of the Valencian Region, 1991-2000* (Martínez-Beneito et al., 2005). That atlas studies the geographical distribution of 28 causes of mortality in

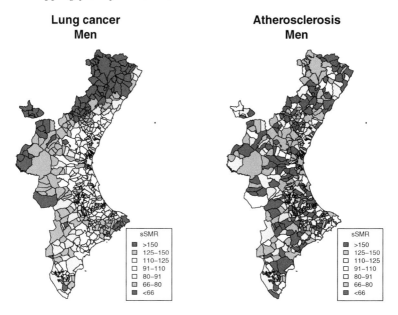

Figure 4.5
Spatial mortality patterns for lung cancer and atherosclerosis in men in the
Valencian Region for the period 1991-2000. Results from the *Mortality Atlas
of the Valencian Region.*

the Valencian Region, 23 of them for men and 24 for women. Among the causes
studied, it is possible to find very different geographical patterns. Below we
review some particularly interesting results published in the Valencian atlas.
Second, we will discuss the results of a specific mortality study carried out
at the Province of Castellón, the northern side of the Valencian Region. The
results of this study clearly illustrate the value of making a thorough statistical
analysis instead of just ending up with naive statistical estimators for the small
area context, like *SMR*s.

The Mortality Atlas of the Valencian Region, 1991-2000

Figure 4.5 shows the *sSMR*s for the BYM model for lung cancer and
atherosclerosis mortality in men. As can be seen, both patterns are completely
different. On one hand, lung cancer mortality shows a clear geographical pattern with a striking risk excess in the eastern gulf of the Valencian Region.
On the other hand, the inland side of the Valencian Region does not show
any risk excess but, on the contrary, it shows in general a protective effect for
this cause of mortality. But surely of more interest to the readers will be the
marked geographical pattern shown by this cause of mortality, the clearest

geographical pattern of all shown in the Valencian atlas. Dependence between spatial units is quite evident for this cause of mortality, being the $sSMR$s of nearby municipalities are very similar in general terms. The BYM model has been able to reproduce this highly dependent geographical pattern, removing the effect of the heterogeneous random effect from the final fit as the dependence of the data surely requires.

On the contrary, atherosclerosis does not show any evident geographical pattern. The atherosclerosis $sSMR$s map resembles a typical map of unsmoothed SMRs full of noise and without a clear underlying signal. Here, the spatial term of the BYM model is cancelled out since data does not show any dependence between nearby sites. The smoothing effect on the $sSMR$s in this case is hardly appreciable and this is an important result. For some epidemiologists SMRs are a kind of 'holy grail', which are the final goal of disease mapping studies and $sSMR$s as a kind of statistical artifacts distorting the 'legitimate' object of interest, the SMRs. In our opinion this is a consequence of confounding the risk of death, the real object of interest for every site, with the SMR, just one risk estimate among many possible estimators. In this sense the statistical term *smoothed* does not really help since it has other different connotations in common language that suggest a statistical artifact underlying the statistical machinery. Nevertheless, the results in the atherosclerosis map have an important lecture in this regard. If the data do advise it, the $sSMR$s are mildly smoothed, allowing $sSMR$s to reproduce the noise in the original data if this was really the main source of variability in the data. In that case the contribution of the spatial term would be removed from the model and we should not be concerned about the presence of this term since it is basically left out from the model by giving it a low posterior standard deviation. Thus, both lung cancer and atherosclerosis maps show that we should not be concerned with the inclusion of both random effects in the BYM model. If some of them were not really needed, they would be ignored by the BYM model.

Figure 4.5 shows the $sSMR$s corresponding to the BYM model for several causes of death with interesting geographical patterns. The first correspond to ischaemic heart disease mortality in men. In general, the spatial distribution of this cause of mortality does not show a clear geographical pattern. Nevertheless, some municipalities at the south-eastern side of the Valencian Region show high $sSMR$s (higher than 150). These sites are among the most touristic municipalities in the Valencian Region (Benidorm, Calpe or Torrevieja). The rest of the most touristic municipalities in the Valencian Region (such as Denia, Altea or Santa Pola) are precisely the rest of high risk sites, $sSMR$s between 125 and 150, around the mentioned municipalities with highest risks. All these geographical units are full of foreign and national retired old people who have settled in this coastal region known as Costa Blanca. These people, when moving to Costa Blanca usually have good living conditions and no serious diseases. People requiring continuous medical attention as a consequence of serious diseases, such as cancer, or highly dependent people, usually stay at their original regions, enjoying easier access to medical resources and they

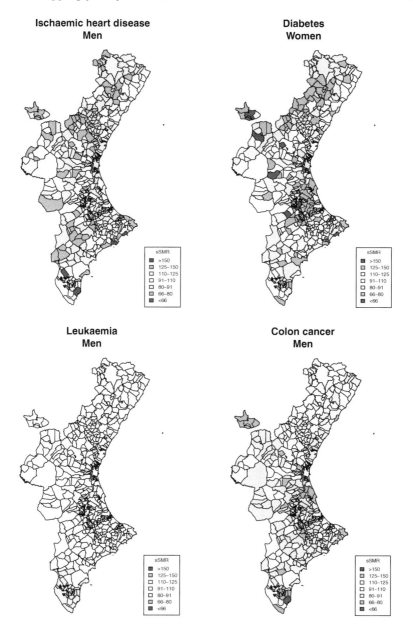

Figure 4.6
Spatial mortality patterns for ischaemic heart disease (men), diabetes (women), leukaemia (men) and colon cancer (men) in the Valencian Region for the period 1991-2000. Results from the *Mortality Atlas of the Valencian Region.*

rarely move to Costa Blanca. Therefore, a high proportion of the old population in these municipalities, those with more chances of dying, lack severe chronic illnesses what make sudden ischaemic heart disease deaths more frequent here than in any other place in the Valencian Region. In fact, Benidorm, the municipality with the highest risk, had 534 observed deaths for this disease in men for 264.3 expected deaths, yielding a smoothed SMR of 195.7. These large numbers make the risk excess for this municipality very evident, and therefore its probability of risk excess virtually equal to 1.

The second interesting map in Figure 4.5 corresponds to diabetes mortality in women. This map shows a clear risk excess of regional scope in the mid-eastern side of the Valencian Region comprised of several adjacent municipalities. The corresponding map with the probabilities of risk excess (map not shown) points out that most of the $sSMRs$ of the municipalities in this region show a high probability (higher than 0,95) of being higher than 100. These results seem even more striking because the spatial pattern of diabetes mortality for men does not show such a clear risk excess around this region, maybe excepting a significant risk excess for the high risk municipality in the centre of this region. At this moment, we do not have a clear idea of the risk factors that may be influencing the diabetes mortality in women in this region; we do not even know whether diabetes incidence is higher in this region or not than in the rest of the Valencian Region. Nevertheless, the high risk region highlighted in the Valencian mortality atlas deserves a closer study surely at an individual level in order to address the underlying reasons of this excess in diabetes mortality.

The third map in Figure 4.5 corresponds to leukaemia mortality for men. The interesting feature of this cause of death is its lack of geographical variability. That is, the risk for this disease is evenly distributed throughout the whole Valencian Region, at least more evenly than for any other cause of death in the Valencian mortality atlas. This (lack of) geographical pattern is also present for leukaemia mortality in women (Martínez-Beneito et al., 2005) and also for the whole of Spain (López-Abente et al., 2006) where this cause of mortality shows hardly any geographical variability. This is a surprising result since leukaemia is usually described as a paradigmatic example of disease tending to show clusters (see Knox (1994); Bradinath et al. (1995); Hoffmann et al. (2007) to cite a few). In our case we do not find any evidence at all, at least at a municipal level and for all ages as a whole, on the trend of this disease to show clusters.

The last map in Figure 4.5 shows the geographical pattern for colon cancer mortality for men. At a first glance, this map does not seem to show any interesting pattern. Nevertheless the three capitals of the three Valencian provinces: Alicante, Castellón and Valencia (see Figure 1.2) are some of the few municipalities with $sSMRs$ higher than 110. These municipalities are distant, placed at the south, north and middle of the Valencian Region (respectively), so their common high risks are not a consequence of geographical dependence. In contrast to these cities, their metropolitan areas do not show any risk excess so they are exclusive of the capitals but not of their surrounding regions. One reason explaining this result would be that colon cancer patients would move to these capitals in order to live close to the hospitals where they are going to get medical attention. Nevertheless, the capitals are not the only municipalities in the Valencian Region hosting hospitals and, on the contrary, no risk excess is appreciated in the rest of municipalities where hospitals are placed. This pattern can also be noticed for this cause of mortality for women in the Valencian Region (Martínez-Beneito et al., 2005) and also for colorectal cancer (both sexes) for the whole of Spain. In the Spanish mortality atlas (López-Abente et al., 2006), it is quite striking to check that several other province capitals (Zaragoza, Huesca, Pamplona, Vitoria, Burgos, etc.) placed at a large low-risk area at the north/north-east side of Spain, are isolated high risk 'islands' within this large region. This result would also deserve a closer study in order to address the underlying effect causing this striking feature of colon cancer mortality.

These kinds of results are the interesting outcomes expected to be obtained in mortality atlases. On one hand, these results provide a better understanding of the diseases studied and give important clues on the risk factors that may be determining their geographical distribution. On the other hand, they allow us to get a deeper knowledge of the health geography of the region studied in the corresponding atlas. This makes it possible to become aware of the regions with systematic health problems for many diseases, and therefore take care of unbearable health inequalities in the region of study that should be further explored.

Chronic Obstructive Pulmonary Disease Mortality in the Castellón Province

The results introduced now correspond to a study that we carried out some years ago. By then, some civic associations of several municipalities in the Castellón Province with presence of ceramic tile industries complained about the impact that the dust of these industrial activities were having on their health. Therefore, the Epidemiology Unit of the Valencian Regional Health Authority was requested to carry out a specific study and to give an appropriate answer to that complaint. As a first approach, we started studying whether or not the mortality in these municipalities by several different respiratory causes was higher than in the rest of the province. We did not find any risk excess in mortality for these causes in the region with tile industries. Nevertheless, before discarding the associations' complaint, we decided to also take a look at incidence data since maybe the tile industries could have increased the incidence of respiratory diseases in the surrounding municipalities but not mortality, which would require a more extreme health impact. In order to carry this second study out, we asked for the hospital admissions database containing the records of the respiratory causes whose mortality we had previously studied.

One of the respiratory causes that we studied was Chronic Obstructive Pulmonary Disease (COPD) in men. Hereafter, we will focus on the incidence study of this specific cause. The upper-left side of Figure 4.7 shows the Standardized Incidence Ratio (the equivalent of the SMR but for incidence data) for COPD. Nothing particularly interesting arises from this map. This is a clear example of unsmoothed $SIRs$ where noise overwhelms any geographical pattern of interest. This map shows lots of municipalities in the more extreme groups as a consequence of the low expected incident cases for most of them. This led us to calculate smoothed $SIRs$, namely by means of the BYM model. The upper-right side of Figure 4.7 shows these smoothed $SIRs$. Much of the variability of the raw $SIRs$ is removed in this map, although some variability remains, namely that which has a statistical relevance. This second map highlights an artifact in the incidence data. The red dots in this map stand for the addresses of the hospitals covering the municipalities of the Castellón province. The smoothed $SIRs$ are in general higher around these dots and lower in those municipalities placed farther from the hospitals. Moreover, this artifact also emerged in the rest of causes studied so this is an effect of incidence data in general. We called this effect 'hospital attraction' and is just the consequence of accessibility to hospitals by simply living closer to them. Basically, people who live far from the hospitals do not frequent them as often as people who live closer. Therefore, it was convenient to fit this effect in order to make the underlying geographical pattern visible.

The lower-left side of Figure 4.7 shows the result of fitting the BYM model with a specific treatment of the hospital attraction. We are not going to give further details on this treatment since ecological regression, the methodology needed to account for additional covariates, will be thoroughly studied in the next chapter of this book. After removing the effect of hospital attraction, the $sSIRs$ are no longer related to the distance of the corresponding municipality to its hospital. This map shows a large low-risk region in the mid-north part of the Castellón province with abrupt changes in risk both in the northern and southern limits of this region. These changes would be more evident if different cutting points were chosen for the categories of the choropleth maps; nevertheless, we have preferred to use the same scale as for the rest of the book. Finally, the lower-right side of Figure 4.7 shows the division of the Castellón province as a function of the hospital (red dots in the upper-right plot) corresponding to each municipality. The limits of the low-risk mid-northern region just mentioned clearly coincide with the borders of the Hospital 2 region in the lower-right plot of Figure 4.7, even though the $sSMRs$ map is smoothed and therefore discontinuities could be blurred. The epidemiologists of the Epidemiology Unit rapidly noticed this coincidence and warned us about this. This convinced us that some artifact was present in the data that was responsible for the lower incidence in the Hospital 2 region. Otherwise, it would not be reasonable that the region of lower incidence exactly matched the limits of that region.

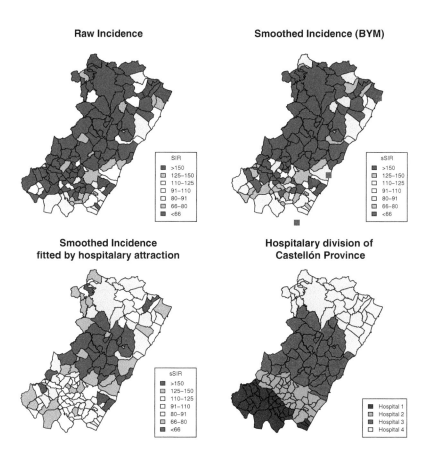

Figure 4.7
COPD incidence spatial analysis. Upper-left: raw municipal Standardized Incidence Ratios. Upper-right: BYM smoothed Standardized Incidence Ratios; red points stand for hospital locations covering the municipalities in the Castellón province. Lower-left: BYM smoothed Standardized Incidence Ratios with specific fitting of "hospitalary attraction" of each municipality. Lower-right: hospital based division of the municipalities in the Castellón province.

Motivated by these results, we asked for an explanation of this artifact to our data providers. They answered that the data of Hospital 2 were retrieved in exactly the same manner as for the rest of the hospitals and no reason was found explaining the lower incidence rates. So, we repeated our analysis seeking for a potential error that could explain the low-incidence region found. Once again, we reproduced exactly the same results so we asked for a reason explaining the results that we were reproducing to our data providers. They reaffirmed that nothing could explain our results and that the low incidence region that we have found should be caused by the presence of a genuine protective factor in that region. Nevertheless, two days later, they said that they have just realized that one of the years of study for Hospital 2 was not included at the reported observed hospital admissions. This explained the results found for the low incidence region corresponding to Hospital 2 in Figure 4.7.

One important conclusion that we draw from this particular study is that the SMRs are no 'holy grail' at all for estimating the underlying risk in disease mapping studies. Although the SMRs are risk indicators widely used and accepted in classic epidemiology, they do not yield any information of interest in our particular study. The gratifying conclusion of our study is that beyond the naive SMRs, statistical modeling allows us to derive alternative risk estimators that, sometimes, make it possible to highlight the underlying risk pattern generating the data. This example shows that making an appropriate statistical analysis of the data (in our case smoothing + controlling hospital attraction) can be a rewarding task, taking the results of epidemiological analyses much more forward than those using naive SMRs, mainly when the units of study are particularly small.

Exercises

1. Check that the MLE for the risks θ_i in the model $o_i \sim Pois(e_i\theta_i)$, $i = 1, ..., I$ are just the corresponding Standardized Mortality Ratios. Additionally, from a Bayesian point of view, show that if a flat $U(0, \infty)$ prior is assumed for the risks θ_i, then the posterior modes for these parameters coincide also with the corresponding Standardized Mortality Ratios.

2. In the supplementary material of the exercises of the book (see https://github.com/MigueBeneito/DisMapBook/tree/master/ Exercises) you will find a shapefile ValenciaCity.zip with the Valencia city census tracts (already used in the exercises of the previous chapter) and a file (COPD.Rdata) with information on chronic obstructive pulmonary disease (COPD) mortality in men for these

census tracts for the 1996-2015 period. The data in this file have been altered in a similar manner to the data available for reproducing the examples in the book, in order to preserve data privacy (see Section 1.1). Our goal with this exercise is putting in practice the content introduced in this chapter for getting reliable visualizations of the geographical distribution of the COPD risk mortality.

- The `COPD.Rdata` file contains the observed counts for COPD mortality in men per census tract (`COPD` object), the age-specific COPD deaths for the whole city (`COPD.age`) and the men population (in person-years) per census tract and age group for the whole period of study (`pop`). This is all the information required for calculating the expected cases per census tract using internal standardization. Calculate those expected values and use them to draw a choropleth map of the Standardized Mortality Ratios for the Valencia city census tracts. Save the expected cases in an `Rdata` file since they will be repeatedly used in the rest of the exercises of this chapter and in those of the following chapters.

- Fit a non-spatial Poisson lognormal model to the data above. Draw a choropleth map of the $sSMR$s derived (their posterior mean) and compare the geographical distribution estimated now with the original SMRs. Draw a second choropleth map with the probability of risk excess for the $sSMR$s drawn for this model ($P(sSMR_i > 1)$).

- Fit now the BYM model to the COPD data above. Use a vague uniform prior distribution on the standard deviation of the random effects in this model. Fit the model with both `WinBUGS` and `INLA` and compare the $sSMR$s estimates and probability of risk excess obtained with both inference tools. For the `WinBUGS` implementation, use the computational tricks introduced in Section 4.3 for speeding up the MCMC inference.

- Consider the PCAR and Leroux's LCAR distribution as an alternative to the BYM model for inducing spatial structure on the $sSMR$s. Compare the $sSMR$s obtained for both models with those of the BYM model.

Part II

Disease mapping: Towards multidimensional modeling

5

Ecological regression

Disease mapping models make it possible to visualize the geographical distribution of risks in a reliable manner, even when the units of study are small in statistical terms. Once that distribution is determined, we may be interested in associating the geographical variations found to some covariates for several reasons. In that case, *ecological regression* is the statistical technique suitable to achieve that goal. In contrast to the main descriptive aim of disease mapping studies, ecological regression has frequently an inferential aim, trying to quantify the relationship, if any, between the geographical distribution of a covariate and the distribution of the risk for a specific disease. Thus, the goals of both techniques are usually, or at least sometimes, quite different.

Ecological regression has its own particularities. The joint consideration of covariates and random effects into a single model is often problematic since both terms will fight to explain the same underlying variability. This will make both terms in the model confounded. Moreover, sometimes one has the temptation of interpreting ecological regression results in individual terms when individual data have not been used to carry out the analysis. This will yield misleading and potentially dangerous conclusions of this kind of analyses. Introducing ecological regression and dealing with its particular aspects is the main goal of this chapter.

This chapter is organized into four sections. Section 5.1 motivates ecological regression as a complementary tool to be used in disease mapping studies. Section 5.2 introduces how to pose ecological regression in statistical terms and introduces several flexible tools for modeling the effect of covariates. This section introduces also some practical issues needed to put ecological regression into practice. Section 5.3 discusses some important issues that should be borne in mind when dealing with ecological regression, such as: confounding between covariates and spatial random effects and a couple of fallacies typically arising when interpreting ecological regression studies that we should know in order to avoid them. Finally, Section 5.4 pays attention to two applications of ecological regression of particular interest in the literature: spatially varying coefficients models and point source models.

5.1   Ecological regression: a motivation

In epidemiology, *ecological studies* are those analyses which 'focus on the comparison of groups, rather than individuals; thus, individual-level data are missing on the joint distribution of variables within groups' (Morgenstern, 1995). Hence, the main feature of ecological studies is that the units of analysis are groups of people instead of single individuals. Ecological regression in particular pursues to determine the association between two, or more, variables by using groups of people as units of study. In our particular disease mapping context, where the groups of population at risk are referred to some geographical division, we will pursue to determine the association between two, or more, geographical patterns: one corresponding to the distribution of the risk of a disease and another one(s) corresponding to the distribution of one(/several) covariate(s). From here on, we will talk in general about ecological regression models with a single covariate, assuming that everything in this chapter can be easily generalized to more than one.

When one wants to explore the relationship between health outcomes and covariates, it would be more natural to do it at an individual level using individual data. Individual data allow us to explore the relationship between the exposure to the covariate and the outcome in a direct manner. Nevertheless, ecological studies are convenient and interesting alternatives to studies at an individual level for a number of reasons. First, ecological data are in general widely accessible and their use typically entails low costs (Morgenstern, 1982; Greenland, 1992). In fact, these data are frequently publicly available (even they are usually available on the Internet) in contrast to individual data whose use and diffusion frequently involve confidentiality issues. Second, sometimes individual exposures are hard to be measured. For example, long-term diet habits are very hard to be quantified at an individual level since this requires a close follow-up of individuals for long periods of time. Individual estimates of exposures in this kind of studies usually accumulate serious biases due to these problems, while in ecological studies those biases are averaged over groups of individuals. Ecological studies, grouping individuals into familiar units or neighbourhoods and estimating their diet habits with supermarket tickets, for example, could be interesting approaches for solving those problems. Environmental exposures are also difficult to be measured at the individual level. For example, Cook and Pocock (1983) or Ferrándiz et al. (2004) are interesting examples of ecological studies exploring the relationship between water hardness and cardiovascular diseases with small areas as units of analysis. Equivalent individual studies would require the disposal of individual covariates, which would entail knowing the drinking habits (consumption of bottled water, liters of water drunk per day, etc.) of a reasonable sample representing the whole population. In contrast, aggregated covariates are easily available for drinking water at municipal or other geographical divisions.

Another interesting example of problems obtaining covariates at an individual level can be found in Lynch and Smith (2005) and Wakefield (2008), who show a case study exploring the relationship between *Helicobacter pylori* (HP) infections during childhood and development of stomach cancer many years after. Studying this relationship at the individual level would require very long follow-ups for the subjects considered. Moreover, information systems of decades ago do not have enough information for monitoring HP infections at individual levels. These authors show an ecological study at country level comparing infant mortality rates per country in 1921-1923 (as a surrogate of HP infections since they are linked to diarrheal disease, one of the main causes of infant mortality then) and stomach cancer mortality rates in those same countries during 1991-1993. Clearly ecological analyses make it possible to explore this relationship even though this is not feasible with individual studies. A final advantage of ecological studies is that they usually have larger populations of study than individual-based analyses, which makes the variability of covariates in general wider than for individual studies. At the end, this increases the statistical power of the relationship between the covariate and outcome that we are seeking to assess (Richardson and Monfort, 2000).

Despite the benefits of ecological regression, it has also some drawbacks that we will discuss later in this chapter that would be convenient to keep in mind. Ecological regression by definition does not use individual data, even though we would typically want to draw conclusions at an individual level. Aggregation of individual information into groups causes information loss that could affect the results drawn. Namely, the information loss produced during the aggregation process precludes the identification of associations of interest at the individual level and, as a consequence, results drawn at the ecological level do not necessarily hold for individuals (Wakefield, 2008). Ecological regression is perfectly suited to make inference on contextual factors (factors inherent to each ecological group instead of individuals) as, for example, for assessing if municipalities with hospitals have lower ischaemic mortality rates than the rest. Nevertheless, when interpreting ecological analysis, the estimates that we derive are not necessarily those which we originally expect at the individual level, yielding misleading interpretations for individuals. Thus, the main problem of ecological analyses is that, quite frequently, researchers try to make inference at the individual level when one does not have the appropriate data to do it.

One particularity that distinguishes ecological regression studies whose groups correspond to different spatial units of other ecological regression studies on sex or racial groups, for example, is that the first will generally exhibit some spatial dependence that should be taken into account in the statistical analysis. Most regression methods assume the data to be independently distributed, given their expected values, which are modeled as a function of a covariate. This assumption will be usually wrong in the spatial ecological regression context, unless an extremely smooth function of the covariate was used to model its effect. In that case, a naive linear or parametric function will be usually insufficient for describing the wiggly geographical variability of risks and we will have to resort to additional tools for modeling the remaining spatial dependence in the residuals. This is also the case of time series analyses where, besides the covariate, a specific acknowledgement is done of temporal dependence since it is hardly sustainable that a covariate alone could have explained all the original temporal dependence in the data. Thus, something similar should be done in spatial ecological regression models if we wanted them to correctly explain the data.

Besides accounting for spatial dependence, there is a second factor in ecological regression models that makes it mostly compulsory to include some further terms into the model, in addition to the plain covariate. As seen in the previous chapter, disease mapping models usually assume Poisson distributions as data likelihoods. One of the features of this distribution is that its mean coincides with its variance so we do not have the same freedom as with, for example, the Normal distribution where these two quantities are in principle independent. As a consequence, the Poisson distribution is much more restrictive and this restriction on the variance has some serious effects. For example, let us assume that the distribution of the risk of a disease depended on a covariate that we did not have available. In that case, if we fitted a Poisson model with a common value for all the geographical units, this value would fit the mean for all the geographical units but it would not be able to fit the unexplained geographical variability of the covariate. This would make the observed counts to be farther apart of their means than they should be. As a consequence, the variance of the observations in this setting would be higher than the mean which would violate the former assumption of Poisson models. This effect is known as *overdispersion* and has an important effect in ecological regression studies, as we will see in the next example. As a consequence, the presence of overdispersion in a model will imply that covariates will tend to be accepted into the model regardless of their real relationship with the outcome. This is a huge problem for spatial ecological regressions that obviously should be controlled in order to generate sensible results.

Example 5.1

This example illustrates the effect of overdispersion in ecological regression studies. We have considered the atherosclerosis municipal mortality data in men for the period 1991-2011; see Figure 4.5. Moreover, we have generated 10 different random covariates as independent Normal draws of mean 0 and variance 1, for each municipality in the Valencian Region. We have run 10 Poisson regression models which explain the log-risks of atherosclerosis mortality as a linear function of each simulated covariate, without any further random effect. A separate ecological regression model has been fitted for each covariate. We have posed these Poisson regression models from a Bayesian

Covariate	Posterior mean	95% Posterior CI
1	0.048	[0.025,0.071]
2	0.059	[0.031,0.086]
3	-0.058	[-0.085,-0.031]
4	0.125	[0.093,0.158]
5	0.087	[0.058,0.117]
6	0.004	[-0.024,0.032]
7	-0.093	[-0.123,-0.063]
8	0.018	[-0.009,0.045]
9	0.031	[0.007,0.056]
10	-0.066	[-0.095,-0.038]

Table 5.1
Posterior summaries (mean and 95% credible interval) of the coefficients of the random covariates in the ecological regression on atherosclerosis mortality.

approach for coherence with the rest of the book, although we could have perfectly posed them from a frequentist point of view. Inference (available in the accompanying material) has been done with INLA.

We would not expect the covariates to have a 'significant' effect in principle on the log-risks, except for some false positives. Thus, in frequentist terms, if we calculated 95% posterior credible intervals for the coefficients of these covariates in the corresponding regression models, then we would expect to find, on average, that 0 or 1 out of the 10 credible intervals would not contain 0 as a value. Table 5.1 shows the posterior mean and 95% credible intervals for the 10 simulated covariates.

As shown in Table 5.1, the estimates of the effect of the covariates do not show any particular bias since their values seem to be distributed around the true value 0. Nevertheless, 8 out of the 10 calculated credible intervals do not contain 0, suggesting that these intervals are tighter than they should be. This result seems surprising at a first glance as the covariates have been generated as random draws without any real relationship with the geographical pattern of atherosclerosis mortality. In order to find some explanation for these results, recall that the geographical pattern for atherosclerosis in men (Figure 4.5) showed a large unstructured variability. This variability makes the observed counts very far apart from those expected when assuming a common risk for the whole region of study. Thus, most of the covariates proposed are welcomed by the model in order to reduce that excess of dispersion that does not fit with the Poisson hypothesis with a common risk for all the observed cases.

This example illustrates why performing a naive linear Poisson regression in a spatial ecological regression context is rarely a good idea for at least two reasons. First, the unaccounted spatial dependence in data makes invalid the independence hypotheses of Poisson regression models given their corresponding means, which would make any inference based on this model unreliable and inaccurate. On the other hand, covariates' effect (namely their variability) would depend on additional factors unrelated to the association between the covariate and the disease that we are trying to measure. Therefore, in such a naive analysis we would be at a serious risk of stating spurious relationships that do not really exist as significant. So, once again, in the spatial ecological regression context, we would be forced to carry out more elaborate studies if we wanted to draw sensible conclusions from our data sets.

As we will see in the next section, ecological regression models in our context will be integrated into disease mapping models since these are appropriate proposals for dealing with small areas and geographical dependence. Nevertheless, in some manner, ecological regression introduces a more inferential aim into disease mapping models, which have a more descriptive purpose focussed on producing reliable depictions of the geographical distribution of risks, even working with small areas. The aim of ecological regression is more inferential since it tries to set the relationship between the covariate and the disease, instead of just depicting a reliable overview of the disease. Thus, ecological regression will be often used as a confirmatory tool of the relationship between covariates and geographical patterns of diseases that could have been suggested by previous disease mapping studies. So, in this sense, the purpose of disease mapping and ecological regression is quite different.

Besides its inferential use on the effect of specific covariates, ecological regression can also be viewed from a second point of view. Disease mapping models, as introduced in the previous chapter, are posed as smoothing devices for the geographical distribution of the risk of some particular diseases. Random effects, bases of functions or some other smoothing tools are used as flexible devices for describing the variability underlying the risk of the corresponding disease. These tools are intended to be used as surrogates of the covariates responsible for the underlying variability, which will be typically unavailable or even unknown. Nevertheless, in case of having a covariate that we suspected could be associated to the variability of the disease, ecological regression would be the appropriate tool for checking its effect or including it in the analysis. The specific inclusion of covariates in disease mapping models in order to achieve enhanced $sSMR$ estimates could be good for several reasons. First, smoothing devices, such as random effects, are flexible tools capable of fitting very complex and different geographical patterns. Nevertheless, they are also prone to overfit the data and therefore to depict random variations that do not really exist in practice. The explicit inclusion of covariates in these models makes the depiction of their effect much more precise than if it is simply modeled by means of very general tools such as those already introduced. Moreover, the inclusion of a covariate into a model would fit its effect if it really existed and would leave the random effects, or whatever smoothing device used for modeling the risk, free for reproducing other sources of variability besides that covariate. This could make these secondary sources of variability fit much more precisely since the effect of the primary confounding covariate would already be fitted. In any case, ecological regression studies make it possible to structure, quantify and separate the sources of variability underlying the geographical distribution of diseases.

All these different motivations make ecological regression studies extend into geographical studies of small areas. Particularly, in the epidemiologic literature, the capability of studies of this kind for summarizing, at a low cost, the effect of a particular covariate on a disease is highly appreciated.

5.2 Ecological regression in practice

As introduced in the previous section, ecological regression studies on small areas can be viewed as an extension of disease mapping analyses either with inferential aim or for enhancing spatial models with the inclusion of covariates. In any case, ecological regression models in this context have a natural formulation as disease mapping models since these solve the issues arising from the use of small units of study. Moreover, most of the disease mapping models already introduced implicitly consider spatial dependence between spatial units as a tool for improving risk estimates, which was one of the issues to be addressed in ecological regression models, as introduced in the previous section. Therefore, disease mapping models are a perfect framework for formulating ecological regression models on small areas. Thus, from an applied point of view, we are going to introduce ecological regression as an extension of the BYM model, or any other disease mapping model that we could have in mind, including the covariate of interest into the linear predictor used to model the log-risks. Therefore, we are going to pose ecological regression models as Poisson mixed regression models including covariates into the linear predictor in addition to the random effects that we already introduced in disease mapping models.

The ecological regression framework for disease mapping can be formulated as follows. Let us assume o_i and e_i to be, respectively, the observed and expected counts for the i-th geographical unit and x_i the value of the covariate of interest x in that same unit. Therefore, a typical ecological regression model assumes:

$$o_i \sim Pois(e_i \cdot \theta_i), \ i = 1, ..., I.$$
$$\log(\theta_i) = \mu + f(x_i, \boldsymbol{\beta}) + g(\boldsymbol{\varphi})_i \qquad (5.1)$$
$$...$$

where φ denotes a vector of random effects implementing a small area smoothing device, which does not depend on the covariate of interest and $g()$ is a suitable transformation. The prior distribution of φ can be either correlated (PCAR, ICAR, BYM, etc.) or simply unstructured, depending on the context. In the usual case that the length of φ is the same as the number of units, $g()$ will be often just the identity function, reproducing the random effects models already introduced in the previous chapter. Nevertheless, $g(\varphi)$ could be also something like $g(\varphi) = \boldsymbol{B}\varphi$ for $\boldsymbol{B}$ a basis of functions, such as piece-wise polynomial functions in the case of spline. So, the $g()$ function makes the model above very general, containing also spatial spline-based models, for example, although we will typically use it with $g()$ being the identity function and φ a vector of spatially structured random effects, with as many components as geographical units.

The second factor in the linear predictor of the expression above $f(x, \boldsymbol{\beta})$ models the contribution of the covariate to the geographical variation of the log-risks of the disease. Now $f()$ denotes a general function, ranging from a simple linear function of the covariate, i.e., $f(x, \beta) = \beta x$ to much more flexible alternatives such as a spline regression model, for example. Note that we have removed the intercept in $f()$ as it was already included in the linear predictor of the model above (μ). A lot of different modeling proposals can be proposed for $f()$, as we will see just below.

Since $f(x, \boldsymbol{\beta})$ in Expression (5.1) accounts for the variability in the log-risks that can be associated to the covariate, $g(\varphi)$ will have a different meaning than the random effects term for traditional disease mapping models. Now $g(\varphi)$ would account instead for the residual variability in the log-risks that cannot be explained by x. As a consequence, the linear predictor in Expression (5.1) splits the log-risks into three additive components, μ, $f(\boldsymbol{x}, \boldsymbol{\beta})$ and $g(\varphi)$ which account for the mean log-risk, the variability associated to the covariate and that which cannot be associated to that factor, respectively. The exponential of this third term is an important byproduct of ecological regression models, since this can be viewed as the estimated $sSMRs$ for each spatial unit leaving out the effect of the covariate x. So this decomposition of the $sSMRs$ allows filtering off the effect of covariates when they are quite strong and do not allow to visualize therefore the effect of any other secondary factors. This can be a very valuable tool from an applied perspective.

We are now going to focus our attention on modeling the covariate effect since the modeling of the spatial residual variability has already focussed enough attention in Chapter 4. In the previous example, a simple linear effect was considered for modeling the effect of covariates on atherosclerosis mortality. Since the observed deaths are modeled as a Poisson regression with logarithmic link, the corresponding linear relationship entails the relative risks to be modeled as an exponential function of the covariates. Nevertheless, more flexible alternatives are available and they should be borne in mind beyond the traditional linear relationship usually assumed. As shown by Natario and

Knorr-Held (2003), the geographical pattern fitted by the random effects in ecological regression models will be very sensitive to the particular functional relationship used to model the covariate. Namely, if an unappropriate fit of the covariate is made, the additional random effects in the regression model will probably reproduce the misfit of the covariate instead of focussing on another additional factor that we might be interested to highlight. Thus, in this sense we would be wasting the opportunity of unveiling additional hidden risk factors that random effects would bring in ecological regression models.

An obvious alternative to assuming a linear relationship between the covariate and the outcome would be to assume instead polynomials of a higher degree or some other parametric functions depending on more parameters. These alternatives would yield more flexible fits. Moreover, the advantage of parametric functions is that their parameters usually have an easier interpretation than those in other modeling devices, such as spline models for example. Nevertheless, the typical problem of parametric functions is that they are usually excessively rigid for describing a wide variety of curves. This problem can be solved resorting to highly parameterized functions, achieving therefore as much flexibility as with non-parametric alternatives (Torres-Avilés and Martinez-Beneito, 2015). Nevertheless, the election of an appropriate set of basis of functions is crucial in this case since the quality of the final fit will critically depend on this issue. However, parametric models make it possible to use basis of functions that could be perfectly suited for the data at hand, such as Fourier bases for cyclic data, which can easily beat any other non-parametric modeling alternative. So, although prone to misfit, some particular features of the data (mainly with a low number of parameters), parametric models in general should not be dismissed as an interesting alternative for modeling covariates in ecologic regression studies.

A second interesting alternative to models which assume a linear relationship between the covariate and the (log-)risks would be to resort to step-wise functions on a partition of the covariate to be modeled (Ferrándiz et al., 2004; Haining et al., 2010; Marí Dell'Olmo et al., 2014). Thus, for a continuous variable x we would categorize its values into discrete groups according to some partition, usually defined by $K - 1$ equispaced points or quantiles $\{Q_1, Q_2, ..., Q_{K-1}\}$. In that case we could define

$$
f(x, \boldsymbol{\beta}) = \begin{cases}
\beta_1 & \forall x: \; x < Q_1 \\
\beta_2 & \forall x: \; Q_1 \leq x < Q_2 \\
\cdots & \cdots \\
\beta_K & \forall x: \; Q_{K-1} \leq x
\end{cases}
$$

Obviously $\boldsymbol{\beta}$ can now define a wide variety of shapes for $f(x, \boldsymbol{\beta})$, including lots of non-linear relationships. An obvious choice as prior for the elements of $\boldsymbol{\beta}$ would be to put improper flat distributions for all of them, i.e., treating those components as fixed effects. This would be an appropriate option for low values of K (let's say lower than 5 or 10) since therefore the estimate of each β_k would be based on a considerable amount of spatial units. Nevertheless, for low values of K, $f(x, \boldsymbol{\beta})$ could depict a step-wise function of large steps, with possibly large discontinuities at $Q_1, \ldots, Q_{K-1}$, which would probably define an unrealistic shape. A possible remedy for this would be to fix a larger value for K and to strengthen $\boldsymbol{\beta}$ estimates by treating its components as random effects. In that case, we could consider for example $\beta_k \sim N(0, \sigma_\beta^2), k = 1, \ldots, K$, for σ_β being an additional variable in the model. The elements of $\boldsymbol{\beta}$ have a natural ordering which would surely induce some kind of dependence and that would be convenient to take advantage of, as we typically do for spatial dependence. Thus, the random effects structure of $\boldsymbol{\beta}$ could reflect that dependence, for example, by considering β_1 to have an improper flat prior distribution and $\beta_k \sim N(\beta_{k-1}, \sigma_\beta^2), k = 2, \ldots, K$. This defines $\boldsymbol{\beta}$ as a first-order random walk that should improve $\boldsymbol{\beta}$'s estimates if its components really showed dependence among nearby intervals of the step-wise function. In this case, the corresponding ecological regression model would not need an additional intercept since $\boldsymbol{\beta}$ itself would be able to reproduce the intercept effect since its components would not be centered at any specific value. Therefore, including an intercept with a first-order random walk structure for $f(x, \boldsymbol{\beta})$, as just defined, would just introduce identifiability problems between that term and $\boldsymbol{\beta}$.

It can be shown (see for example Section 3.3.1 of Rue and Held (2005)) that the first-order random walk process just introduced could be also alternatively defined by making $\beta_k = \mu + \gamma_k$ where μ follows an improper flat prior distribution and $\boldsymbol{\gamma}$ follows an ICAR distribution. In that case, the k-th component of $\boldsymbol{\gamma}$ should be considered as neighbour of the $(k-1)$-th and $(k+1)$-th component, for $1 < k < K$. Thus, step-wise modeling with ICAR random effects on its parameters is an alternative smoothing procedure for the relationship between the covariate and outcome in ecological regression. Nevertheless, although both implementations of first-order random walks (conditionally defined random walks and ICAR-based) yield the same dependence structure they are not completely equivalent. ICAR distributions are usually subject to some restrictions, namely a sum-to-zero restriction in WinBUGS, while the conditionally defined random walk is completely unrestricted. This makes it necessary to include the separate intercept term μ into models including ICAR-based random walks but not for the conditional formulation. This gives to the ICAR-based models an additional degree of freedom compensating the sum-to-zero restriction that conditional first-order random walk models do not have.

Besides first-order random walks, further dependence structures can be set for the components of $\boldsymbol{\beta}$ in step-wise functions. Thus, a second-order random walk structure could be also defined for $\boldsymbol{\beta}$ by making $\beta_k \sim N(2\beta_{k-1} - \beta_{k-2}, \sigma_\beta^2), k = 3, \ldots, K$. In other words, β_k's mean is $\beta_{k-1} + (\beta_{k-1} - \beta_{k-2})$ so that it is not located at the last available observation of the series, but it takes also into account the last observed evolution between consecutive observations $(\beta_{k-1} - \beta_{k-2})$. If β_1 and β_2 are considered to have improper flat distributions, and $\beta_3, \ldots, \beta_K$ to have a second-order random walk structure as defined above, then this would be equivalent to assume $\boldsymbol{\beta}$ to follow an ICAR distribution with precision matrix (see Section 3.4.1 in Rue and Held (2005))

$$\Sigma^{-1} = \sigma^{-2} \begin{pmatrix} 1 & -2 & 1 & & & & & \\ -2 & 5 & -4 & 1 & & & & \\ 1 & -4 & 6 & -4 & 1 & & & \\ & \ddots & \ddots & \ddots & \ddots & \ddots & & \\ & & 1 & -4 & 6 & -4 & 1 & \\ & & & 1 & -4 & 5 & -2 & \\ & & & & 1 & -2 & 1 & \end{pmatrix}.$$

This matrix is also of the form $\boldsymbol{D} - \boldsymbol{W}$, for $\boldsymbol{W}$ being sparse and $\boldsymbol{D}$ diagonal with terms equal to the sum of the rows in $\boldsymbol{W}$. Thus, also in the second-order random walk we find a parallel between the conditional modeling of $\boldsymbol{\beta}$ and its modeling by means of ICAR random effects. In that ICAR formulation each observation β_k in $\boldsymbol{\beta}$ would be a neighbour of the $k-2, k-1, k+1, k+2$-th elements of that vector with different weights. An implementation of this second-order random walk effect (and one for the first-order random walk too) with ICAR distributions can be found in Example 9 of the `GeoBUGS` help manual (menu `Map>Manual`) of `WinBUGS`.

Neither for the second-order random walk, the conditionally defined and ICAR-based formulations are completely equivalent. Namely, the matrix Σ^{-1} of this model has rank $n-2$ instead of $n-1$, the rank for the first-order random walk. As a consequence, ICAR-based second-order random walks should be ideally subject to two restrictions: a sum-to-zero restriction (so that it is orthogonal to the intercept), and a second orthogonality restriction with respect to linear terms, i.e., $\boldsymbol{\beta}$ should be orthogonal to the vector $(1, 2, \ldots, K)$. These two constraints, which make $\boldsymbol{\beta}$ orthogonal to the dimensions corresponding to the rank deficiency of $\boldsymbol{\Sigma}^{-1}$, should be compensated by the inclusion of an intercept and a linear term into the linear predictor of the model. However, `WinBUGS` only imposes the sum-to-zero restrictions for ICARs so the implementation of the second-order random walk in this software is problematic. Therefore, we advise to use `INLA` for models using that dependence structure for $\boldsymbol{\beta}$. The two constraints on $\boldsymbol{\beta}$ can be imposed in `INLA` by including the arguments `constr=TRUE, extraconstr=...` into the corresponding $f(...)$ argument(s) in the model; see for example the supplementary material of Marí Dell'Olmo et al. (2014) for an example of this procedure.

Assuming either a first- or a second-order random walk for modeling the effect of covariates can make a substantial difference in terms of the fit of the effect of the corresponding covariate. Second-order random walks will generally define substantially smoother relationships than first-order random walks (Rue and Held, 2005; Schrödle and Held, 2011b). Moreover, first-order random walks will shrink the effect of the covariate towards the overall mean, while second-order random walks will shrink that effect towards a line fitting the relationship between the covariate and the outcome. Therefore, if forecasting was an issue (if the covariate was time, for example) the performance of both models could be very different and therefore the choice between these two models should be made with much care (Knorr-Held and Rainer, 2001).

There are some more alternatives available for modeling a covariate effect beyond step-wise functions with random walks. Auto-regressive or moving average models for $\boldsymbol{\beta}$ are obvious alternatives to random-walks for $\boldsymbol{\beta}$. Namely, first-order auto-regressive modeling could also be reproduced by a PCAR auto-regressive distribution in a similar manner as random-walks can be reproduced by means of ICAR distributions. Therefore, we can notice how the same tools that have been used for spatial smoothing can also be used for structuring, in a non-parametric way, the relationship between covariates and outcomes in ecological regression. For first-order auto-regressive modeling of $\boldsymbol{\beta}$ the corresponding covariance matrix is not rank-deficient so we would not have to care about this. As a consequence, a conditionally defined and PCAR-versions of the first-order auto-regressive model would be completely equivalent. The good thing about auto-regressive models is that they can tune the strength of dependence between consecutive observations and therefore, in this sense, they are more flexible than random walks. In general, auto-regressive models will fit more wiggly relationships than random walks, which could also make an evident difference in terms of prediction.

We have previously highlighted that discontinuities in step-wise functions are one of the most important disadvantages of using that tool for modeling the effect of covariates. Joinpoint analyses (Kim et al., 2000, 2009) are a different modeling approach solving that problem that could also be used within ecological regression models. In contrast to stepwise functions, joinpoint analyses consider very few (although unknown) points where the functional form of the covariate changes. In fact, the main goal of joinpoint analyses is determining how many change points are necessary for explaining the effect of the covariate and where those change points should be placed (Martinez-Beneito et al., 2011). The epidemiological relevance of these questions makes joinpoint analyses a powerful tool very appreciated under an applied point of view. In its simplest version, joinpoint analyses consider

$$f(x, \boldsymbol{\beta}, \eta) = \begin{cases} \beta_1 + \beta_2 x & \forall x : x < \eta \\ \beta_3 + \beta_4 x & \forall x : x \geq \eta \end{cases}$$

for $f()$ constrained to be continuous at every point of its domain, in particular for η. Thus, in this sense, joinpoint analysis is a much more satisfactory alternative than stepwise functions. More complex alternatives could also be formulated by introducing more changepoints and/or more complex (non-linear) functions between them. Bayesian hierarchical models are a very convenient framework for fitting these models since they perfectly accommodate the unknown character of η into the model and incorporate its uncertainty into the inference of the rest of parameters in the model (Carlin et al., 1992; Martinez-Beneito et al., 2011). If we had particular interest in quantifying the number or location of changepoints when describing the effect of a covariate, joinpoint modeling would be the appropriate tool.

A hybrid tool fusing the ideas of step-wise functions and joinpoint analyses would be the modeling of covariates by means of spline. Spline are a particular case of modeling based on bases of functions, in this case piecewise polynomial functions defined over a collection of nodes splitting the range of observed values of the covariate. As for joinpoint models, spline are typically restricted to be continuous everywhere; indeed further continuity restrictions on the derivatives of spline are typically imposed in order to define more smooth functions. Spline modeling makes it possible to reproduce non-linear effects of the covariate by performing a linear combination of the piecewise polynomial basis of functions, which make the fit of the model computationally much more convenient. Nevertheless, spline are not the only the basis of functions suitable for linearizing a non-linear function. Thus, Gaussian radial functions, for example, could be also a reasonable alternative to spline to be used as basis of functions for fitting the effect of the covariate. Therefore, although the use of step-wise functions is very common in ecological regression studies, the use of other typical regression tools as those mentioned in this paragraph would be also advisable in that context. A large number of specialized literature on these modeling tools is available on this topic (Faraway, 2016; Wood, 2017) which in general could also be used for ecological regression.

Example 5.2

For illustrating ecological regression, we are going to use a different data set than that which we have been using throughout most of the book. In this case we are going to consider a data set on AIDS mortality in men throughout Valencia city, the capital of the Valencian Region. The period of study extends for 12 years (1996 to 2007), and observed and expected deaths are retrieved for that period for the 553 census tracts that compound the city. In addition to those observed and expected deaths we have a covariate available, a deprivation index calculated at the census tract level which summarizes the social environment of each census tract. This index is centered at 0, has a variance of 1 and takes high values for those areas showing more deprivation. More information on the calculation of the deprivation index and of the MEDEA Project in general, the project that this data set belongs to, can be found in Borrell et al. (2010). Our goal with this example is to explore the association between that deprivation index and the risk for AIDS mortality.

We have fitted three ecological regression models in this study. The first model assumes a linear relationship between the deprivation index and the log-risks for each census tract; the second model assumes a step-wise function of 5 levels; and the third model assumes a step-wise function of 25 levels. The cut-points for defining the step-wise functions for the second and third models are the percentiles of the deprivation index that split that variable in groups with the same number of census tracts. The values of the components of β for the stepwise functions have been modeled as a fixed effect with improper flat distributions for the second model and as an ICAR random effect (RW1) vector for the third one. In addition to the deprivation index, we have considered spatial and heterogeneous random effects (BYM spatial structure) modeling the residual variability that cannot be explained by deprivation.

The coefficient for deprivation in the Poisson regression model has a posterior mean of 0.52 and a 95% credible interval of $[0.42, 0.64]$. This means that deprivation is directly associated with high risks for AIDS mortality, being the relative risk equal to $1.68 (= \exp(0.52))$ for each unit of increase of deprivation. Taking into account that the highest difference in the deprivation index between census tracts is 5.80, then the relative risk of the region with the highest deprivation as compared to that with the lowest is of 20.92. The upper-left plot of Figure 5.1 shows the relationship between deprivation and the log-risks for all three models fitted. As shown, that relationship is close to linear even for the step-wise functions, so ecological regression models with non-linear relationships do not seem to outperform that assuming a linear relationship. This is confirmed also by the DICs since the linear model attains the lowest value (1,453.1) followed by the model with 25 levels (1,457.0) and the model with 5 levels (1,469.7). Thus, it becomes clear that the large steps in the step-wise function with 5 steps damage the fit of the ecological regression model. We will focus from now on the results of the model assuming a linear relationship for the log-risks and deprivation.

The top-right plot in Figure 5.1 shows the $sSMR$s fitted for AIDS mortality for the census tracts of Valencia city. That plot shows substantial variability, pointing out many census tracts in the groups with extreme risks. Specifically it points out several hot spots scattered throughout Valencia city which in general correspond with the most deprived neighbourhoods of the city. Thus, this factor does not allow to see the presence of further risk factors beyond deprivation. Fortunately, the different terms in the linear predictor of ecological regression models allow to split the variability in the $sSMR$s into two parts: one associated with deprivation and another one which cannot be associated with that factor. This second part corresponds with the variability accounted for the random effects in the model. The two maps in the bottom row of Figure 5.1 correspond to these two factors. The $sSMR$s map is proportional to the product of the values of these two maps since $\log(\theta_i) = \mu + \beta x_i + \varphi_i$ and therefore $sSMR_i = \exp(\mu) \exp(\beta x_i) \exp(\varphi_i)$ for $i = 1, ..., I$. The standard deviation of the deprivation component is 0.53, while that for the residual variability is 0.57, therefore deprivation explains a $46\% (= 100 \cdot 0.53^2/(0.53^2 + 0.57^2))$ of the total variance in the log-SMRs. The deprivation component reproduces most of the hot spots mentioned of the $sSMR$s map which correspond to deprived neighbours. Nevertheless, the map of the residual variability shows additional features that were not highlighted in the original $sSMR$s map. Thus, the downtown of the city has high risk levels that would not correspond to the values of the deprivation index in that area. In particular, once deprivation is controlled, this area shows a high risk excess in comparison to the rest of the

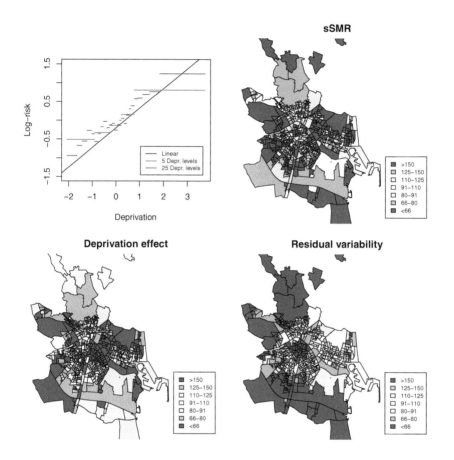

Figure 5.1
Top-left: relationship between deprivation and log-risks for all three models
fitted. Top-right: $sSMR$s for the model assuming a linear effect for deprivation. Bottom-left: Effect of deprivation on the $sSMR$s. Bottom-right: Residual
variability on the $sSMR$s that cannot be explained by deprivation.

city. Downtown Valencia city is a heterogeneous neighbourhood with the most affluent census tracts in the city, but also with deprived areas. The variables composing the deprivation index do not seem to be sensitive to these deprived areas and consider all the downtown as an affluent zone. The residual variability seems to highlight this misfit of the deprivation index that could be due to the index itself or some other factors that make the downtown to be different than the rest of the city. The residual term also points out a risk excess in the eastern side of Valencia, close to the port side that cannot be explained by deprivation and to which it would be surely worth paying particular attention.

5.3   Some issues to take care of in ecological regression studies

5.3.1   Confounding

In the previous two sections we have shown that the use of random effects in ecological regression is almost compulsory in practice. Random effects avoid overdispersion under the usual Poisson assumption of disease mapping models. Nevertheless, the joint inclusion of covariates and random effects into a single model entails its own problems since these two components may compete for explaining the same effect, causing a kind of confounding between them. This problem is particularly likely when introducing spatial random effects into a model, since the distribution of covariates often shows also geographical dependence and therefore the confounding between these two factors would be even more likely.

The discussion on spatial confounding dates back to at least Clayton et al. (1993) who noticed a substantial change in the fixed effects estimates of ecological regression models when introducing spatial random effects. In order to explain that confounding, let us assume an ecological regression model with BYM spatial structure, which accounts for a covariate x with a linear effect. That is, the linear predictor for this model would be

$$\log(\boldsymbol{\theta}) = \beta_0 \mathbf{1}_I + \beta_1 \boldsymbol{x} + \boldsymbol{\varphi} + \boldsymbol{\psi} \tag{5.2}$$

where $\boldsymbol{\varphi}$ and $\boldsymbol{\psi}$ are vectors of heterogeneous and spatial (ICAR) random effects, respectively. It is clear that the term $\boldsymbol{\varphi}$ can also be put as $\boldsymbol{I}_I \boldsymbol{\varphi}$, i.e., the design matrix corresponding to this term is just an identity matrix. It is also evident that the matrix $[\boldsymbol{x} : \boldsymbol{I}_I]$ is of rank I and therefore the effect of the covariate could be also reproduced by the heterogeneous random effect term by simply setting $\boldsymbol{\varphi} = \beta_1 \boldsymbol{x}$. In other words, $\boldsymbol{x}$ and $\boldsymbol{\varphi}$ will be collinear, which makes the data unable to distinguish their effects and they can only be identified through the shrinkage of their prior distributions. Typically β_1 will have a flat prior distribution which does not induce any shrinkage on this parameter but, on the contrary, the prior distributions of φ do constrain their values through the common variance of all their components, which will make it possible to distinguish the effect of these two factors. Nevertheless, as σ_φ^2 approaches to ∞, both β_1 and φ will become progressively unidentifiable and confounding may appear between these two terms. A similar confounding effect would also hold for the intercept term (β_0) and φ. For σ_φ^2 approaching to ∞, the intercept will become unnecessary since it can be replaced by simply increasing or decreasing all the components of φ which will be hardly penalized by their random effects structure.

This confounding effect will be typically more important for the spatial random effect ψ. Informally, ψ is an I-vector constrained by a sum-to-zero restriction; therefore, it spans an $(I-1)$-dimensional space: the hyperplane of $\mathbb{R}^I$ orthogonal to $\mathbf{1}_I$, since all the elements are orthogonal to this vector. That restriction makes confounding between β_0 and ψ avoidable. Therefore, this term jointly with the intercept of the model, will span the whole $\mathbb{R}^I$ and, as a consequence, x will be collinear with these terms. Specifically, the effect of the covariate x can be reproduced once again by setting $\beta_0 = \beta_1 \bar{x}$ and $\psi = \beta_1(x - \bar{x}\mathbf{1}_I)$, which fulfills the sum-to-zero restriction of ψ. Nevertheless, in contrast to the heterogeneous case, ψ's spatial prior distribution, the device in charge of identifying the values of this vector, favours it following a spatial dependent pattern, which the covariate might also be supposed to show. As a consequence, the separation of x and ψ effects by means of ψ's prior distribution will be more difficult and therefore x and ψ might be confounded. Hodges and Reich (2010) point out that this effect is not exclusive to ICAR spatial random effects, but it would also be present if a (geostatistical) Gaussian random field (Wakefield, 2007; Paciorek, 2010), penalized spline (Hodges and Reich, 2010) or other alternative CAR distributions (Lee, 2011; MacNab, 2014), for example, were used to structure the spatial dependence in ψ. That confounding effect between a covariate and a spatial random effect is known as *spatial confounding*. A more technical and detailed explanation of this informal introduction to (spatial) confounding in ecological regression can be found in Reich et al. (2006), Hodges and Reich (2010) or Chapter 10 in Hodges (2013).

Confounding could also occur between φ and ψ; in fact identifiability problems in random effects could also modify the effect of covariates (MacNab, 2014). Namely, φ spans the whole $\mathbb{R}^I$ while, as mentioned, ψ spans a hyperplane of $\mathbb{R}^I$, so the effect of the spatial random effect for any value of ψ can be also reproduced by φ since the latter is unconstrained. Data can only identify the sum of both random effects, but their separate individual values can be only (weakly) identified by the shrinking effect of their prior distributions. This problem would be particularly worrisome for small lattices where everything is relatively close and, therefore, distinguishing between spatial dependence and heterogeneous variability is especially challenging. In contrast to the case of confounding with a covariate, the confounding between random effects is expected to be lower because of the shrinking effect of the prior distribution of both terms. Nevertheless, the separate inference on these two random effects instead of its sum is discouraged in general. Confounding between random effects is a different issue than confounding with a covariate, which goes beyond ecological regression models. This kind of confounding has been further studied in MacNab (2011) where a reparameterization of the BYM model is proposed in order to alleviate this effect. We will treat more in depth this issue in Chapter 6 and, for the rest of this section, we will focus on the spatial confounding between covariates and spatial random effects.

Reich et al. (2006) and subsequent works of these authors describe some interesting results on spatial confounding in ecological regression that may help us to understand better the cause, effect and scope of this artifact. We start by identifying some settings where we should expect to find substantial confounding in ecological regression studies. Specifically, Reich et al. (2006) show that a necessary condition for a spatial unit to have a large impact on β_1 is that the covariate takes a very different value in that unit, in comparison to their neighbours (see also Paciorek (2010) for some related results). This result illustrates how ecological regression distinguishes between the effect of the covariate and that of the spatial random effect. Basically, if for these locations the relative risk of the disease is close to those in their neighbours (despite their large differences on the covariate), this would be a sign of a high contribution of the spatial random effect on the outcome. If, on the contrary, the risk in this unit is very different than those in its neighboring units, in a manner conforming with the covariate under study, this would mean that the covariate is mainly responsible for the variation on the relative risks. As a consequence, if x showed a smooth spatially correlated pattern, it would be convenient that, despite that dependence, the covariate also showed some degree of heterogeneity, i.e., some of the units do not closely follow the hypothetical spatial pattern. Otherwise, the model will not have spatial units allowing to distinguish between the covariate and the spatial effect, therefore favouring confounding between these two terms.

Additionally, Reich et al. (2006) show also that different spatial distributions of the covariate could yield confounding problems of different magnitude. They show that these confounding problems will be particularly evident when the covariate is highly correlated with some of the eigenvectors corresponding to the lowest non-zero eigenvalues of $D - W$, the precision matrix of ψ. These eigenvectors are a kind of canonical spatial pattern that ψ will be a linear combination of. The coefficients of that linear combination will be random effects of variances inversely proportional to the corresponding eigenvalues, so the patterns corresponding to the lowest eigenvalues will be in general more influential on ψ. Thus, confounding may be more worrisome when the covariate is similar to one of those eigenvectors, particularly those with lower eigenvalues since they will be less constrained by their prior distribution. As an illustration, Figure 5.2 shows the three lowest non-zero eigenvectors of $D - W$

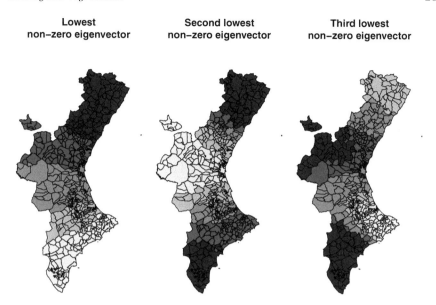

**Lowest
non–zero eigenvector**

**Second lowest
non–zero eigenvector**

**Third lowest
non–zero eigenvector**

Figure 5.2
First three non-zero eigenvectors of the precision matrix of an ICAR distribution $(D - W)$ on the Valencian Region. Light, respectively dark, municipalities stand for negatives values, respectively positive, of the corresponding eigenvector.

for the Valencian Region, using adjacency as criterion for building the adjacency matrix W. That figure shows how these three eigenvectors correspond respectively to linear, quadratic and cubic patterns along the north-south axis of the Valencian Region. As a consequence, ecological regressions on this region, with covariates mainly varying from north to south, will show more confounding in general than those with covariates varying mainly from east to west. This is a consequence of the geometry of this particular region which induces a particular dependence structure on the spatial random effects with larger variability along the north-south axis, the longest axis crossing through the Valencian Region. This performance is quite general, as shown by Hodges and Reich (2010), making confounding particularly likely if the covariate varies mainly along the longest axis crossing the region of study.

Once we have an intuition on when to expect important confounding issues in ecological regression, we wonder now, what is the expected effect of spatial confounding on β_1's estimation? Spatial confounding is the effect of the collinearity of x and some of the eigenvectors of $D - W$, which are a basis for the linear space where ψ takes values. Collinearity, in general, makes the variances of estimates inflated, so this is the main effect that we would expect to notice on β_1's posterior distribution when the corresponding model contains a spatial random effect. Indeed if ψ was not smoothed at all (σ_ψ^2 was infinite), this would make the posterior variance of β_1 become infinite, making that value unidentifiable. Therefore, in the specific case of the Valencian Region, we would expect that introducing a spatial random effect into the ecological regression model would increase β_1 posterior variance, particularly if x varied mainly from north to south. This variance inflation will alleviate the effect of overdispersion, which made us find much more significant results in Example 5.1 than we ought, achieving in principle more reasonable results.

Beyond variance inflation, Hodges and Reich (2010) show that including spatial random effects in ecological regression studies also produces some bias in β_1's estimate. Specifically, they show that including random effects in ecological regressions also modifies β_1's estimate, although in an unknown direction. That is, if $\widehat{\beta}_1$ and $\widehat{\beta}_1^*$ corresponded to the posterior mode of the effect of x in a Poisson regression model with and without, respectively, random effects then $\widehat{\beta}_1$ could be either lower or higher than $\widehat{\beta}_1^*$, depending on the specific data at hand. As a consequence, introducing random effects into ecological regression models does not necessarily have either a reducing or amplifying effect on β_1's estimation, on the contrary its effect could be qualified as haphazard. Richardson (2003) also reaches this conclusion from a more empirical point of view in contrast to, for example, Clayton et al. (1993) who qualifies introducing spatial random effects into ecological regression models as a dilution of the effect of the covariate. Additionally, Hodges and Reich show that if no further covariate besides x had an influence on the distribution of the relative risks, the spatial random effects would modify $\widehat{\beta}_1^*$ even though it was not required, which seems an unpleasant performance that we would like to avoid.

Our goal when dealing with confounding would be to avoid the effect (bias) of ψ on $\hat{\beta}_1^*$ while fitting for overdispersion and spatial dependence in the data. For achieving this goal in Gaussian ecological regression models, Reich et al. (2006) propose to impose ψ to be orthogonal to the covariate x. This restriction, when applied to the intercept term, is equivalent to the frequently assumed sum-to-zero restriction on ψ that allows us to identify the effect of the intercept in the linear term of the BYM model. The proposal of Reich and Hodges would be to apply also that procedure to the new covariate x. These constraints could also be applied to φ although, as we exposed above, the confounding between the covariate and the heterogeneous term would be expected to be milder. In the Poisson-based case, the orthogonality restriction becomes imposing orthogonality between $C^{1/2}x$ and $C^{1/2}\psi$, where C is a diagonal matrix with $C_{ii} = Var(o_i|\beta, \psi, \varphi) = e_i\theta_i$ (Reich et al., 2006). This yields instead the following weighted orthogonality constraint on ψ: $x'C\psi = 0$. In a similar manner, that constraint, with regard to the intercept, would yield the expression: $1_I'C\psi = 0$. A drawback of imposing this constraint in WinBUGS is that it necessarily assumes the typical (unweighed) sum-to-zero restriction on ψ so two orthogonality constraints would be associated to the intercept. Additionally, C depends on the relative risks θ, which depend themselves on β, ψ and φ; therefore, the weights in the weighted constraints above would be also stochastic, which induces additional estimation difficulties. As a consequence, some simplifying assumptions should be imposed in practice in order to implement that restriction (see the next example). Imposing restrictions of this kind in order to reduce confounding leads to a particular kind of ecological regression proposal known as *restricted spatial regression.*

Restricted spatial regression attributes the competing explanatory effect between x and ψ to the covariate. Although in principle there is not a clear reason for this, indeed this procedure is controversial (Paciorek, 2010; Prates et al., 2018; Hanks et al., 2015), it may be justified in several ways. First, random effects are usually conceived as smoothing devices trying to reproduce either the underlying variability in the relative risks that cannot be explained by the available covariates or the spatial dependence shown by the data that once fitted these covariates. Under this point of view, random effects are of secondary importance as compared to covariates and therefore the inference on the spatial random effect would be subordinated to a good estimation of the effect of the covariate. Hence imposing a restriction here on the random effects would seem justified. This is different from ordinary fixed effects regression where it is usually hard to justify that some covariates are less important than others. Moreover, in case that a secondary unobserved variable was influencing the spatial distribution of the log-relative risks, we would not have any guarantee that the spatial random effect would fit its effect (Hodges and Reich, 2010). Thus, in that case, we would be forced to admit that if an unaccounted covariate could have been missed in the model, then the estimation of x's effect could be therefore biased, as would occur for any other traditional fixed effects regression model. Thus, bearing in mind that we cannot assume a miraculous effect of ψ if there was an influential missing covariate (Hodges and Reich, 2010), we can just aspire to fit spatial dependence and overdispersion in the model with ψ trying to interfere as less as possible in β_1's estimate. This is what restricted spatial regression is supposed to do.

Although with a different aim, restricted spatial regression has also been considered for modeling the non-linear effect of covariates (Marí Dell'Olmo et al., 2014). In that case, a basis of functions is considered in order to model the non-linear effect of the covariate and the spatial random effect is considered to be orthogonal to the space spanned by that basis of functions. Likewise, if more than one covariate was to be included into the model, a separate orthogonality restriction should be imposed for any of the covariates considered in order to avoid spatial confounding.

From a practical point of view, Hodges and Reich have made available their routines implementing restricted spatial regression (`https://www4.stat.ncsu.edu/~reich/Code`). These are R routines implementing an MCMC algorithm for fitting this model for both Gaussian and count data. Basically, for the Gaussian case, this algorithm reparameterizes Expression (5.2) as

$$\log(\boldsymbol{\theta}) = \beta_0 \mathbf{1}_I + \beta_1 \boldsymbol{x} + \boldsymbol{L}\boldsymbol{\psi}^* + \boldsymbol{\varphi} \qquad (5.3)$$

where $\boldsymbol{L}$ are the $I-1$ non-zero eigenvectors ($I-k$ if $\boldsymbol{x}$ was a matrix containing k covariates) of $\boldsymbol{P} = \boldsymbol{I}_I - \boldsymbol{x}(\boldsymbol{x}'\boldsymbol{x})^{-1}\boldsymbol{x}'$, the projection matrix on the orthogonal space to $\boldsymbol{x}$. The last eigenvector of $\boldsymbol{P}$, with eigenvalue equal to 0, has been removed from the $\boldsymbol{L}$ matrix since it is proportional to $\boldsymbol{x}$; otherwise, this term would be collinear with the covariate. Now $\boldsymbol{\psi}^*$ will be a $(I-1)$-vector as a consequence of the dimension reduction arising from the orthogonality constraint imposed. $\boldsymbol{\psi}^*$ will follow a $N_{I-1}(\mathbf{0}_{I-1}, \sigma^2_{\psi^*}(\boldsymbol{L}(\boldsymbol{D}-\boldsymbol{W})\boldsymbol{L}')^{-1})$ prior distribution. Therefore, with this reparameterization, restricted spatial regression is now posed as a saturated mixed model with as many covariates as observations, with coefficients shrunk towards 0 by their prior distribution. Note that $\boldsymbol{\psi}^*$'s prior precision matrix is no longer a sparse matrix, which makes restricted spatial regression much less convenient from a computational point of view than the unrestricted alternative. Hughes and Haran (2013) proposed an alternative, and computationally much more convenient, formulation of restricted spatial regression. Hughes and Haran use $\boldsymbol{M}$ as an alternative matrix to $\boldsymbol{L}$ in (5.3) but with $q << I-1$ columns. This $\boldsymbol{M}$ matrix takes into account the geographical structure of the region of study, which makes it possible to use only $q \approx I/10$ eigenvectors in the model without a significant loss in practical terms. This computationally convenient implementation of ICAR-based models in general has its own interest beyond ecological regression models as it provides a computationally convenient MCMC-based proposal for making inference in challenging large data sets.

Alternative implementations of restricted spatial regression can also be done in WinBUGS and INLA as we illustrate in the following example. The WinBUGS implementation of the (unweighed) orthogonality restriction, with respect to the covariate, could be done by simply adding the following lines of code to an ecological regression model:

```
zero ~ dnorm(sum.psi,prec.restr)
sum.psi.x<-inprod2(psi[],x[])
```

where zero=0 should be given to the model as data and prec.restr is also provided as data and should take a high value, as for example 100 or 1,000. This piece of code imposes a stochastic restriction, i.e., we are imposing $\sum x_i \psi_i$ to follow a zero mean Normal distribution with low variability. In that manner, we ensure $\sum x_i \psi_i$ to be very close (although not necessarily equal) to zero. Alternative exact restrictions could be coded, as for example including psi[i]-inprod2(psi[],x[])/sum(x[]) instead of psi[i] in the linear predictor. Nevertheless, in our experience, these alternatives slow down substantially the computation, making the models unfeasible in practice. Although ideally prec.restr should be set as high as possible, this would affect the performance of the MCMC so in our experience we advise choosing moderate values for this parameter, such as 100 or 1,000, in order to avoid those problems. Weighted constraints could also be implemented in `WinBUGS` by substituting `sum.psi.x` in the code above by `<-inprod2(psi[],xweights[])` for `xweights[i]<-x[i]*weights[i]` for suitable `weights`. For imposing a restriction of this kind on the intercept, we should change x by the vector $\mathbf{1}_I$.

Restrictions are imposed in `INLA` by simply using the `extraconstr` argument in the corresponding $f()$ term defining the BYM vector of random effects (Schrödle and Held, 2011b). The argument `extraconstr` should be assigned a list with arguments `A` and `e`, for `A` being a matrix of dimensions $K \times I$ and `e` a vector of length K, where K is the number of linear restrictions to be imposed. This argument imposes the K linear constraints $\boldsymbol{A}_k.\boldsymbol{\omega} = e_k$, $k = 1, ..., K$ on the BYM vector of random effects $\boldsymbol{\omega}$ defined by $f()$. Additionally, the argument `rankdef` should account for the rank-deficiency in the covariance matrix of the random effects arising from the constraints imposed. One example of formula for making `INLA` to perform a restricted spatial regression with a linear term for the covariate $\boldsymbol{x}$ could be the following

```
A=matrix(x,nrow=1); e=0
form.RSR= 0 ~ x + f(sp.unit,model="besagproper",graph="foo.
inla",
constr=TRUE,extraconstr=list(A=A,e=e),rankdef=2)
```

The argument `rankdef=2` accounts for the sum-to-zero restriction (implemented by the implicit `constr=TRUE` argument) and the additional orthogonality restriction on the covariate. Note that `bym` models contain $2 \cdot I$, where I is the number of spatial units in the region of study. Thus, for `bym` models, the matrix `A` above should have $2 \cdot I$ columns instead. More detailed examples of the implementation of restrictions of this kind can be found in the literature for more complex ecological regression models (see the supplementary material of (Marí Dell'Olmo et al., 2014)) and spatio-temporal models (Schrödle and Held, 2011b; Ugarte et al., 2014).

Example 5.3

With this example we are going to illustrate the confounding effect on a linear covariate in ecological regression studies. First, we have considered our usual oral cancer data set in men on the Valencian Region and we have used as covariate the latitude of the centroids of the units of study. We expect to find important confounding problems for this covariate, as it has a smooth spatial structure and it varies from north to south, the main axis of variation of the spatial random effect for the Valencian Region lattice as we mentioned above. The analyses shown in this example have been made with `INLA` since the handling of constraints in this package is better than in `WinBUGS`. In particular, we can leave out the sum-to-zero constraint on the spatial random effects and substitute it by an alternative constraint. This is something that we will want to do specifically in our example.

We have fitted several ecological regression models and we have focussed our attention on the coefficient of the latitude covariate on those ecological regressions. Note that we have standardized our covariate in order to avoid further confounding between the intercept and the covariate. First, we have fitted a naive Poisson regression model (*Model 1*) including just an intercept and the covariate. Second, we have fitted the same model including a spatial (ICAR) and a heterogeneous random effect in order to fit potential remaining overdispersion (*Model 2*). This model is only restricted by the typical sum-to-zero restriction of ICAR random effects. Third, we have fitted the same model but restricting the spatial random effect in the latest model to be orthogonal also to the covariate (*Model 3*). That is, *Model 3* would be a restricted spatial regression model with a raw (unweighted) orthogonality restriction between the spatial random effects and the covariate. As fourth and fifth models, we have implemented the second model above removing the sum-to-zero restriction on the spatial term and including two additional constraints on the spatial random effects. These weighted orthogonality constraints are two different versions of the restrictions for the Poisson case introduced above. These are $\mathbf{1}_I'\hat{\mathbf{C}}\boldsymbol{\psi} = 0$ and $\mathbf{x}'\hat{\mathbf{C}}\boldsymbol{\psi} = 0$ for $\boldsymbol{\psi}$ the spatial random effect fitted within the model. The diagonal matrix $\mathbf{C}$ should have in its diagonal terms: $C_{ii} = Var(o_i|\boldsymbol{\beta},\boldsymbol{\gamma}) = E(o_i|\boldsymbol{\beta},\boldsymbol{\gamma})$. This last term could be approximated in two different ways. First, $\hat{C}_{ii} = E(o_i|\boldsymbol{\beta},\boldsymbol{\gamma}) \approx e_i$ which will be a reasonable approximation if the variability in the expected cases is substantially higher than that in the relative risks. The weighted orthogonality restrictions arising from this approximation are those corresponding to the fourth model implemented (*Model 4*). Finally, a second approximation is reasonable for the diagonal terms in $\mathbf{C}$, this is $\hat{C}_{ii} = E(o_i|\boldsymbol{\beta},\boldsymbol{\gamma}) = e_i\hat{\theta}_i$ where $\hat{\boldsymbol{\theta}}$ is the vector of risk estimates (posterior modes as suggested by Reich et al. (2006)) derived from any of the previous models. We have considered as $\hat{\boldsymbol{\theta}}$ the risk estimates derived from *Model 2*, although we have checked that, excepting for the first model those estimates hardly vary between models. The fifth model run in our study (*Model 5*) corresponds to that implementing the weighted constraint with this latest weighting. In practice, the implementation of *Model 5* will always require the previous running of an alternative model in order to plug in a risk estimate $\hat{\boldsymbol{\theta}}$.

Table 5.2 summarizes the results obtained for the coefficients of the intercept and latitude for these 5 models. Specifically, it shows for all 5 models the posterior mean and standard deviation for those coefficients. Regarding the posterior mean of the intercept, we see how *Models 2* and *3* have a substantially different estimate in comparison to the rest of models. These models implement a sum-to-zero restriction so the Poisson specific constraints seem to bias the intercept estimates in a much lower extent than the Poisson specific alternatives. In terms of the posterior standard deviation for the intercept, all

Model	Post. mean β_0	Post. sd β_0	Post. mean β_1	Post. sd β_1
Model 1	-0.015	0.017	-0.051	0.017
Model 2	-0.156	0.034	-0.057	0.150
Model 3	-0.158	0.033	-0.128	0.035
Model 4	-0.058	0.027	-0.049	0.022
Model 5	-0.028	0.030	-0.053	0.024

Table 5.2
Posterior summaries for the intercept (β_0) and covariate (β_1) coefficient for all 5 models run.

4 models with random effects inflate the variance of the intercept estimates in a similar extent, possibly a bit more for *Models 2* and *3*. Regarding the posterior mean of the covariate's effect, we see how *Model 3* yields results markedly different from the rest of the models. Thus the non-Poisson-specific constraint seems to have an important effect in this case in terms of bias, as for the intercept. Alternatively, regarding the posterior standard deviation of this coefficient, we see how *Model 2* is by far the alternative with more distinct results. Note that this model does not implement any constraint for the random effects in relation to the covariate. Thus the huge variance inflation for this model is a consequence of the confounding between these two unconstrained factors. That variance inflation is more or less controlled for the models implementing some specific restriction between the random effects and covariate. The models with the Poisson-specific constraint show little change in the covariate effect estimate as compared to the model without random effects (*Model 1*). Moreover, these models effectively inflate the posterior variance of the coefficients, although much less than that without any particular constraint (*Model 2*), whose variance is overinflated as a consequence of confounding. Note finally that the results of *Models 4* and *5* are quite comparable, at least for this data set where the variability of the expected cases is far higher than that of the relative risks.

We have run also all 5 models above on 45 additional combinations of mortality causes and sexes in the Valencian Region. The goal now is to explore the generality of the previous results on a wide collection of causes instead of just for oral cancer in men. Table 5.3 summarizes the results for the covariate effect (β_1) for all the mortality causes analyzed. This table shows, for each model, the relative change for β_1 measured as $|\widehat{\beta}_1^i - \widehat{\beta}_1^1|/\widehat{\beta}_1^1$ where $\widehat{\beta}_1^i$ denotes the posterior mean for β_1 according to *Model i*. Additionally, Table 5.3 summarizes also the variance inflation produced for β_1 for each model, measured as the quotient of posterior standard deviations for β_1 for each model divided by that in *Model 1*. Results in this table basically reinforce those conclusions drawn in Table 5.2. The biases between the models with Poisson-specific intercepts and the model without random effects are quite low (around 18%) in comparison to

Comparison	Relative difference	Variance inflation
Model 2 vs *1*	0.81	8.70
Model 3 vs *1*	1.09	1.93
Model 4 vs *1*	0.18	1.73
Model 5 vs *1*	0.17	1.74

Table 5.3
Comparison of β_1 estimates for all models, in comparison to *Model 1*, for a set of 45 different causes of death.

the rest of the alternatives. Moreover, the variance inflation is just moderate for them in contrast to the unconstrained *Model 2*. Finally, the results of both Poisson-specific models are once again quite similar so they seem mostly equivalent in practical terms, at least in data sets with substantial variability in the expected cases. Therefore, *Model 4* which is easier to implement than *Model 5*, which requires a previous run of a model for estimating $\boldsymbol{\theta}$, seems a convenient implementation in practice.

Finally, we have run *Model 4* for all 10 simulated data sets in Example 5.1 (results not shown are available at the online supplementary material). For all of them, the resulting 95% credible intervals for the covariate's coefficients contained the value 0, in agreement with the nominal probability level of those intervals. Therefore, the variance inflation performed by *Model 4*, around 73% according to Table 5.3, seems enough for controlling false positives for these simulated covariates.

Spatial confounding is becoming a very active field which is attracting considerable attention. MacNab (2014), Hanks et al. (2015), Goicoa et al. (2018b), and Prates et al. (2018) are just some recent papers dealing with this issue and paying it the attention that it surely deserves. For sure, many more enlightening works on this field will be published in the next few years.

5.3.2   Fallacies in ecological regression

In addition to confounding, there are a couple of interpretation misunderstandings in ecological regression studies that we should try to avoid. It is important to be aware of these problems as a first step to avoid them; that is why we introduced them here in detail.

5.3.2.1   The Texas sharpshooter fallacy

Disease mapping is frequently used as a statistical tool for observational studies without a planned statistical design. As a consequence, ecological regression is often used as a confirmatory tool for evidencing or fitting the relationship between the geographical pattern highlighted in a previous disease mapping study and a covariate whose geographical distribution resembles that of the previously depicted health outcome. This is a dangerous procedure prone to lead to false associations between covariates and health outcomes known as the *Texas sharpshooter fallacy* (see Kulldorff (1999) or page 251 of Waller and Gotway (2004), for example). The name of this fallacy comes from a tale of someone who shoots a bullet to a wall and later draws a bull's eye around the bullet hole. Obviously, the success rate of this procedure is disparately high, regardless of the skill of the shooter. Something similar happens with the ecological regression procedure just described. If a covariate is proposed for ecological regression based on its similarity with a health outcome's geographical distribution, we will probably end up qualifying that covariate as influential on the health outcome, regardless of whether it was really taking an effect or the geographical resemblance of both factors was only due to chance or other external factors. The Texas sharpshooter fallacy is most frequently noticed in the cluster detection literature, where the covariate would be the proximity to a place causing potentially risk excess. In this case, it would be very easy to set a visual link between the presence of some potentially hazardous facility(/ies) and the presence of a high risk area for some causes of mortality. Nevertheless, this effect applies also to ecological regression in general with more general covariates which do not necessarily summarize proximity to some specific location.

If the geographical distribution of a health outcome resembled that of a specific covariate and we wanted to check that association; ideally, it would be convenient to perform that confirmatory ecological regression with new data, possibly corresponding to a different period or region of study. Frequently, it would not be possible to have this secondary source of data available since disease mapping studies typically include as many years of study as possible. In that case the alternative is waiting for some few years in order to have more data available, although this is not usually a reasonable option. In any case, if we were forced to perform the mentioned ecological regression with the original data, it would be convenient to keep in mind this fallacy when interpreting the corresponding results, and we should be very cautious in stating association between the covariate and the health outcome.

The Texas sharpshooter fallacy is related to the occurrence of false positives in general, which is also a common problem in ecological regression that has focussed scarce attention, mainly in the epidemiological literature. It is common to find works in the literature performing ecological regressions for different covariates in order to set which of them, if any, are related to the health outcome under study. Sometimes the amount of covariates considered is high as, for example, when studying the potential effect of point sources of different types: metal-related industries, paper related industries, chemical industries, etc. Moreover, sometimes, several different health outcomes are regressed against these sets of covariates in order to explore which exposures could be linked to a collection of health problems. Obviously, a false positive error protection mechanism should be used in this setting, since otherwise a considerable number of spurious relationships between covariates and health problems would be stated. It would be convenient to avoid this in our studies and to be conscious of its existence in order to avoid the literature to reproduce these false positives that will not be possible to find again in subsequent studies.

5.3.2.2   The ecological fallacy

Ecological regression assesses the relationship between covariates and outcomes but at an aggregate level, i.e., both exposure and outcome are summaries for each of the units of study available. This is perfectly right if inference on those relationships is pursued at the corresponding aggregate level for some particular reason, such as being interested in the contextual effect of the covariate instead of its individual effect. Nevertheless, ecological analyses are often performed because of data availability and not for a particular interest of researchers on drawing conclusions at the aggregate level. In those cases, drawing individual conclusions from ecological regression studies performed at an aggregate level is a risky procedure that, as we will explain now, should be avoided.

Although statistical relationships found at the aggregate level could also hold for individuals, this is not necessarily true in general. Leaving aside the potential effect of unconsidered confounding covariates, there is in general a difference between the effect estimates derived at individual studies as compared to those derived at the aggregate level. This gap between the aggregate and individual effect estimates is known as *ecological bias*, which makes effects found at the aggregate level not hold at the individual level (Morgenstern, 1982; Freedman, 2001). The *ecological fallacy* will be the product of the error produced by ecological bias when drawing conclusions at the individual level from ecological studies. The ecological fallacy is a general effect which applies to regression studies on aggregate data in general, whatever is the origin of the aggregation: sex, age, race, municipalities, etc. Nevertheless, obviously, in our particular context we will be mostly interested in the ecological bias coming from the aggregation of individuals in geographical groups.

An important source of ecological bias is what is known as *pure specification bias* (Greenland, 1992), which is an exclusive bias of ecological studies. This issue arises as a consequence of the behaviour of non-linear transformations under data aggregation. In more detail, let us assume that we had the deaths from a disease, at an individual level, for a population. This binary outcome would follow a Bernoulli distribution of probability $q(\boldsymbol{x}, \boldsymbol{\theta})$, where $\boldsymbol{x}$ denotes a vector of covariates for the corresponding individuals and $\boldsymbol{\theta}$ denotes a vector of parameters that we would like to learn of. For the individuals of the j-th geographical unit, R_j from now on, we will assume the covariate $\boldsymbol{x}$ to be distributed according to $P(\boldsymbol{x}|\boldsymbol{e}_j)$, with $\boldsymbol{e}_j$ being a vector of parameters. If, given the probabilities $q(\boldsymbol{x}, \boldsymbol{\theta})$, individuals died for that cause independently, then the expected number of deaths in region j would be

$$Q_j(\boldsymbol{e}_j, \boldsymbol{\theta}) = \int_{R_j} q(\boldsymbol{x}, \boldsymbol{\theta}) P(\boldsymbol{x}|\boldsymbol{e}_j) d\boldsymbol{x}, \qquad (5.4)$$

where this integral would be understood as a finite sum if we had individual information on all the individuals in R_j. Since, typically, we will not have individual information on the individual deaths, but just the aggregated cases, the only available tool for making inference on $\boldsymbol{\theta}$ is through Expression (5.4). We would assume a model linking the observed deaths for each spatial unit and the corresponding $Q_j(\boldsymbol{e}_j, \boldsymbol{\theta})$ and we will derive an estimate $\hat{\boldsymbol{\theta}}^i$ of $\boldsymbol{\theta}$ according to this model. We will refer to this estimate as $\hat{\boldsymbol{\theta}}^i$ in order to stress its individual character. For example, if the individual relationship between the covariates and probability of death was assumed to be linear, that is $q(\boldsymbol{x}, \boldsymbol{\theta} = (\alpha, \beta)) = \alpha + \beta\boldsymbol{x}$, we would have:

$$Q_j(\boldsymbol{e}_j, \boldsymbol{\theta}) = \int_{R_j} (\alpha + \beta\boldsymbol{x}) P(\boldsymbol{x}|\boldsymbol{e}_j) d\boldsymbol{x} = \alpha + \beta E_{R_j}(\boldsymbol{x}|\boldsymbol{e}_j)$$

therefore, for the linear case we could estimate $\boldsymbol{\theta} = (\alpha, \beta)$ by assuming also a linear relationship between the covariate and the probabilities of death at an aggregate level. Maximum likelihood, Bayesian methods, etc. could be used for estimating $\hat{\boldsymbol{\theta}}^i$ in this case.

In ecological regression studies, the expected cases for the j-th unit of study are usually assumed to be equal to $q(E_{R_j}(\boldsymbol{x}|\boldsymbol{e}_j), \boldsymbol{\theta})$, instead of Expression (5.4), where $E_{R_j}(\boldsymbol{x}|\boldsymbol{e}_j)$ denotes the mean value of the covariate in unit j. That is, in a typical ecological regression model, the outcome is directly regressed against some summary of the covariate for the set of units of study considered. Thus, in ecological regression studies $\boldsymbol{\theta}$ is usually estimated according to the relationship between expected cases and covariates given by the latter expression, which would yield a new estimate $\hat{\boldsymbol{\theta}}^e$, where the superscript e stresses now its ecological character. For example, for the linear case above we would have $\hat{\boldsymbol{\theta}}^e$, to be an estimate of a model assuming the relationship:

$$q(E_{R_j}(\boldsymbol{x}|\boldsymbol{e}_j), \boldsymbol{\theta}) = \alpha + \beta E_{R_j}(\boldsymbol{x}|\boldsymbol{e}_j),$$

which coincides with the expression also used for deriving $\hat{\boldsymbol{\theta}}^i$. Thus, for the linear case $\hat{\boldsymbol{\theta}}^i = \hat{\boldsymbol{\theta}}^e$ and therefore no pure specification bias would hold then.

Regretfully, the previous situation does not hold in general. Let us consider now the typical setting in spatial ecological regression with a Poisson data likelihood. In that case, a log-linear relationship is usually considered between the expected deaths and the covariate at an aggregate level or, in other words, $q(E_{R_j}(\boldsymbol{x}|\boldsymbol{e}_j), \boldsymbol{\theta}) = \exp(\alpha + \beta E_{R_j}(\boldsymbol{x}|\boldsymbol{e}_j))$. On the other hand, at the individual level, an equivalent model would assume $q(\boldsymbol{x}, \boldsymbol{\theta}) = \exp(\alpha + \beta\boldsymbol{x})$. If a Normal distribution of the kind $P(\boldsymbol{x}|\boldsymbol{e}_j = (\mu_j, \sigma_j^2)) = N(\boldsymbol{x}|\mu_j, \sigma_j^2)$ was assumed for the covariate for each spatial unit, then the exponential relationship above would yield (Plummer and Clayton, 1996; Richardson and Monfort, 2000):

$$Q_j(e_j, \boldsymbol{\theta}) = \exp(\alpha + \beta\mu_j + 0.5\beta^2\sigma_j^2) \neq \exp(\alpha + \beta\mu_j) = q(E_{R_j}(\boldsymbol{x}|e_j), \boldsymbol{\theta}).$$

As a consequence, $\hat{\boldsymbol{\theta}}^e \neq \hat{\boldsymbol{\theta}}^i$ producing therefore pure specification bias. Note that if the covariate $\boldsymbol{x}$ had no variability within the geographical areas, then $\sigma_j^2 = 0$ for all j, and therefore no pure specification bias would hold in this case. Therefore, in the very general case of using a logarithmic link for modeling the expected cases in ecological regression studies, it would be convenient to make geographical units as homogeneous as possible in order to avoid pure specification bias as much as possible. This is one of the reasons why broad-scale studies have been partially shifted to local small areas analyses (Richardson and Monfort, 2000). Note also that if β takes values close to 0, i.e., the covariates have a low effect on the outcome, then $Q_j(e_j, \boldsymbol{\theta})$ will be similar to $q(E_{R_j}(\boldsymbol{x}|e_j), \boldsymbol{\theta})$, resulting then in a low ecological bias. As a consequence, when a covariate has hardly any effect on the outcome, β's estimate will show hardly any pure specification bias (Wakefield, 2007).

Although the results above rely on the Normality of $P_j(\boldsymbol{X}|e_j = (\mu_j, \sigma_j^2))$ they can also be derived for non-Normal distributions adding higher order moments of the corresponding distribution to the expression of $Q_j(e_j, \boldsymbol{\theta})$ (Plummer and Clayton, 1996). Wakefield (2007) studies the case of a binary covariate when an exponential individual relationship is assumed which results, at the aggregate level, in a linear model for the mean depending on the proportion of people showing one of the values of the covariate. Lasserre et al. (2000) study the individual/ecological relationship for the case of two categorical covariates and Richardson et al. (1996) for the case of continuous variables, proposing some alternatives to inference instead of considering the individual relationship between covariates and outcomes also at an ecological level. Salway and Wakefield (2005) makes a thorough study of ecological regression assuming a logistic link for $q(\boldsymbol{x}, \boldsymbol{\theta})$. Regretfully, the implementation of most of the proposals of this kind usually require either assuming some simplifying hypotheses which will rarely be possible to contrast or knowing the distribution (or some specific statistic) of the covariate within the geographical units, when this information will not be generally available.

Beyond pure specification bias, a well-known example of ecological fallacy is *Robinson's Paradox* (Robinson, 1950) who studied, at an aggregate level, the relationship between the illiteracy rate and the presence of foreign-born population in the United States. Robinson calculated the correlation for these two variables, at an ecological level, being equal to -0.53. Therefore, according to the ecological character of the analysis, we should just conclude that the higher the foreign-born population of a state, the lower its illiteracy rate. Nevertheless, this relationship reverses when studied at an individual level (correlation at the individual level equal to 0.12), i.e., in practice a foreign-born population is less literate than the native U.S. population. This counterintuitive effect can be explained because foreign-born populations tended to settle in places of higher income levels, which showed also lower illiteracy rates. Therefore, in this situation, the aggregate relationship found does not apply at all to an individual level. This occurs because variation within and between areas follow different processes that cannot be disentangled working with just one of these disaggregation levels. The aggregate level is sensible to both sources of variation and if variability between areas overwhelms individual variation within areas, the estimates at the aggregate level can be very different, even opposed, to those at the individual level. Indeed, some authors (Wakefield, 2003) argue that more effort should be placed on the modeling of within-areas variability in ecological regression studies rather than other aspects of these models, such as the spatial dependence of observations.

Figure 5.3 illustrates Robinson's Paradox in graphical terms. The left plot in that figure shows how for each of the groups in the study the relationship between covariate and outcome shows, at an individual level, clear positive correlation meanwhile, at an aggregate level, the group-based estimates (bold symbols) depict a negative correlation. The plot in the right illustrates also this idea in a second simulated example. This plot shows for 40 individuals (10 individuals per age group), all of them smokers, the relationship between the number of daily cigarettes smoked and the number of visits to their doctor during the 3 subsequent years. At the individual level, controlling the age group effect, people who smoke more cigarettes use more healthcare services since for each group the data describe a positive relationship between both variables. In contrast, at the aggregate level, data point out negative dependence. In this case, age plays a confounding effect: older people smoke less in general and visit doctors more frequently. This effect can be controlled at the individual level emerging then the real individual relationship between both variables. At the group level, this relationship is clearly reversed. Thus, this effect, and Robinson's Paradox in general, are particular cases of specification bias, related with the distribution of the covariate within the different groups in the study, which produces this particular kind of ecological bias.

A related example of ecological fallacy is *Simpson's Paradox* (Simpson, 1951), which is indeed a version of Robinson's Paradox for discrete covariates. This paradox, originally formulated for contingency tables in general, states that if two variables are dependent and a third variable comes into the analysis disaggregating the data further, then the original dependence between the first two variables can be even reversed once considered the third factor. Under the disease mapping perspective, Simpson's Paradox can also be considered as a kind of *modifiable areal unit problem* which also states that the relationship between variables will in general depend on the disaggregation level chosen to perform the corresponding analysis (Cressie, 1996). Hence, Robinson's Paradox can be seen as a direct consequence of Simpson's Paradox, that is, when interpreting ecological regression studies we should bear in mind that their conclusions will not generally be valid for another different

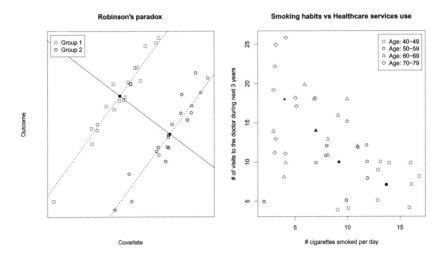

Figure 5.3
Left: General illustration of Robinson's Paradox. Right: Robinson's Paradox in a simulated example on the relationship of smoking habits and healthcare services use. Points are jittered in the right plot. Bold symbols represent the mean of the corresponding groups for both figures.

aggregation level. In particular, results derived at an aggregate level should not be extrapolated to an individual level.

In summary, ecological regression is an extremely useful tool, which due to the general availability of aggregated covariates makes it possible to perform a large number of low-cost epidemiological studies. Inference in ecological regression studies is perfectly legitimate if the covariate represents a contextual variable instead of a summary of individual variables. For example, if we wanted to study the effect of green areas, as purifying environmental devices, or soil composition on the health of people living around, ecological regression would be the adequate tool to measure that effect. Nevertheless, if our main intention is deriving individual estimates of the effect of covariates from ecological studies, we should take extreme care since ecological estimates may not be the outcome that we really expected. It is not reasonable to pretend to draw conclusions at an individual level when we lack information at that level. Deriving individual conclusions should require individual data and the effect of the loss of information when only aggregate data are available may have very distinct consequences. We should be very aware of this limitation of ecological studies.

5.4 Some particular applications of ecological regression

To conclude this chapter, we are going to talk about a couple of particular applications of ecological regression models: spatially varying coefficient models and point source modeling. The first of these settings can be viewed as an enhanced case of ecological regression, while the second is a particular application of that kind of model to a particular problem, the assessment of hazardous facilities with potential damage to health. Both settings have focussed substantial attention in the spatial epidemiology literature, so we are going to review them briefly now.

5.4.1 Spatially varying coefficients models

Varying Coefficient Models date back to Hastie and Tibshirani (1993). These models are regression models where the coefficient(s) of some covariate(s) varies as a smooth function of some other factor(s) in the model. In this manner, these models implicitly assume an enhanced interaction between the covariate of interest and the factor mentioned. Therefore, these models are particularly useful when an effect modifier of the covariate is present and should be controlled. Hastie and Tibshirani introduced Varying Coefficient Models in a more general context where the coefficients varied by means of, for example, kernel smoothers (Fan and Zhang, 1999; Park et al., 2015) or linear combinations of spline (Hastie and Tibshirani, 1993; Huang et al., 2002) depending on a covariate. Nevertheless, from now on, we will focus on Spatially Varying Coefficient Models (SVCMs) where the effects of some covariate vary for each spatial unit (Assunçao, 2003; Gelfand et al., 2003; Mu et al., 2018).

Ecological regression models with a BYM spatial term, in its simplest formulation, have been stated as mixed Poisson regression models where the linear predictor is of the form

$$\log(\boldsymbol{\theta}) = \beta_0 \mathbf{1}_I + \beta_1 \boldsymbol{x} + \boldsymbol{\varphi} + \boldsymbol{\psi} = (\beta_0 \mathbf{1}_I + \boldsymbol{\varphi} + \boldsymbol{\psi}) + \beta_1 \mathbf{x}.$$

In this expression, the random effects have been merged into the intercept, which makes it vary smoothly between spatial units. Therefore, traditional ecological regression models can be seen as regression models with a common slope for the covariate of interest, but with a different intercept for each spatial unit. In the same manner that ecological regression models allow the intercept to vary between spatial units, we could consider the effect of the covariate $\boldsymbol{x}$ to vary also between spatial units. In that case the corresponding SVCM (with

BYM spatial structures) could be formulated as

$$
\begin{aligned}
o_i &\sim Pois(e_i\theta_i) \ i = 1, ..., I \\
\log(\boldsymbol{\theta}) &= \gamma_0 + \gamma_1 \boldsymbol{x} \\
\gamma_0 &= \beta_0 + \varphi_0 + \psi_0 \\
\gamma_1 &= \beta_1 + \varphi_1 + \psi_1 \\
\beta_0, \beta_1 &\sim U(-\infty, \infty) \\
(\varphi_0)_i &\sim N(0, \sigma^2_{\varphi_0}), (\varphi_1)_i \sim N(0, \sigma^2_{\varphi_1}) \ i = 1, ..., I \\
\psi_0 &\sim ICAR(\sigma^2_{\psi_0}), \psi_1 \sim ICAR(\sigma^2_{\psi_1})
\end{aligned}
$$

where once again β_1 stands for the overall effect of the covariate for the set of spatial units in the region of study. Nevertheless, the effect of the covariate will show additional structured variability between spatial units as a consequence of the interaction covariate-spatial units that SVCMs implicitly assume.

It is easy to find examples where the effect of a covariate could vary depending on each particular location or depending on some other factors. For example, mosquitoes are frequent vectors transmitting infectious diseases in humid areas. Presence of mosquitoes, and therefore of the corresponding diseases, in these areas could heavily depend on rainfalls since they determine the presence of standstill waters along a region of study. Nevertheless, the effect of rainfalls could be very different on locations close to the borders of permanent repositories of water, such as rivers or lakes, than for places lacking those repositories. Rainfalls will be much more influential on the presence of the disease in the second case, since they will only host the vector of the disease in humid periods. On the contrary, the disease will be endemic for locations nearby to rivers or lakes where the effect of rainfalls will be much milder. Therefore, rainfall effect would be appropriately modeled in this setting by means of a SVCM.

Gelfand et al. (2003) show also a clear example of this spatially varying effect of covariates in a real estate market case study. In this context, it is clear that the effect of the age of a home in its selling price could be very different depending on its particular location. Thus, old homes in downtowns could be expensive as they could be historical buildings but, on the contrary, old homes in general would be cheaper in many other locations of a city. For all these settings, SVCMs would be the appropriate methodology, whereas naive ecological regression models, with a common effect for the covariate, would yield misleading results.

SVCMs, as posed above, will show in general identifiability problems. When introducing the BYM model, we mentioned identifiability problems between the heterogeneous and spatial random effects since only their sum may be identified. Specifically, the values of these two vectors of random effects may only be identified through their prior structures since the likelihood function only provides information on the sum of both vectors. For SVCMs this problem is more serious since, when assuming BYM structures for the intercept and the slope of the covariate, we have 4 random effects for each observation. So the identifiability problems of the naive BYM model are multiplied in this case. As a consequence, we advise to center the covariate in SVCM models. In that manner, the design matrix of both two terms in the model will be orthogonal, which will favour the identifiability of their coefficients. On the contrary, if the intercept and covariate were highly collinear, any change in the random effects in the intercept could be compensated with another change in those random effects in the covariate. As a consequence, high standard deviations for one of these random effects would be allowable if the other random effect takes also a high standard deviation, producing then dependence in their posterior distributions or even potential posterior impropriety problems. These problems could be prevented by making both terms orthogonal as suggested above. Anyway, Banerjee et al. (2014) (see Section 9.6 of that book) find unappealing some consequences of that orthogonalization and propose some alternative procedures. Specifically, they propose to orthogonalize the design matrix just for the fixed effects in the intercept and covariate terms but not for the random effects. As seen, we prefer to orthogonalize it for all the effects in the model for the reasons exposed.

The identifiability problems pointed out would be alleviated in case of having a vector of observations per spatial unit, with distinct values of the covariate, instead of a single outcome (Assunção et al., 2002; Assunçao, 2003; Congdon, 2007a). In that case all those observations for each spatial unit would contribute to determine the corresponding regression line which will be based on several data points. As a consequence we would not have just a single observation for each 4 random effects per spatial unit. Those several observations per areal unit could be for example the observed deaths for different time periods. In that case, the corresponding SVCM would yield a spatio-temporal model as those developed in Chapter 7. Bernardinelli et al. (1995b), Sun et al. (2000), Assunção et al. (2001), Torres-Avilés and Martinez-Beneito (2015) are some examples of spatio-temporal models defined as SVCMs that we will introduce in that chapter.

The implementation of SVCMs with multiple spatially varying covariates requires particular care. First, confounding problems in models of this kind are exacerbated for the same reasons that we pointed out for SVCMs of a single covariate. If in that case we suggested to make the covariate orthogonal to the intercept as a potential remedy, we should now propose making all the covariates (including the intercept) mutually orthogonal. Regretfully, in that case the original interpretability of the covariates would be lost, making the interpretation of the results much more cumbersome. Moreover, assuming smoothly varying coefficients on covariates which do not have a clear interpretation (orthogonalized variables) may not make too much sense. SVCMs with multiple spatially varying covariates have also motivated the use of multivariate spatial priors, as those introduced in Chapter 8, for the set of spatially varying coefficients (Assunção et al., 2002; Assunçao, 2003; Congdon, 2007a; Banerjee et al., 2014). That is, in this case, the vectors γ_0, γ_1 ... will be assumed to follow a joint prior distribution inducing spatial dependence and covariance for all of them. In this manner, dependence between coefficients, typically arising from the collinearity of covariates, would be taken into account. Besides the adequacy of this assumption for explaining the data, considering a multivariate spatial prior may also improve the performance of MCMC algorithms making them converge better. Thus, the use of those multivariate spatial priors seems, for several reasons, a particularly good idea.

SVCMs can be easily implemented in WinBUGS as a straightforward extension of regular ecological regression models. The implementation of those models in WinBUGS does not require any particular care, except for the identifiability problems already pointed out. Beyond WinBUGS, Gamerman et al. (2003) describe some MCMC algorithms particularly suited for SVCMs. Finally, SVCMs can be also easily implemented in INLA, see for example Franco-Villoria et al. (2018) for some code illustrating the fitting of those models with this function.

5.4.2 Point source modeling

Diseases naturally tend to cluster around specific places, that is why we perform disease mapping studies in order to know which places are showing a higher mortality of the corresponding disease. That clustering, or simple variability in risk, is the consequence of the heterogeneous distribution of determinants of the disease around the study region which makes the distribution of the mortality non-uniform. Nevertheless, despite that natural variability of the disease, there are sometimes locations that contain specific hazardous facilities such as nuclear power plants (Hoffmann et al., 2007), incinerators (Wakefield and Morris, 2002) or foundries (Lawson and Williams, 1994) that could potentially harm the health of people living nearby. In that case, the assessment of the risk caused by those facilities would be also of particular interest. The aim in these problems is quite different to that of general disease mapping problems since, for the first, we are interested in the variations (usually increases) of the risk in some particular places in contrast to the natural geographical variability of the disease. If our aim in a study is highlighting the impact of a hazardous facility, a point source analysis will be much more advisable than a traditional disease mapping study. The latter will smooth the risk pattern all around, including the neighbourhood of the corresponding facility, in contrast to the point source analysis which is specifically devised to make evident the associated risk excess at that precise location.

The assessment of the increase in risk around one or several potential sources is known in the epidemiological literature as *focussed clustering* (Besag and Newell, 1991) and this is the main object of interest of this subsection. Focussed clustering analyses can be posed as either point based or as areal studies as for traditional disease mapping analyses. Point based focussed clustering studies are typically posed as case-control studies where the distribution of these two populations are compared by considering them as point processes. In that case, particular interest is paid to the different distribution of those two populations in the surroundings of the potential risk source (Diggle, 1990; Biggeri and Lagazio, 1999; Diggle et al., 2000).

We will focus henceforth on areal based focussed clustering studies. The assessment of a point source on areal data has focussed considerable attention in the epidemiological literature. Indeed, substantial literature on statistical tests for this purpose has been previously developed (see Stone (1988); Cuzick and Edwards (1990); Waller and Lawson (1995); Bithell (1995); Hoffmann and Schlattmann (1999), for just a few examples). Nevertheless, these tests find important problems for taking into account particular features of the data sets of study, such as fitting the presence of overdispersion or the presence of a confounding effect that should be controlled. As a consequence, model-based point source modeling seems to be a much more flexible alternative for these studies and therefore has focussed more attention in the literature for the last few years.

Model-based point source studies are just a simple particular case of ecological regression models. In this case the covariate of interest would be the exposure to the focus, which is typically summarized as the distance of each areal unit to the potential risk source or some non-linear function of that distance. For measuring that distance, usually the centroid of each areal unit is considered or even a population weighted centroid of each unit. We will denote henceforth as $d = (d_1, ..., d_I)$ the vector of distances of each areal unit to be the focus of interest. We will restrict ourselves from now on to the case of having a single risk source of interest in our study. In case of having more than one risk source in our region of study, the changes to be made to the proposals below would be straightforward (see for example Morris and Wakefield (1999)). Nevertheless, it is usually quite convenient to have several risk sources scattered around the region of study in order to avoid some confounding effect that a single point source could show with the particular conditions of its surrounding region. In case of having several risk sources in our study, those particular conditions will be averaged in general and therefore the potential confounding will be reduced.

A typical formulation of a Bayesian point source model with areal data could be that introduced by Wakefield and Morris (2002). That proposal is a traditional Poisson regression model where the observed cases for each area depend on the corresponding expected cases, and the relative risk is modeled as:

$$\log(\theta_i) = \mu + f(d_i, \gamma) + \varphi_i + \psi_i.$$

This is a typical ecological regression model with intercept (μ), spatial (ψ) and heterogeneous (φ) random effects and a term depending on the covariate d. In this case, $f()$ denotes a non-linear transformation of the covariate, of parameters γ. The presence of the random effects becomes mostly compulsory for point source models, as for ecological regression models in general, since they would control overdispersion and residual spatial dependence if any of them were present. Anyway, attention should be put in order to avoid confounding between the point source effect and the random effects in the analyses as for ecological studies in general. In this sense, centering of the exposure effect could be also a good idea in this context although the use of informative priors for the model parameters have also been proposed as an alternative procedure (Wakefield and Morris, 2002).

Considerable attention has been paid to the functional form of $f()$ in point source models. The adequacy of that functional relationship to the shape of the effect of a point source may have important consequences on the power of the model for detecting that effect. Maybe the simplest, but possibly the most common, choice for $f()$ is considering a far-near scheme where $f(d_i, \gamma) = \gamma_0$ if $d_i < \delta$ and $f(d_i, \gamma) = \gamma_1$ otherwise, for a fixed parameter δ. This radial step-wise definition of $f()$ can be easily generalized to more than 2 discs/rings (Hoffmann and Schlattmann, 1999) allowing for enhanced non-parametric dosis/response relationships. Other authors (Diggle et al., 1997) have also proposed to smooth the step between rings by proposing interim decreasing functions for some rings of $f()$ instead of uniform flat functions for each of those rings. For example, Diggle et al. propose to model the risk in the outer ring as a function of the kind $f(d_i, \gamma) = \gamma_0 \exp(-\gamma_1(d_i - \delta)^2)$, which makes the risk function continuous in the border of the two regions considered. Despite the popularity of this approach, the use of step-wise radial functions for assessing point source exposures shows evident problems. First, the term δ defining the border where the risk changes is generally arbitrary; therefore, it could be easily chosen in order to maximize the significance of the studied point source. As a consequence, a kind of Texas sharpshooter fallacy could easily occur with the arbitrarity introduced with this parameter. Moreover, due to the discrete nature of data, the results could be heavily sensible to the choice of those parameters. Additionally, in case of using step-wise radial functions with more than 2 steps, multiple testing should be borne in mind in order to avoid false positives to flourish in our analyses.

Beyond step-wise radial functions, several enhanced parametric alternatives have been proposed for modeling the relationship between the distance to the focus and its effect on mortality. Thus, for example, Wakefield and Morris (2002) propose to define $f()$ as:

$$f(d_i, \gamma) = \log\left(1 + \gamma_0 \exp\left(-\gamma_1 d_i^2\right)\right). \tag{5.5}$$

In this manner $f()$ will increase up to $\log(1 + \gamma_0)$ as we approach to the focus and the effect of the distance to the focus will tend to 0 as we move farther away. On the other hand, γ_1 controls the range of distances for which the focus has an influence. The authors report inference problems for this function and strong prior sensitivity for γ_0 since the data has very little information on this local parameter for which very few areal units provide some information.

As a consequence, Wakefield and Morris (2002) advocate to not overparameterize the exposure function $f()$ according to that comment. For example, Lawson (1993) proposes an anisotropic function $f()$ which considers different exposures for equidistant points to the focus as a function of their relative position. According to Wakefield and Morris's comment, it would be advisable to avoid such complex functions unless we had a good reason to include them in the model, such as substantial evidence of wind influence on exposure to the point source.

Alternative simple $f()$ functions have been proposed such as $f(d_i, \gamma) = \gamma d_i$ or $f(d_i, \gamma) = \gamma/d_i$ (Morris and Wakefield, 1999). According once again to Wakefield and Morris's comment, selecting a suitable $f()$ will be difficult, as the data provides scarce information on the shape of that exposure function. Nevertheless, the exposure functions mentioned are qualitatively very different, what could guide us for choosing one of them. Thus, the exposure function defined in Expression (5.5) is differentiable and finite in the point source, while $f(d_i, \gamma) = \gamma d_i$ is just finite and $f(d_i, \gamma) = \gamma/d_i$ is neither finite nor differentiable. Moreover, for the first and third of these functions the effect of the point source completely vanishes as we separate from the point source. On the contrary, for $f(d_i, \gamma) = \gamma d_i$, with $\gamma < 0$ (the expected effect of the point source), the risk function will tend to 0 all around as we separate from the point source. As a consequence, this function kills the risk variability, even that of the random effects, for all distant locations to the point source, in contrast to the other two alternatives. Therefore, we can appreciate how the assumptions of the exposure function chosen could be very influential on the risk pattern fitted and we should take particular care in choosing this issue in point source models.

Finally, we would like to finish this section by stressing a typical misuse of point source studies. Sometimes, this kind of study is applied to the massive crossing of point source data sets against mortality data sets comprehending many causes of death. The massive crossing of both data sets is sometimes done in order to find some unknown relationship between different kinds of exposures and mortality for some specific cause. Nevertheless, this procedure is prone to produce also massive false positives as a consequence of multiple testing. Basically, if the amount of different point sources and causes of mortality is large enough, we will usually find positive results unless specific care is taken on multiple testing and error protection. Otherwise, for any point source that we could think of, we will usually find a cause of death associated to the presence of those point sources and, conversely, for any cause of death we will usually find a point source associated to risk excesses for that cause. It is convenient to be aware of this dangerous procedure in order to avoid it and also avoid stating results that will not be replicable in additional posterior studies (Ioannidis, 2005).

Exercises

1. The adjacency matrix of the Valencia city census tracts was already calculated as a Chapter 3 exercise. According to the eigendecomposition of that matrix, what particular spatial pattern(s) should have a covariate for showing a strong confounding effect with an ICAR spatial random effect?

2. The `Deprivation.Rdata` file contains the value of a deprivation index for each of the Valencia city census tracts. That index is based on the 2001 National Spanish Census and negative values of the index mean higher socioeconomic deprivation. Perform an ecological regression model where the log-relative risks are modeled as a linear function of the mentioned deprivation index. Introduce also a spatial term within the model in order to fit additional residual variability and ignore, for now, any possible confounding problem between the covariate and the spatial random effect for this analysis. Do you find association evidence between deprivation and COPD mortality? Describe the spatial pattern associated to deprivation and the remaining residual variability explained by the random effects in the model? Which percentage of the whole variance in the $sSMR$s do these components explain?

3. Compare the linear fit performed in the previous issue with some other non-linear alternative. For example, divide the deprivation index into decile groups and model the effect for this set of groups by means of a random walk process. Do you find evidence of a non-linear relationship? Which model do you prefer for describing the effect of deprivation on COPD mortality?

4. Assess the magnitude of confounding between the deprivation index and the spatial random effect in the linear version of the previous analysis. Does the deprivation index posterior effect and uncertainty substantially change when the spatial random effect is removed from the model? How does the posterior effect and uncertainty of the deprivation index modify when orthogonality restrictions are imposed between that term and the spatial random effects? Assess the impact of all three orthogonality restrictions considered in Example 5.3.

5. The `Deprivation.Rdata` file contains also a second covariate `confound`, which would be expected to show a high confounding effect with the spatial random effect, according to the first exercise of this chapter. Fit now an ecological regression model considering a linear effect of this variable. Assess the confounding for this variable by considering: (i) an ecological regression model with

just this covariate (no additional random effects), (ii) an ecological regression model including this covariate and additional spatial random effects (assume a BYM structure for the random effects), and (iii) the same model as in (ii) but including an orthogonality restriction. Once again consider for (iii) all three orthogonality restrictions in Example 5.3. Do the posterior effect or uncertainty of the covariate effect vary substantially for all these models?

6

Alternative spatial structures

Most of the spatial models previously introduced in this book induce dependence by means of CAR random effects. There are many more options available for inducing spatial dependence that would be convenient to know. This chapter seeks to explore those alternatives to CAR random effects. There is surely no model which is the best option for any possible setting. Particular features of each specific data set such as presence of excessive zeroes, discontinuities or lack of spatial dependence among units will make some models particularly suited for some settings but not for other ones. Knowing the scope of models available will allow choosing always at least a good model for each setting. This is the main goal of this chapter.

Several works have been published comparing disease mapping models with different spatial structures. Among these we find Lawson et al. (2000), Best et al. (2005), Ugarte et al. (2006), Lee (2011), and MacNab (2011). We find particularly relevant the study undertaken in Best et al. (2005) due to the wide variety of (Bayesian) models compared, all of them using very different spatial structures. Richardson (2003) provides also a good review of spatial structures used in the disease mapping literature.

This chapter has been structured according to the main modeling approaches previously followed for inducing spatial dependence in the disease mapping literature. Not all modeling proposals previously published fit within any of the categories in this division. Those works could be considered a sort of isolated proposals which, for now, do not have substantial related works in the literature developing further their ideas. Among those works we find for example: Thurston et al. (2000), Mugglin et al. (2000), Kottas et al. (2007), Nathoo and Ghosh (2013), Rodrigues et al. (2014), Papageorgiou et al. (2015), and Smith et al. (2015). The value of these approaches is not lower than that of the works introduced in the next sections, but we have preferred to focus our attention on the description of the main lines of development followed in the disease mapping literature for the last years. Those popular approaches correspond in our opinion to the next sections of this chapter.

The rest of this chapter is structured as follows: Section 6.1 discusses some additional features (possibly advanced topics) of CAR-based spatial structures that have not been yet addressed in this book. These features have not been previously introduced as they were not essential for the formulation of CAR-based models, which was the main purpose of the previous chapters.

Moreover, most of the topics to be introduced now are a bit more technical than the level used in the previous chapters, so we have preferred to introduce them now that you are more experienced users of these tools. In any case, an appropriate knowledge of these issues will help us get a better knowledge of CAR distributions and associated models which, as already seen, are the default modeling tool for disease mapping. Section 6.2 introduces geostatistics as an alternative tool for modeling spatial dependence in disease mapping studies. Section 6.3 introduces moving-average processes as a third tool for structuring dependence and a series of different proposals for implementing these ideas for spatial modeling. Section 6.4 introduces the use of spline as a convenient low-dimensional smoother for modeling local variations of risks. Finally, Section 6.5 introduces the modeling of some specific features of some data sets that should require particular treatment. Section 6.5 is split into two parts: the modeling of risks by means of partition and discontinuities models, which are appropriate for data sets showing these particular features and the modeling of data sets with zero excesses, a specific kind of overdispersion particularly prevalent in disease mapping studies.

6.1   CAR-based spatial structures

An interesting alternative representation of ICAR random effects that allows a deeper insight of those terms is the following. Let $\sigma^{-2}(\boldsymbol{D} - \boldsymbol{W}) = \boldsymbol{U}\boldsymbol{L}\boldsymbol{U}'$ be the eigendecomposition of the precision matrix of an ICAR distribution, where $\boldsymbol{L} = \sigma^{-2}diag(l_1, ..., l_I)$ contains the corresponding eigenvalues sorted in decreasing order. Therefore, the eigendecomposition of the covariance matrix in the ICAR distribution should be $\sigma^2(\boldsymbol{D} - \boldsymbol{W})^{-1} = \boldsymbol{U}\boldsymbol{L}^{-1}\boldsymbol{U}'$. Then, any ICAR distributed vector φ could be alternatively reexpressed as $\varphi = \boldsymbol{U}\boldsymbol{\epsilon}$ with $\epsilon_i \sim N(0, \sigma^2 l_i^{-1})$. That is, the original ICAR-distributed vector φ can be seen as a linear combination of a set of orthogonal vectors ($\varphi = \sum_j \epsilon_j \boldsymbol{U}_{\cdot j}$), the eigenvectors of its precision matrix. The coefficients $\boldsymbol{\epsilon}$ in that linear combination, although independent, do not take non-informative priors. On the contrary, they are random effects whose variances depend on a common unknown factor σ^2, that should be estimated, and each variance has a different scaling factor l_i^{-1}, implicitly given by the geometry of the region of study. Thus, those coefficients corresponding to the eigenvectors associated to the lowest eigenvalues of $\boldsymbol{D} - \boldsymbol{W}$ will have more variability than those corresponding to the higher eigenvalues. As a consequence, the linear combination $\boldsymbol{U}\boldsymbol{\epsilon}$ will overweigh the eigenvectors corresponding to the lower eigenvalues of $\boldsymbol{D} - \boldsymbol{W}$ and underweigh the rest of their components. As pointed out in Figure 5.2, the eigenvectors whose components in $\boldsymbol{\epsilon}$ have higher variance for the Valencian Region describe linear, quadratic or cubic trends from north to south, having minor variance the components with higher polynomial degree.

As described in Hodges (2013) this performance is very general since polynomial terms of low degree along the largest axis across the region of study usually correspond to those eigenvectors with lowest eigenvalues in $\boldsymbol{L}$. Thus, in terms of Section 5.2.2. of Hodges (2013) (citation slightly modified to adapt it to the notation of this book): "Columns of $\boldsymbol{U}$ (eigenvectors of $\boldsymbol{D} - \boldsymbol{W}$) describing low-frequency or large-scale trends have coefficients that are shrunk least among all the coefficients, so variation in the space of these columns is mostly retained in the fit. Columns of $\boldsymbol{U}$ describing high-frequency or small-scale features have coefficients that are shrunk most among all the coefficients, so variation in the space of these columns is mostly pushed into error". This illustrates how the smoothing procedure in ICAR distribution proceeds; it filters out the variability in the more noisy columns of $\boldsymbol{U}$ while it retains the variability of the more smooth sources of variation according to the geometry of the region of study. This explains and provides a deeper insight on the smooth patterns typically reproduced by ICAR random effects.

As mentioned in Section 4.3, leaving aside the precision term σ^{-2}, the precision matrix of the ICAR distribution $\boldsymbol{D} - \boldsymbol{W}$ is just semidefinite positive. This matrix accomplishes $(\boldsymbol{D} - \boldsymbol{W})\mathbf{1}_I = \mathbf{0}_I$, so $I^{1/2}\mathbf{1}_I$ is an eigenvector of that precision matrix and therefore one of the columns of $\boldsymbol{U}$. As $\boldsymbol{D} - \boldsymbol{W}$ is semidefinite positive all its eigenvalues will be higher than or equal to 0, then $I^{1/2}\mathbf{1}_I$ is the eigenvector $\mathbf{U}_{\cdot I}$ associated to its lowest eigenvalue $l_I = 0$. Similarly, if the region of study was composed of $k > 1$ isolated connected components $\mathcal{C}_1, ..., \mathcal{C}_k$, then the multiplicity of the eigenvalue $l_I = 0$ will be also k and a basis of the eigenvector space corresponding to that eigenvalue would be $\{\boldsymbol{V}_1, ..., \boldsymbol{V}_k\}$ where $(\boldsymbol{V}_k)_i = 1$ if $i \in \mathcal{C}_k$ and 0 otherwise (see Section 5.2.1 in Hodges (2013)). In that case we would have $\mathbf{U}_{\cdot(I-(k-1)):I} = [\boldsymbol{V}_1 : ... : \boldsymbol{V}_k]$. Turning back to the decomposition in the previous paragraph, we had that $\epsilon_i \sim N(0, \sigma^2 l_i^{-1})$, but $l_{I-(k-1)} = ... = l_I = 0$ making the distribution of the latest k elements in $\boldsymbol{\epsilon}$ ill-defined. The infinite variance in these components is precisely the factor making ICAR distributions improper, unless some restriction(s) is imposed on $\boldsymbol{\epsilon}$. Sum-to-zero restrictions for the connected components $\mathcal{C}_1, ..., \mathcal{C}_k$ on ICAR-distributed vectors simply constrain $\boldsymbol{\epsilon}$'s variability on the directions which make its prior distribution improper. That is, these restrictions fix $\epsilon_{I-(k-1)}, ..., \epsilon_I$ to 0 so the decomposition of $\boldsymbol{\varphi}$ in the paragraph above could have been formulated simply as

$$\boldsymbol{\varphi} = \boldsymbol{U}_{[\cdot, 1:(I-k)]} \cdot \boldsymbol{\epsilon}_{1:(I-k)}, \qquad (6.1)$$

which is a low-dimensional representation of the constrained vector $\boldsymbol{\varphi}$. Obviously, this new (constrained) expression for $\boldsymbol{\varphi}$ has a proper prior distribution since the prior distributions of $\boldsymbol{\epsilon}_{1:(I-k)}$ are also proper. This expression makes clear the geometry of the $I - k$ dimensional subspace, embedded into $\mathbb{R}^I$, that contains any random vector corresponding to an ICAR distribution.

Besides an enhanced comprehension of ICAR random effects, expression (6.1) has also an interesting use for ICAR distributed vectors. That expression provides a manner to generate samples from this distribution (see Section 3.2

in Rue and Held (2005)) for carrying out for example simulated studies. Thus, for simulating from an ICAR distribution of variance parameter σ^2 it would be enough to simulate a vector $\boldsymbol{\epsilon}_{1:(I-k)}$ with $\epsilon_i \sim N(0, \sigma^2 l_i^{-1})$ and apply Expression (6.1) for obtaining an ICAR-distributed vector.

Another use of Equation (6.1) would be obtaining a low-dimensional representation of ICAR random effects. Namely, $\boldsymbol{\varphi}$ could be approximated as $\boldsymbol{U}_{[\cdot, J:(I-k)]} \cdot \boldsymbol{\epsilon}_{J:(I-k)}$ for $J \gg 1$. This would remove those terms in $\boldsymbol{U}$ with a lower contribution (the elements corresponding to $\boldsymbol{\epsilon}$ with a lower variance) to the spatial pattern in $\boldsymbol{\varphi}$. Something similar has been proposed in the context of ecological regression by Hughes and Haran (2013) as a computationally efficient way to avoid confounding between fixed and spatial random effects. Hughes and Haran use a different $\boldsymbol{U}$ matrix that takes into account the geometric arrangement of the region of study and in principle makes it possible to achieve appropriate low-dimensional representations with few dimensions. Namely, retaining just 10% of the columns in their $\boldsymbol{U}$ matrix would be enough according to these authors. Nevertheless, according to Hughes and Haran's proposal, the prior distribution of $\boldsymbol{\epsilon}_{J:(I-k)}$ should be multivariate Normal with a dense covariance matrix, what could be a problem for large I. Nevertheless, beyond ecological regression, the low-dimensional representation above, with a diagonal covariance matrix for $\boldsymbol{\epsilon}$, could be a computationally convenient approach to disease mapping. However, the selection of an appropriate number of dimensions to be used to approximate the ICAR random effects is something to be further explored.

A similar eigenvector decomposition could be done of the precision matrix of other CAR distributions, such as PCAR. Nevertheless, in that case, the set of eigenvectors $\boldsymbol{U}(\rho)$ and the variability of the coefficients $\boldsymbol{\epsilon}(\rho)$ would depend on the eigendecomposition of $\boldsymbol{D} - \rho\boldsymbol{W}$ and therefore on the unknown value ρ. Then the interpretation of this eigendecomposition will be less clear than for the ICAR case. Regarding the PCAR distribution, Assunçao and Krainski (2009) find also strong connections between many of the statistical properties of PCAR distributed vectors and the eigenvalues/eigenvectors of the matrix $\boldsymbol{D}^{-1}\boldsymbol{W}$. Specifically, they interpret this matrix as the transition matrix of a Markovian stochastic process on the lattice of study, thus $(\boldsymbol{D}^{-1}\boldsymbol{W})^k$ could be also interpreted as the k-steps-ahead transition matrix of that Markovian process. They further use the following identity

$$
\begin{aligned}
(\boldsymbol{D} - \rho\boldsymbol{W})^{-1} &= (I - \rho\boldsymbol{D}^{-1}\boldsymbol{W})^{-1}\boldsymbol{D}^{-1} \\
&= (I + \rho\boldsymbol{D}^{-1}\boldsymbol{W} + \rho^2(\boldsymbol{D}^{-1}\boldsymbol{W})^2 + \rho^3(\boldsymbol{D}^{-1}\boldsymbol{W})^3 + ...)\boldsymbol{D}^{-1}
\end{aligned}
\tag{6.2}
$$

in order to obtain an analytic approximation of the variance-covariance matrix of PCAR distributions. This is an interesting result since variance-covariance matrices of general PCAR distributions on irregular lattices do not have analytical known closed forms. Thus this result gives us substantial intuition on those unknown matrices. A straightforward consequence of Expression (6.2) is that the covariance structure of PCAR vectors cannot be simply explained by just first-order neighbours, but it also depends on the paths of higher order that link any two areal units. This explains many of the alleged problems of PCAR distributions according to Wall (2004) such as different marginal variances or correlations for units which have the same number of neighbours. Those features could be explained by the overall structure of the graph instead of the local position of the units with regards to their neighbours. Interestingly, Assunçao and Krainski find analytically (for Gaussian likelihoods) that most of the non-intuitive features in the covariance matrix of PCAR random effects raised in Wall (2004) are mitigated in their posterior distribution.

The series expansion in Expression (6.2) converges for $\|\rho\| < 1$. Moreover, its rate of convergence depends mainly on the magnitude of l_2, the second larger eigenvalue of $\boldsymbol{D}^{-1}\boldsymbol{W}$ (the first larger eigenvalue is always $l_1 = 1$). The authors find that for smaller values of l_2, the rate of convergence of the series is faster; therefore, the corresponding variance-covariance matrix could be reasonably approximated by a few elements in the series. As a consequence, variances and covariances of the elements of $\boldsymbol{\varphi}$ depend mainly on just their closer neighbours. On the contrary, if l_2 is larger, those properties depend strongly on more distant units. Thus l_2 strongly determines the covariance in $\boldsymbol{\varphi}$, whether this is more local or depends more on the overall structure of the graph of the region of study. Additionally, Assunçao and Krainski (2009) show also that for many typical lattices used in disease mapping l_2 is usually quite high, making the spatial dependence of PCAR distributions on those lattices to be not so local as could be thought according to their conditional definition. As a consequence, the overall geometric configuration of the region of study plays usually an important additional role on these random effects beyond the local arrangement of each unit of study.

MacNab (2014) makes a parallel view of Expression (6.2) but for Leroux et al.'s LCAR distributions. Specifically, she finds that the correlation between any two units for the LCAR distribution is always larger than that for the PCAR distribution when a common value is set to the correlation parameters of both distributions. Thus, LCAR induces stronger correlation structures than PCAR for the same value of the dependence parameter. This alleviates one of the alleged problems of the PCAR distribution, the low spatial dependence for most of the possible values of ρ. MacNab (2014) shows also that, for a common spatial dependence parameter ρ, the correlation between areal units tends to 0, as a function of distance between units, at a slower speed for this distribution than for PCAR. Thus the range of dependence for LCAR distributions is, for a same ρ, larger than for PCAR. Additionally, Rodrigues et al. (2014) also use Expression (6.2) for the study of the theoretical properties of the spatial model of LeSage and Pace (2007), based on an exponential matrix representation. Rodrigues et al. evidence some pathological features of the covariance structure of this model that were previously unnoticed. In our opinion, studies of this kind exploring covariance structures of spatial models and their relationship with the structure of the graph of the region of study should be encouraged. These studies undoubtedly provide an enhanced understanding of the details of those dependence structures.

Expression (6.2) has a final interesting consequence. The matrices in that series expansion are sparse, sparser for the first components. Specifically, the k-th of these matrices will have a non-null element in its (i,j) cell if there is a path through k (or less) units in the region of study joining units i and j. Thus, if i and j are distant units, the first matrices in the series expansion in (6.2) will not contribute anything to their covariance. Moreover, the non-null elements of the matrices in that expansion will be all positive. Thus, covariance matrices for both PCAR and LCAR distributions will have all their cells positive and tending to 0 as long as the distance between units increases. Therefore, in this sense, the covariance matrices for these two random effects have a similar performance to that of geostatistical models (Diggle et al., 1998), which seems a very sensible performance.

Although they seem very similar at a first glance, the correlation structure of the ICAR distribution is very different from that of the PCAR and LCAR distribution. As the series expansion in Expression (6.2) converges for $\|\rho\| < 1$ it may not be applied to the study of ICAR distributed vectors. Thus, we do not have any parallel version of that expression for the ICAR distribution, which would provide also analytic insight on its covariance matrix. Nevertheless, some works have shown some unpleasant features on the covariance structure of ICAR vectors (MacNab, 2011; Botella-Rocamora et al., 2012). Those features are summarized in Figure 6.1. All correlations shown in that figure have been drawn from the Moore-Penrose generalized inverse of $\sigma^{-2}(D - W)$ for both studies considered. We will justify at the end of this section why this matrix should be used as covariance matrix for ICAR-distributed vectors. The upper side of Figure 6.1 studies the correlation between different sites for a linear shaped region composed of 51 consecutive units, where unit i has units $i-1$ and $i+1$ as neighbours for $i = 2, ..., 50$. The red, blue and green curves correspond, respectively, to the correlation function of the 13-th, 26-th and 51-th positions in the linear lattice considered. Each of these curves depicts the correlation of the corresponding unit with the rest of the positions in the lattice. The first unappealing feature in that plot is that all three correlation functions become negative for distant units. This is a consequence of the sum-to-zero constraint imposed on the ICAR vector which implicitly makes the observations for some sites to necessarily have opposite performances, otherwise that constraint would not be fulfilled. Obviously, those more distant locations would be the appropriate pairs for having that opposite performance, consequently their correlation becomes negative. In principle, the performance of the correlation functions for PCAR or LCAR distributions seems much more reasonable as, for these, the correlation for any pair of sites tends to 0 for higher distances. This performance would be in accordance with independence between distant regions, which seems a more reasonable assumption than having an opposite performance. Negative correlations between distant regions imply that an increase in the risk in a specific site of the map should decrease the risk for the opposite far region of the map, which does not seem to have any epidemiological sense.

The lower side of Figure 6.1 performs a similar correlation analysis for an irregular spatial lattice, the Valencian Region. Specifically, the lower-left side of the figure shows the correlation between Castellón (dark green region in the northeast) and the rest of the municipalities in the Valencian Region for an ICAR distributed vector. The lower-right side shows the correlation between Valencia (dark green region in the east) and the rest of the municipalities. For this irregular lattice, distant regions show once again negative correlations reproducing the previously described effect in the linear lattice. Nevertheless, the irregularity of the region of study causes some less intuitive results. Thus, for the lower-right map, the regions at the south of Valencia with negative correlations are much closer geographically to this municipality than those in the north. Moreover, we can also find some municipalities in the south of the lower-left map with low negative correlations when they are surrounded of municipalities with high negative correlations. All these municipalities with low correlations have very few neighbours, making their conditional variances to be higher. Thus, the information from their neighbours is low in comparison to their variability, what makes their correlation to be closer to 0.

Figure 6.1 shows also a second unpleasant feature. ICAR random effects depend on a single parameter that controls their variance and therefore correlations cannot be tuned or modified for any of the plots in that figure. As a consequence, correlations with respect to a particular place are positive for approximately one half of the units for all cases considered. This feature of the ICAR distribution can be inappropriate in many cases. For example, if a disease showed spatial dependence of very short range in the Valencian Region, such as dependence for at most one or two neighbours away (otherwise units would be independent), then the ICAR would necessarily induce dependence of longer range. Nevertheless, this could be worse if the region of study was larger. In national instead of regional studies, using an ICAR distribution for random effects would implicitly assume spatial positive dependence for units separated much farther away than for studies in the Valencian Region. This is a strong assumption, linked to the region of study used, that the ICAR distribution does not allow to modify. Moreover, Botella-Rocamora et al. (2012) show (for the linear-shaped case) that this performance of ICAR is not alleviated by using the BYM proposal instead. The BYM model, by introducing a heterogeneous term, makes the correlation functions in the upper side of Figure 6.1 flatter. Nevertheless, the shapes of those functions are basically maintained: they cancel at exactly the same places and they are positive, respectively negative, at exactly the same units as ICAR. Thus, in contrast to PCAR or LCAR, which allow to modulate the range of spatial dependence, both ICAR and BYM are fairly rigid in this sense.

An appropriate understanding of the correlation structure of the main distributions used for disease mapping, such as ICAR, LCAR or PCAR, is very

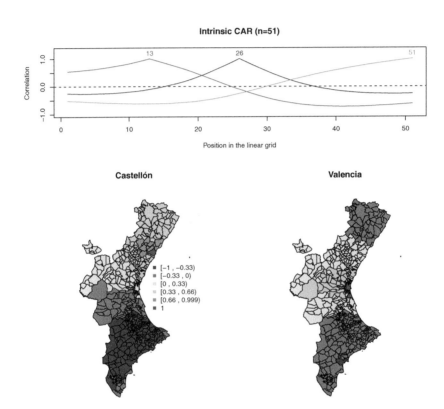

Figure 6.1
Correlation structure of the ICAR distribution for specific locations of a linear-shaped lattice composed of 51 consecutive units (upper plot), the Valencian Region (lower plots).

important. Thus, it is usual to set out simulation studies in order to compare the ability of these (or another) tools to model different simulated spatial patterns (Best et al., 1999; Martinez-Beneito et al., 2008; Lee, 2011). However, some specific simulation procedures will be particularly suited for some of these tools, possibly producing then biased results and conclusions. For example, imposing positive spatial dependence for all the risks in a region of studying could be particularly convenient for LCAR or PCAR distributions, which induce positive spatial dependence between any two spatial units. We should bear these considerations in mind in order to avoid to yield biased results favouring, by design, one of these (or other) options.

A number of variants have been proposed of traditional CAR-based disease mapping models, mainly for BYM (MacNab, 2011; Simpson et al., 2017). Thus, MacNab (2011) reformulates the log-risks for the BYM model as

$$\log(\boldsymbol{\theta}) = \mu \mathbf{1}_I + \sqrt{\lambda}\boldsymbol{\varphi} + \sqrt{1-\lambda}\boldsymbol{\psi}$$

for $\boldsymbol{\varphi} \sim ICAR(\sigma^2)$, $\boldsymbol{\psi} \sim N(\mathbf{0}, \sigma^2 \boldsymbol{I}_I)$ and $\lambda \sim U(0,1)$, although she carries out a sensitivity analysis for several alternative prior distributions of λ. For this parameterization the variance-covariance matrix of the log-risks would be

$$\boldsymbol{\Sigma} = \sigma^2 (\lambda (\boldsymbol{D} - \boldsymbol{W})^- + (1-\lambda)\boldsymbol{I}_I)$$

i.e., a mixture of the variance-covariance matrices of the ICAR and heterogeneous random effects. As explained by MacNab, the reasoning for this parameterization is favouring the identifiability of the components (mainly the variances) in the BYM model and avoiding some of the inference problems associated with the lack of identifiability in its original formulation (Eberly and Carlin, 2000). In that original formulation, the variances of the two random effects involved in the model, σ_φ^2 and σ_ψ^2, competed to explain a single source of variability identifiable by the data, the variance of $\log(\boldsymbol{\theta})$. For this new formulation, λ balances the weight of these two sources of variance, favouring then their identifiability. So, instead of having two variables competing for a single identifiable term, MacNab's proposal has a single variable σ^2 explaining the whole variability of $\log(\boldsymbol{\theta})$ and an additional variable λ modeling the spatial/heterogeneous character of the geographical pattern. Riebler et al. (2016) propose a scaling of the ICAR precision matrix in this context in order to set additional sensible prior distributions on λ.

MacNab's BYM reparameterization is in some sense similar to the BYM reparameterization used throughout this book, which puts the standard deviations of the random effects as multiplicative factors in the linear predictor of the Poisson regression. We have found great computational advantage, at least in the `WinBUGS` implementation of this model, when putting these parameters out of the random effects; this is mainly why we opt for this parameterization. Nevertheless, there is a second feature that we also like of our proposed alternative. In our case, we have a clear control of the prior distributions of the standard deviations of the random effects, which are intuitive variables measured in the same scale as the data. This makes us feel relatively safe and comfortable. Specifically, we put uniform vague priors on those standard deviations as recommended by some other authors in the literature (see Chapter 4 for a more detailed discussion on this). MacNab's proposal would be equivalent to putting standard deviations of $\sqrt{\lambda}\sigma$ and $\sqrt{1-\lambda}\sigma$ respectively, for both random effects in the model. If a uniform vague prior distribution was assigned to σ and $\lambda \sim U(0,1)$ this would imply a decreasing prior distribution for both standard deviations with modes in 0 in contrast to the uniform prior distribution used by other authors. The influence of this prior choice could be important since λ has been found to be weakly identifiable and prior sensitivity has been also reported for it (MacNab, 2014).

Other different reparameterizations of the BYM model have also been proposed for different purposes. Thus, Congdon (2007b) proposes the following reparameterization of the log-risks

$$\log(\boldsymbol{\theta}) = \mu\mathbf{1}_I + \boldsymbol{\eta} \circ \boldsymbol{\varphi} + (\mathbf{1}_I - \boldsymbol{\eta}) \circ \boldsymbol{\psi}$$

for $\boldsymbol{\varphi}$ and $\boldsymbol{\psi}$ being ICAR and heterogeneous random effects, respectively, of different variances and $\eta_i \sim Beta(h,h)$. The operator $\circ$ in the expression above denotes the component-wise product of two vectors, as defined in Chapter 1. Congdon's proposal is similar to that of MacNab but with different weights for the spatial and heterogeneous effects for each unit and without square roots on those weights. Congdon (2007b) motivates this reparameterization of BYM as a flexibilization of that model allowing a spatially adaptive balance between both random effects in the model. Nevertheless, the identification of the parameters of this model can be quite problematic as the log-risk for each areal unit depends on three parameters. Moreover, two of them are spatially heterogeneous, which makes the transferring of information between neighbouring units, and therefore available, more limited.

A second modification of the BYM model proposed also by Congdon (2007b) would consider

$$\log(\boldsymbol{\theta}) = \mu\mathbf{1}_I + \boldsymbol{\varphi} + \boldsymbol{\delta} \circ \boldsymbol{\psi}$$

for $\boldsymbol{\varphi}$ and $\boldsymbol{\psi}$ being, once again, ICAR and heterogeneous random effects and $\delta_i \sim Bernoulli(\gamma)$, where γ is an additional parameter in the model. This makes heterogeneity present only for some specific locations where it could be specifically needed. Congdon warns about identifiability problems on γ and suggests the use of informative prior distributions for the precisions of $\boldsymbol{\varphi}$ and $\boldsymbol{\psi}$ in order to alleviate those problems. He suggests to run two previous versions of the model, pure spatial and pure heterogeneous, in order to estimate both precisions and use those estimates for setting up informative priors.

Lawson and Clark (2002) also propose a variation of the BYM model, specifically, they propose to model the log-risks as:

$$\log(\boldsymbol{\theta}) = \mu\mathbf{1}_I + \boldsymbol{\psi} + \boldsymbol{\eta} \circ \boldsymbol{\varphi} + (\mathbf{1}_I - \boldsymbol{\eta}) \circ \boldsymbol{\phi}$$

where φ and ψ are ICAR and heterogeneous random effects, as usual. Now, ϕ is an ICAR vector of spatial random effects but based on conditional Laplace distributions instead of Normal distributions (see Section 4.3 for a more in-depth description of this distribution). Besides, the components of $\boldsymbol{\eta}$ are assumed to have independent $Beta(h, h)$ distributions with h fixed to either 0.5 or 1. The vector ϕ is better suited than φ for modeling discontinuities in the risk surface. Thus, the motivation for this proposal is having an adaptive model able to choose between a continuous or discontinuous performance at each site. If continuity is considered more convenient, the corresponding η_i will take a value close to 1, giving higher weight to the Normal ICAR component; on the contrary, if a discontinuity is found more convenient for that unit, the corresponding η_i would be close to 0. Note, however, the high number of parameters of this model, which uses 4 specific variables for modeling each log-risk. In fact, Lu and Carlin (2005) report that they had to fix $\eta_i = 0.5$ for achieving identifiability in this model. All three previous modifications of BYM can be easily implemented in `WinBUGS`; however, to our knowledge their implementation is not so straightforward (if possible) in `INLA`.

Some other modifications of popular CAR-based models have also been proposed yielding sensible models. Thus, Congdon (2008) proposed a spatially adaptive modification of the LCAR distribution with different spatial correlation parameters for each areal unit. In case of using an adjacency criterion for defining relations between neighbors, Congdon's proposal could be defined as:

$$\varphi_i | \boldsymbol{\varphi}_{-i}, \sigma, \boldsymbol{\lambda} \sim N\left(\frac{\lambda_i}{1 - \lambda_i + \lambda_i n_i} \sum_{j \sim i} \lambda_j \varphi_j, \frac{\sigma^2}{1 - \lambda_i + \lambda_i n_i}\right),$$

where n_i is the number of neighbours of unit i. If $\boldsymbol{\Lambda} = diag(\lambda_1, ..., \lambda_I)$ is a diagonal matrix with the spatial correlation parameters for each unit, this ensemble of conditional distributions yields a multivariate Normal distribution for $\boldsymbol{\varphi}$ with precision matrix $\sigma^{-2}(\boldsymbol{\Lambda Q} + (\boldsymbol{I}_I - \boldsymbol{\Lambda}))$ for $Q_{ii} = n_i$, $Q_{ij} = -\lambda_j$ if $j \sim i$ and 0 otherwise. The weighting of the non-diagonal cells of $\boldsymbol{Q}$ as a function of the correlation parameters makes symmetric the resulting precision matrix. This model, as the original Leroux et al. (1999) proposal is able to reproduce either ICAR distributions for $\boldsymbol{\Lambda} = \boldsymbol{I}$ or i.i.d. Normal random effects for $\boldsymbol{\Lambda} = \boldsymbol{0}_I$. In addition, and in contrast to the original LCAR, this model is also able to reflect different degrees of spatial dependence for each location of the region of study. Different prior distributions are proposed for the spatial correlation parameters such as beta, logit-Normal or probit-Normal Congdon (2008). The two latter options are more suitable to be modeled than the beta distribution, which can be an advantage, as that distribution is used as a prior for a long vector of variables. See the example in the original paper for several specific modeling proposals having logit-Normal prior distributions. This proposal can be easily implemented in `WinBUGS` by coding the conditional distributions reproduced above, as for the implementation of the original LCAR.

The intrinsic CAR distribution is sometimes alternatively formulated (Besag et al., 1991) as a function of pairwise differences between neighbours as

$$P(\varphi|\sigma) \propto \exp\left(\frac{-1}{2\sigma^2}\sum_{i=1}^{I}\sum_{\{j\sim i:j>i\}} w_{ij}(\varphi_i - \varphi_j)^2\right). \tag{6.3}$$

This relationship is made evident by considering that the precision matrix of any ICAR process $D - W$ can be expressed as $\sum_{i=1}^{I}\sum_{\{j\sim i:j>i\}} Q_{ij}$, for Q_{ij} being an $I \times I$ matrix with $(Q_{ij})_{ii} = (Q_{ij})_{jj} = w_{ij}$, $(Q_{ij})_{ij} = (Q_{ij})_{ji} = -w_{ij}$ and 0 otherwise. Therefore,

$$P(\varphi|\sigma) \propto \exp\left(\frac{-1}{2\sigma^2}\varphi'\left(D - W\right)\varphi\right)$$

$$= \exp\left(\frac{-1}{2\sigma^2}\varphi'\left(\sum_{i=1}^{I}\sum_{\{j\sim i:j>i\}} Q_{ij}\right)\varphi\right)$$

$$= \exp\left(\frac{-1}{2\sigma^2}\sum_{i=1}^{I}\sum_{\{j\sim i:j>i\}}\varphi'Q_{ij}\varphi\right)$$

$$= \exp\left(\frac{-1}{2\sigma^2}\sum_{i=1}^{I}\sum_{\{j\sim i:j>i\}} w_{ij}(\varphi_i - \varphi_j)^2\right).$$

For adjacency-based neighbours, every w_{ij} would be simply equal to 1 in this expression. Therefore, if φ were time-referenced variables instead of being referred to as spatial locations, such as for the upper side of Figure 6.1, then units i and j would be neighbours if and only if $|i-j| = 1$. In that case, Expression (6.3) would trivially yield a first-order random walk process. Therefore, in this sense the intrinsic CAR distribution is considered a generalization to irregular spatial lattices of the first-order random walk time process (Besag and Newell, 1991; Botella-Rocamora et al., 2012). Expression (6.3) makes that relationship evident.

Expression (6.3) makes also particularly evident the impropriety of ICAR distributions. That expression yields the same probability to any vector φ and to $\varphi + \mu\mathbf{1}_I$ for any value of μ. This is because μ cancels out the differences in the right-hand side of Expression (6.3). As a consequence, the ICAR distribution does not change the probability of vectors when we increase (or decrease) all their components in a same amount, this makes the integral of its density function to be infinite as it does not decrease when moving along that direction. Sum-to-zero restrictions make that if $\sum_i \varphi_i = 0$ for a certain vector φ then $\sum_i(\varphi_i + \mu) = \sum\varphi + I\mu = I\mu$, which is zero only for $\mu = 0$. That is, the sum-to-zero constraint restricts the possible values of φ along the direction that makes the ICAR distribution improper, fixing therefore that impropriety.

Another reformulation of ICAR distributions as a function of pairwise differences of elements of φ is the following: for any two neighbouring units i

and j with $j > i$ just assume $\varphi_i - \varphi_j \sim N(0, w_{ij}^{-1}\sigma^2)$. This would yield the following joint distribution

$$\prod_{i=1}^{I} \prod_{\{i \sim j : j > i\}} \exp\left(\frac{-1}{2\sigma^2} w_{ij}(\varphi_i - \varphi_j)^2\right),$$

which is obviously equivalent to Expression (6.3). The main advantage of this latter formulation is that it admits a convenient matrix expression. Thus, the independent Normal distributions above on $\varphi_i - \varphi_j$ for $i \sim j$ can be reexpressed as $\boldsymbol{C\varphi} = \boldsymbol{\epsilon}$, where $\boldsymbol{\epsilon} = N(\boldsymbol{0}, \sigma^2 diag(\boldsymbol{w}^{-1}))$ and $\boldsymbol{w}$ denotes the vector containing the non-zero weights w_{ij} of $\boldsymbol{W}$ for an (irrelevant) specific ordering. Matrix $\boldsymbol{C}$ in the expression above is of dimension $m \times I$, for m being the total number of neighbours for the region of study. Each row of $\boldsymbol{C}$ corresponds to a pair of neighbours, i and j, in the graph defining the region of study. Each row in $\boldsymbol{C}$ will have all its cells equal to 0 except for the i-th and j-th positions which are respectively equal to 1 and -1. Obviously, the order for the rows of $\boldsymbol{C}$ and the components of $\boldsymbol{w}$ should be the same.

Note that the diagonal elements of $\boldsymbol{C'C}$ are simply the number of neighbours of each unit and the non-diagonal terms are equal to -1 if units i and j are neighbours and 0 otherwise. Thus, if adjacency was the neighbouring criterion for building the graph of the region of study, then $\boldsymbol{C'C}$ would be equal to $\boldsymbol{D} - \boldsymbol{W}$. More generally, for a weighted neighbouring criterion, $\boldsymbol{C'}diag(\boldsymbol{w})\boldsymbol{C}$ would be then equal to $\boldsymbol{D} - \boldsymbol{W}$ for $\boldsymbol{W}$ being now a weighted matrix. This identity allows a deeper understanding of the matrix $\boldsymbol{C'}diag(\boldsymbol{w})\boldsymbol{C}$, which can be decomposed as $\boldsymbol{C'}diag(\boldsymbol{w})\boldsymbol{C} = \boldsymbol{ULU'}$, where $\boldsymbol{U}$ and $\boldsymbol{L}$ are the matrices with the eigenvectors and eigenvalues of $\boldsymbol{D} - \boldsymbol{W}$. As a consequence, $\boldsymbol{C'}diag(\boldsymbol{w})\boldsymbol{C}$ is not of full rank and has (at least) one eigenvector associated to the eigenvalue 0. That eigenvalue $\boldsymbol{U}_{\cdot I}$ is proportional to $\boldsymbol{1}_I$, thus we can put

$$\boldsymbol{C'}diag(\boldsymbol{w})\boldsymbol{C} = \sum_{i=1}^{I} l_i \boldsymbol{U}_{\cdot i}(\boldsymbol{U}_{\cdot i})' \tag{6.4}$$

with $l_I = 0$, this expression will be used in a couple of paragraphs. For the next few paragraphs, we will assume that the region of study has a single connected component; so, therefore, the eigenvalue $l_I = 0$ has multiplicity 1 and $\{l_i : i = 1, ..., I-1\}$ will all be positive. This will save us from introducing specific comments throughout for the case of having more than one connected component.

The formulation above defines the ICAR distribution through a set of linear combinations $(\boldsymbol{C\varphi})$ of the original vector of variables $\boldsymbol{\varphi}$. These linear combinations follow independent Normal distributions. Under this approach imposing linear restrictions, such as sum-to-zero restrictions, and studying their effect on the resulting covariance matrix of ICAR vectors is quite easy. Specifically, an overall sum-to-zero restriction could be imposed by considering $\boldsymbol{C^*} = [\boldsymbol{C'}, \boldsymbol{1}_I]'$ instead of $\boldsymbol{C}$ and $\boldsymbol{C^*\varphi} = \boldsymbol{\epsilon^*}$, where $\boldsymbol{\epsilon^*} = (\boldsymbol{\epsilon}, 0) \sim N(\boldsymbol{0}, \sigma^2 diag((\boldsymbol{w}^{-1}, 0)))$. This expression will allow us to derive the variance-covariance matrix of any ICAR distributed vector constrained by a sum-to-zero restriction.

The good thing about $\boldsymbol{C}^*$ is that $(\boldsymbol{C}^*)'diag((\boldsymbol{w},a))\boldsymbol{C}^*$ is invertible for any $a > 0$, in contrast to $(\boldsymbol{C})'diag(\boldsymbol{w})\boldsymbol{C}$. Let's see this

$$
\begin{aligned}
(\boldsymbol{C}^*)'diag((\boldsymbol{w},a))\boldsymbol{C}^* &= \begin{pmatrix} \boldsymbol{C}' & \boldsymbol{1}_I \end{pmatrix} \begin{pmatrix} diag(\boldsymbol{w}) & \boldsymbol{0} \\ \boldsymbol{0} & a \end{pmatrix} \begin{pmatrix} \boldsymbol{C} \\ \boldsymbol{1}'_I \end{pmatrix} \\
&= \boldsymbol{C}'diag(\boldsymbol{w})\boldsymbol{C} + a\boldsymbol{1}_I\boldsymbol{1}'_I \\
&= \sum_{i=1}^{I} l_i \boldsymbol{U}_{\cdot 1}(\boldsymbol{U}_{\cdot 1})' + a I \boldsymbol{U}_{\cdot I}(\boldsymbol{U}_{\cdot I})' \\
&= \sum_{i=1}^{I} l_i^* \boldsymbol{U}_{\cdot i}(\boldsymbol{U}_{\cdot i})'
\end{aligned}
$$

where $l_i^* = l_i$ for $i = 1, ..., I - 1$ and $l_I^* = aI > 0$. Thus $(\boldsymbol{C}^*)'diag((\boldsymbol{w},a))\boldsymbol{C}^*$ share eigenvectors with $\boldsymbol{D} - \boldsymbol{W}$ but, in contrast to this matrix, has all positive eigenvalues so it is therefore invertible.

Turning back to the expression $\boldsymbol{C}^*\boldsymbol{\varphi} = \boldsymbol{\epsilon}^*$ of the ICAR distribution, now we can make, for any $a > 0$

$$
\begin{aligned}
\boldsymbol{\varphi} &= ((\boldsymbol{C}^*)'diag((\boldsymbol{w},a))\boldsymbol{C}^*)^{-1}(\boldsymbol{C}^*)'diag((\boldsymbol{w},a))\boldsymbol{C}^*\boldsymbol{\varphi} \\
&= ((\boldsymbol{C}^*)'diag((\boldsymbol{w},a))\boldsymbol{C}^*)^{-1}(\boldsymbol{C}^*)'diag((\boldsymbol{w},a))\boldsymbol{\epsilon}^*.
\end{aligned}
$$

Bearing in mind that $\boldsymbol{\epsilon}^* \sim N(\boldsymbol{0}, \sigma^2 diag((\boldsymbol{w}^{-1},0)))$ the variance-covariance matrix of $\boldsymbol{\varphi}$ results

$$
\begin{aligned}
&((\boldsymbol{C}^*)'diag((\boldsymbol{w},a))\boldsymbol{C}^*)^{-1}(\boldsymbol{C}^*)'diag((\boldsymbol{w},a)) \cdot \sigma^2 diag((\boldsymbol{w}^{-1},0)) \cdot \\
&\quad diag((\boldsymbol{w},a))\boldsymbol{C}^*((\boldsymbol{C}^*)'diag((\boldsymbol{w},a))\boldsymbol{C}^*)^{-1} \\
&= \sigma^2((\boldsymbol{C}^*)'diag((\boldsymbol{w},a))\boldsymbol{C}^*)^{-1}(\boldsymbol{C}^*)'diag((\boldsymbol{w},0))\boldsymbol{C}^* \\
&\quad \cdot((\boldsymbol{C}^*)'diag((\boldsymbol{w},a))\boldsymbol{C}^*)^{-1} \\
&= \sigma^2((\boldsymbol{C}^*)'diag((\boldsymbol{w},a))\boldsymbol{C}^*)^{-1}\boldsymbol{C}'diag(\boldsymbol{w})\boldsymbol{C}((\boldsymbol{C}^*)'diag((\boldsymbol{w},a))\boldsymbol{C}^*)^{-1} \\
&= \sigma^2 \left(\sum_{i=1}^{I}(l_i^*)^{-1}\boldsymbol{U}_{\cdot i}(\boldsymbol{U}_{\cdot i})' \right) \left(\sum_{j=1}^{I} l_j \boldsymbol{U}_{\cdot j}(\boldsymbol{U}_{\cdot j})' \right) \left(\sum_{k=1}^{I}(l_k^*)^{-1}\boldsymbol{U}_{\cdot k}(\boldsymbol{U}_{\cdot k})' \right) \\
&= \sigma^2 \left(\sum_{i=1}^{I}(l_i^*)^{-1}l_i(l_i^*)^{-1}\boldsymbol{U}_{\cdot i}(\boldsymbol{U}_{\cdot i})' \right) = \sigma^2 \left(\sum_{i=1}^{I-1} l_i^{-1}\boldsymbol{U}_{\cdot i}(\boldsymbol{U}_{\cdot i})' \right).
\end{aligned}
$$

The latter expression corresponds to the Moore-Penrose generalized inverse of $\sigma^{-2}(\boldsymbol{D} - \boldsymbol{W})$. Thus, it is interesting to check that among all the generalized inverses of $\sigma^{-2}(\boldsymbol{D} - \boldsymbol{W})$, the variance-covariance matrix of $\boldsymbol{\varphi}$, when this is constrained by a sum-to-zero restriction, is precisely its Moore-Penrose generalized inverse. This has been the covariance matrix used for reproducing the graphs in Figure 6.1. Note that this covariance matrix is also rank deficient as it has the same number of null eigenvalues than the precision matrix of the ICAR distribution.

Note that the identities used for developing the expression of the covariance matrix of φ hold regardless of the value chosen for $a > 0$, thus this value has no significant contribution to the final expression. Note also that those identities are valid since the sum-to-zero restriction imposed has made the expression $(\boldsymbol{C}^*)'diag((\boldsymbol{w}, a))\boldsymbol{C}^*$ used in there invertible, in contrast to $\boldsymbol{C}'diag(\boldsymbol{w})\boldsymbol{C}$. Thus, the Moore-Penrose generalized inverse of $\sigma^{-2}(\boldsymbol{D} - \boldsymbol{W})$ would not be necessarily the variance-covariance matrix of φ unless the sum-to-zero restriction on this vector was not imposed. Thus, imposing that restriction has been essential for determining which one of the generalized inverses of the precision matrix is suitable as covariance matrix for φ.

6.2   Geostatistical modeling

An alternative way of inducing geographical dependence on the $sSMR$s is by means of *geostatistical methods*, also known as *Kriging*, mostly in the frequentist literature. Geostatistics (see for example Chilès and Delfiner (2012) for a comprehensive monograph on this topic) use correlated Gaussian (non-Markovian) Random fields for inducing dependence between observations as a function of the geographical distance of the points where those data have been observed. In contrast to Gaussian Markov Random Fields (GMRF) that take advantage of the neighbourhood structure of the region of study for inducing conditional dependence between geographical units, Gaussian Random fields used in Geostatistics ignore that graph structure. In contrast, they model the cells of the variance-covariance matrix of the observations for the set of units available as a function $f(D_{ij})$, for $\boldsymbol{D} = (D_{ij})_{i,j=1}^{I}$ being the distance matrix between units. Several $f()$ functions, typically known as *covariograms*, could be used for defining the variance-covariance matrix as a function of distances between units. Nevertheless, care should be taken so that $f()$ yields valid symmetric, positive-definite matrices. Several families of functions guarantee those conditions so any of them could be used in practice, see Section 2.1.3. in Banerjee et al. (2014), for example, for a collection of suitable covariogram functions.

Diggle et al. (1998) pioneered the use of geostatistical ideas in Bayesian hierarchical models. They proposed the use of generalized linear models with underlying correlated Gaussian random fields. This proposal has become very popular for modeling spatially correlated point referenced data and the hierarchical setting provides a convenient and flexible framework for fitting any additional specific feature that the data at hand could show. Thus, geostatistical Bayesian hierarchical models for disease mapping easily allow to fit the observed counts as Poisson variables and to use a logarithmic link for the $sSMRs$ inducing correlation between units as a function of their distance. This makes them a straightforward alternative to GMRF-based models.

Specifically, geostatistical Bayesian hierarchical modeling for disease mapping would proceed as follows. The number of observed cases for the i-th areal unit would follow a $Pois(e_i\theta_i)$ distribution, with e_i the corresponding expected observations and θ_i the relative risk to be modeled. The log-relative risks would be modeled as $log(\theta_i) = \mu + \varphi_i$ with $\varphi \sim N_I(\mathbf{0}, \mathbf{\Sigma})$. In this case the use of a spatially independent term is no longer needed since heterogeneity can be induced in φ by simply inflating the diagonal $\mathbf{\Sigma}$ by a common value. The variance-covariance matrix $\mathbf{\Sigma}$ is usually modeled as $f(\mathbf{D})$ for $\mathbf{D}$ a matrix with the distances between centroids of the areal units; see for example Christensen and Waagepetersen (2002), Best et al. (2005), and Mohebbi et al. (2014) for some centroid-based dependence structures. These works set $\mathbf{\Sigma} = \sigma^2 \exp(-\phi\mathbf{D})$ for the first two references and $\mathbf{\Sigma} = \sigma^2 \exp(-\phi\mathbf{D}^2)$ for the third one, with ϕ and σ being additional random variables also fitted within the model. The fit of ϕ is in general quite problematic in these kinds of models since the data contain little information about it, making its estimation in general inconsistent (Zhang, 2004). Thus informative prior distributions are usually set or suggested for this parameter. These two covariograms, known as exponential and Gaussian respectively, differ in the exponent of $\mathbf{D}$ which controls the smoothness of the geographical pattern fitted, yielding the Gaussian covariogram more smooth patterns than the exponential alternative. Thus, the term in the exponent of $\mathbf{D}$ (which should be interpreted as a cell-wise instead of a matrix operation), could be considered as an additional variable κ in the model (`WinBUGS` allows for this option), but this makes the identifiability problems for ϕ even worse and identification of κ is also very problematic, so κ is usually considered as fixed.

A nice feature of the geostatistical approach is that the vector φ is a realization of an underlying continuous Gaussian process $\varphi(\mathbf{x})$ evaluated at the centroids of the areal units $\{\mathbf{x}_1, ..., \mathbf{x}_I\}$. Inference on this continuous spatial process $\varphi(\mathbf{x})$ is made according to the information available in $\varphi = (\varphi_1, ..., \varphi_I)$ and that information can be later extrapolated to any collection of points with locations $\mathbf{x}^*$. The predictive distribution of $\varphi(\mathbf{x}^*)$ follows a multivariate Normal distribution with a larger contribution of the components of φ which are placed closer to those locations in $\mathbf{x}^*$ (Diggle et al., 1998). Specifically,

$$\varphi(\mathbf{x}^*)|\boldsymbol{\theta} \sim N(\mathbf{\Sigma}'_{12}(\mathbf{\Sigma}_{11})^{-1}\varphi, \mathbf{\Sigma}_{22} - \mathbf{\Sigma}'_{12}\mathbf{\Sigma}_{11}^{-1}\mathbf{\Sigma}_{12})$$

for $\mathbf{\Sigma}_{11} = Cov(\varphi(\mathbf{x}), \varphi(\mathbf{x})) = \mathbf{\Sigma}$, $\mathbf{\Sigma}_{12} = Cov(\varphi(\mathbf{x}), \varphi(\mathbf{x}^*))$ and $\mathbf{\Sigma}_{22} = Cov(\varphi(\mathbf{x}^*), \varphi(\mathbf{x}^*))$. By drawing this predictive distribution for a comprehensive grid of points $\mathbf{x}^*$ over the region of study, we could estimate the continuous distribution of the spatial process φ for that region, making it possible to plot that continuous estimate underlying pattern, which is known as an *isopleth map*. These isopleth maps can be used as an alternative to choropleth maps, which are sometimes distorted by the different shapes and sizes of the areal units of study, producing misleading views of the geographical distribution of the risk. Nevertheless, care should be taken for not overinterpreting local variability in isopleth maps. Data may only provide information on the underlying process for distances, at least, above the minimum distance between observed sites so local variability may just respond to modeling artifacts or being just simple random correlated noise.

The geostatistical models above concentrate all the mass of the areal units in their centroids for setting the correlation between areas. This is a strong simplification, mainly for those areal units with large extensions, that ignores the size, shape and relative position of the spatial units. Kelsall and Wakefield (2002) propose an alternative model solving this issue. This proposal assumes the observed counts to be Poisson distributed, as usual, and models the log-risks as the sum of an intercept and a vector φ whose i-th component is defined as $\varphi_i = |A_i|^{-1} \int_{A_i} \varphi(x)dx$ for $\varphi(x)$ being a continuous random field on the region of study and A_i the geographical region corresponding to the i-th unit. Instead of making the covariance matrix depend on the distance between centroids they define $Cov(\varphi_i, \varphi_j) = \int_{A_i} \int_{A_j} Cov(\varphi(x), \varphi(y))dxdy$ with $Cov(\varphi(x), \varphi(y))$ being equal to $f(d(x, y))$ for a given covariogram, a cubic function in the original paper. The point-wise covariogram $f()$ induces a joint distribution on the aggregate $(\varphi_1, ..., \varphi_I)$, which is derived from standard properties of the multivariate Normal distribution. The integrals used for defining covariance between units are sensible to the shape, size and relative position of the units of analysis, so the resulting covariances between components of φ will be also. In the case that we had information available on the geographical distribution of the population ($P(x)$ for every point x in the region of study), Kelsall and Wakefield propose to include that information on the calculation of $\varphi_i = |A_i|^{-1} \int_{A_i} \varphi(x)P(x)dx$ and $Cov(\varphi_i, \varphi_j) = \int_{A_i} \int_{A_j} Cov(\varphi(x), \varphi(y))P(x)P(y)dxdy$. This is a nice feature of this model, as it is able to take into account the variability of both the risk function and that of the population within the units of study.

Geostatistical modeling in disease mapping has also focussed considerable attention from the frequentist point of view, possibly even more than under the Bayesian approach. One of the main problems that frequentist geostatistical models face in disease mapping studies is the heteroscedasticity of the observations in these problems. Counts are well modeled by Poisson distributions with spatially varying means, whose variances are implicitly equal to those means. This makes the observations have markedly different variances. This heteroscedasticity requires specific attention for applying traditional geostatistical frequentist techniques. Berke (2004) proposes a two-step smoothing procedure. First, rates are smoothed by means of an empirical Bayes (non-spatial) smoothing model since this procedure has a variance-stabilizing effect on the rates. Second, a geostatistical procedure is applied on the smoothed rates in order to draw a spatially dependent estimate of the underlying continuous risk function. In our opinion, the use of two smoothing methods for deriving risk estimates could oversmooth the geographical patterns.

Poisson Kriging (Goovaerts, 2006) is a frequentist alternative approach to geostatistical disease mapping. This proposal estimates a smoothed SMR for each areal unit as a linear combination of the raw SMRs for a set of neighbouring units. These linear combinations may take into account the spatial correlation between sites for all the locations composing each areal unit (Area to Area Poisson Kriging) or simply that same correlation between the centroids of those units (Point Poisson Kriging). The first of these options incorporates the size and shape of the spatial units when computing their correlation, but the latter is a much simpler alternative from a computational perspective. Both options do not generally show big differences in real terms (Goovaerts, 2006), although these differences are more evident when the areal units are more heterogeneous (very different shapes or sizes). Some works (Goovaerts and Gebreab, 2008) state some particular advantages of Poisson Kriging as compared to Bayesian alternatives (BYM), such as less smoothing and more flexibility for modeling the spatial structure. Nevertheless, for the comparison in Best et al. (2005) (Bayesian) geostatistical models attain very modest results with substantially larger DICs than the most competitive proposals, suggesting that these models do not provide enough information on the spatial structure.

CAR-based disease mapping models define the joint distribution of the log-$sSMR$s through its conditional distributions. Those conditional distributions depend on a series of weights usually defined in an arbitrary and simplistic way by modelers and without a clear guidance on the effect of that choice over the correlation structure of the log-$sSMR$s. Therefore, important factors for geographic dependence of the diseases such as the size, relative position or shape of the units of study are usually ignored under that conditional approach. Moreover, the structure of those distributions depends mainly on the conditional graph of the region of study, whose division does not meet in general health-related arguments but to very different administrative criteria. As a consequence, the overall result of all these factors on the joint distribution of the random effects used to induce geographic dependence is at least unclear. On the contrary, geostatistical models ignore the graph arising from the administrative division of the region of study so they are less dependent on this aspect of the modeling with obscure consequences on the geographical pattern fitted. Moreover, geostatistical models make it quite easy to incorporate some specific features of spatial dependence such as directional differences in the dependence between units (*anisotropy*), which can be incorporated into the distance matrix used for building the covariogram.

A second important difference between using geostatistical or CAR-based random effects is the different geographical dependence that they induce. For CAR-based models, the conditional distributions used yields a joint Gaussian distribution with a well-defined and sparse precision matrix. So the use of CAR random effects implies an implicit modeling of the corresponding precision matrix. On the contrary, geostatistical random effects induce dependence by directly modeling the variance-covariance matrix instead. Both ways of defining dependence may seem reasonable, even though they are clearly different. Precision and covariance matrices are inverse of each other; since matrix inversions produce in general non-intuitive transformations, the use of CAR models will yield non-intuitive correlation matrices (mainly for irregular lattices as usually done) and therefore weird correlation structures. Similarly, geostatistical models will yield non-intuitive relationships between units under a conditional point of view. More specifically, the division of one of the units of study into two units, for example, changes the whole correlation structure of the random effects in a CAR-based model, even for units very far apart from those which are split. This seems an undesirable feature of CAR-based models. Thus, the choice between either CAR or geostatistics for inducing spatial dependence would not be clear in principle, since both seem coherent under their specific point of view. In theory it may be as reasonable to model the variance-covariance matrix (marginal dependence) as the precision matrix (conditional dependence between units). In any case, geostatistics is a modeling alternative to CAR random effects for inducing spatial dependence that should be borne in mind.

A third important difference between geostatistics and CAR modeling comes from the computational side. CAR random effects model the corresponding precision matrix by making it sparse due to the assumed Markovianity. This sparsity makes the conditional distributions of their components particularly simple, which yields considerable computational benefits. On the contrary, geostatistical models do not use in general any computationally convenient structure for the variance-covariance matrix, so they are much less computationally convenient, particularly for long vectors of random effects. MCMC inference can be particularly painful for geostatistical models since it entails the inversion of the variance-covariance matrix for each iteration of the algorithm which is generally large and lacking a computationally convenient structure. Geostatistical Bayesian hierarchical models can be in general easily coded in `WinBUGS` although, as mentioned, they will be typically slow for even mid-sized data sets. Some specific efficient algorithms have been proposed for doing inference in geostatistical Bayesian hierarchical models (Christensen and Waagepetersen, 2002), although regretfully they may not be used within `WinBUGS`. On the contrary, `INLA` seems particularly suited for dealing with these models. It uses the Stochastic Partial Differential Equation (SPDE) approach (Lindgren et al., 2011) which approximates the geostatistical process by a more computationally convenient GMRF (CAR distributed vector) that takes explicit advantage of its sparse formulation. Thus `INLA` is a much more computationally appealing tool for working with geostatistical models.

6.3   Moving-average based spatial dependence

A second alternative for inducing spatial dependence in disease mapping models is by using moving average processes. We have already mentioned that ICAR distributions can be seen as the spatial generalization to irregular lattices of first-order random walks. In a similar manner, PCAR distributions can be also considered as spatial generalizations of first-order auto-regressive process typically used for time series modeling (Botella-Rocamora et al., 2012). Thus, a third obvious way to induce spatial dependence in disease mapping models is by generalizing the moving average process of time series to the discrete irregular spatial domain. Several efforts have been made in that direction. We review now some of those approaches.

Ickstadt and Wolpert (1999) model the spatial variation of risks along a region of study as a kernel smoothing, i.e., a local weighted average, of an underlying continuous gamma random field. For the discrete version of this proposal, also introduced in Ickstadt and Wolpert (1999) and further developed in Best et al. (2000a) and Best et al. (2000b), a gamma random field with discrete support γ is assumed on a fine partition of the region of study. This partition could be, for example, a quadrat division of the whole region of study and each element γ_j of the gamma random field $\gamma = (\gamma_j)_{j=1}^{J}$ would correspond to each of these quadrats. The observed cases for each unit of study would be modeled as:

$$o_i \sim \quad Pois(e_i\theta_i) \qquad i = 1, ..., I$$
$$\theta_i = \quad \beta_0 + \sum_{j=1}^{J} k_{ij}\gamma_j$$

where $k_{ij} = k(d(i, j))$ is a kernel function depending on the distance between the i-th and j-th quadrat. The authors define $k(d(i, j))$ as a zero-mean Normal function of the corresponding distance, although more alternatives could be suitable. The variance of the kernel function $k()$ could also be set as an additional variable in the model controlling the smoothness of the risk surface fitted. Thus, $k()$ acts as a device mixing the noise in the independent underlying gamma process and therefore inducing local spatial dependence between nearby spatial units. Covariates could also be included in this model as described in Best et al. (2000a). The elements in γ are assumed to follow a $Gamma(\alpha_\gamma, \beta_\gamma)$ distribution and both $\alpha_\gamma, \beta_\gamma$ and the prior distribution of β_0 (which is also a gamma distribution) are set out following informative arguments (see for example Best et al. (2000b) for more detail on those arguments).

This proposal, the *Poisson-gamma model* from now on, has an identity link for the risks θ, in contrast to most of the Poisson regression models used in disease mapping. This feature could be particularly useful if the risk surface that had spots (point sources) that increase the risk around them in an additive manner, i.e., the increase is independent of the basal risk surface without spots. The vector of risks $\boldsymbol{\theta}$ would be the cumulative local effect of the spots, or local variability, placed around each specific location. Hence, depending on the problem, additive risk surfaces could be particularly suitable and Poisson-gamma models would be particularly appropriate in that case.

A second interesting feature of this proposal is that it estimates an underlying risk surface with a different support to that corresponding to the administrative division of the data. Although typical choropleth maps on the original administrative division could also be made just mapping the vector $\boldsymbol{\theta}$, we could also plot the vector $\boldsymbol{\gamma}$ on the alternative finer division used as support for this vector. As already mentioned, this new division is usually a regular collection of quadrats so the display of the risks will be more attractive and less prone to visual artifacts that usually arise when representing choropleth maps in irregular lattices. This visual advantage is similar to that produced by isopleth maps when using geostatistics based methods. Indeed, there is a close connection between kernel smoothing and geostatistical methods (Higdon, 2002). Thus, the properties of Poisson-gamma models would be in theory equivalent to those of geostatistics-based smoothing models which, according to Best et al. (2005), seemed to be a bit rigid for modelling the spatial variability of risk patterns. Indeed, geostatistical models and the Poisson-gamma model were those modeling proposals achieving worst results in general in the comparative study developed in that paper.

The Poisson-gamma model can be estimated in `WinBUGS`. Indeed, this could be directly programmed using the `BUGS` language, but the version 1.4 of `WinBUGS` incorporates a specific function for fitting this process `pois.conv()`. This function internally uses a data augmentation process in the inference in order to exploit the Poisson-gamma conjugacy for the components of $\boldsymbol{\gamma}$. In theory, this particular built-in distribution should produce improved convergence as compared to the raw coding of the Poisson-gamma model. More information on this function can be found on the `Map> Manual> Spatial distributions` menu of `WinBUGS`.

Choo and Walker (2008) propose also a moving-average spatial model with two particular features. First, the underlying random field also follows a gamma distribution instead of being Gaussian, as typically assumed. Thus, this model is called *multivariate Poisson-gamma* (MPG) in terms of the authors. Second, the underlying random field has as support the edges of the graph (neighboring units) representing the region of study. Namely, let us consider $\boldsymbol{R}$ a vector of length equal to the number of edges of the graph of the region of study. Choo and Walker define the risk for unit i as

$$\theta_i = \mu + n_i^{-1} \sum_{j \in A_i} \psi_j$$

where n_i is the number of neighbours of region i and A_i is the set of edges that have unit i as one of their nodes. The elements of $\boldsymbol{\psi}$ are assumed to be random effects with distribution $Gamma(\alpha, \alpha)$ and α is an additional parameter in the model having a vague gamma prior distribution.

Leaving out the intercept μ, the vector $\boldsymbol{\psi}$ marginally induces on each component θ_i a $Gamma(n_i\alpha, n_i\alpha)$ distribution, which makes $E(\theta_i) = 1$ and $Var(\theta_i) = (n_i\alpha)^{-1}$; therefore, that variance is inversely proportional to the number of neighbours as in the ICAR distribution. Hence, the $sSMRs$ in this model have gamma prior distributions as in Clayton and Kaldor (1987) but, in contrast to that model, $Cov(\theta_i, \theta_{i'}) = n_i^{-1}n_{i'}^{-1}Var(\psi_j) = (n_in_{i'}\alpha)^{-1}$ if $i \sim i'$, and 0 otherwise. This covariance comes from ψ_j where j is the edge linking i and i', which contributes to both θ_i and $\theta_{i'}$ making them dependent. In contrast to other tools inducing spatial dependence, the $sSMRs$ for this proposal corresponding to non-neighbouring units do not show any correlation at all. This makes the spatial dependence under this model very local, what could be a serious drawback when studying diseases with spatial dependence of long range or with very small spatial units since strength will be pooled in the estimates just for strictly neighboring units. Thus, in summary, Choo and Walker's proposal has an underlying gamma process instead of the usual lognormal alternative but, in contrast to Clayton and Kaldor (1987), it shows spatial dependence, which is not so straightforward to induce as for Normal distributions. The MPG model can be easily implemented in `WinBUGS`, but not in `INLA` since it does not rely on any underlying GMRF.

Botella-Rocamora et al. (2012) propose another moving-average based model, Spatial Moving Average Risk Smoothing (SMARS) in terms of the authors. In this case the link for modeling the risks is logarithmic, as frequently assumed, and they are modeled with an underlying independent Gaussian random field. Following the spirit of time series ARIMA models, this random field has support on the set of geographical units in the region of study so, the underlying random field of this model $\boldsymbol{\phi}$ has the same length as the vector of observed counts. Thus, in this sense, this model is much less overparameterized than, for example, MPG or BYM models. In SMARS, the log-$sSMRs$ for the i-th geographical unit is defined as:

$$\log(\theta_i) = \mu + \lambda_i^{-1}\left(\omega_0\phi_1 + \omega_1(\sum_{j\sim_1 i}\phi_j) + ... + \omega_m(\sum_{j\sim_m i}\phi_j)\right).$$

In this expression μ stands for the intercept of the log-$sSMRs$, $\boldsymbol{\phi}$ the underlying vector of independent Gaussian random effects and $\boldsymbol{\omega}$ a vector of positive values representing a non-parametric kernel. This vector weighs the random effects of the neighbouring units to spatial unit i as a function of the distance to that unit. The expression $\cdot \sim_k i$ stands for the k-th order neighbours of unit i, i.e., those units whose shortest path to unit i goes through k or less units. Note that under this definition if a unit is k-th order neighbour of unit i it is also k' order neighbour for any $k' > k$. As a consequence the random effects of k-th order neighbours are weighted by $\sum_{i=k}^{m}\omega_i > \sum_{i=k'}^{m}\omega_i$. Therefore, those units that are farther apart from unit i are weighed less in the expression of θ_i

than those that are closer, i.e., the contribution of the underlying random effects to the log-$sSMR$s is a decreasing function of the distance between units. The parameter λ_i in the expression above is a variance stabilizer quantity making the variance of the units in the center of the region of study (with a higher number of neighbours) have the same variance than those closer to the borders of that region. Basically, that parameter depends on $\boldsymbol{\omega}$ and the number of neighbours of each unit.

Since $\boldsymbol{\omega}$ can be seen as a vector of positive weights (weighing the contribution of the random effects $\boldsymbol{\phi}$ to the log-$sSMR$s as a function of their distance), they are given a Dirichlet prior of parameter $\mathbf{1}_m$. This is a uniform distribution in the simplex containing $\boldsymbol{\omega}$, once imposed that their elements should sum 1 and to be larger than 0. The weights $\boldsymbol{\omega}$ are imposed to sum 1 since the scale of $\boldsymbol{\theta}$ is explained by the standard deviation of $\boldsymbol{\phi}$ thus, if $\boldsymbol{\omega}$ was unrestricted, it would compete with $\boldsymbol{\phi}$ for explaining the variability of the log-risks, inducing therefore identifiability problems.

SMARS weights the contribution of the underlying random field $\boldsymbol{\phi}$ up to m units away. Similar proposals to SMARS have been proposed with m fixed to 1 (Langford et al., 1999; Congdon, 2007b; Moraga and Lawson, 2012). Nevertheless, for SMARS the parameter m is also considered as a random variable that the model makes inference on, determining its posterior distribution. Note that this parameter also determines the length of $\boldsymbol{\omega}$ so the number of variables in the model depends itself on the model, therefore trans-dimensional MCMC, such as Reversible Jump (see Section 2.3), is required to sample from its posterior distribution model. The authors developed specific code in R in order to carry inference out of this model. That code is available at the web page: https://www.uv.es/mamtnez/SMARS.html.

As pointed in Botella-Rocamora et al. (2012), one of the main drawbacks of the ICAR distribution, also mentioned in Section 6.1, is that the distance between units where the correlation vanishes depends on the geometry of the region of study and not on the data. This means that for a lattice following a linear ordering, i.e., all units i except the first and last have exactly two neighbours: units $i-1$ and $i+1$, positive correlations are necessarily achieved for about one half of all the units, as shown in Figure 6.1. This may seem excessive in some occasions such as for diseases showing very local dependence (a couple of neighbours away) in very large data sets. In this case, the dependence fitted by the ICAR distribution could have a dependence range much larger than that really needed. Regretfully, this is not alleviated by the introduction of the independent random effect in the BYM model. Other models such as the MPG model introduced just above have the opposite performance, its range of dependence is quite local, just one unit away. Thus these proposals are not adaptive in terms of the range of dependence, in contrast to SMARS. The m parameter in that model, which is itself determined by the data, controls this feature of the geographical pattern fitted so it may fit spatial patterns of very different kind.

A second unpleasant effect of the ICAR distribution, also pointed out in Section 6.1, is that for units placed very far apart the correlation between the corresponding random effects becomes negative. This means that if high risks are fitted in a border of the map, the risks at very distant regions will tend to be low, and vice versa, when in theory those risks should be independent. SMARS, like PCAR or geostatistics based models for example, does not show this effect since, unless m gets very high, very distant units will not share any common underlying random effect so their risks will be completely independent. Thus, for SMARS, correlations will vanish to 0 for distant units, meanwhile for ICAR based models those correlations will become negative. This is in our opinion a nice feature of SMARS.

6.4   Spline-based modeling

Although spline models have been frequently used in spatio-temporal disease mapping, their use in simpler spatial models has been scarcer (Goicoa et al., 2016a). Nevertheless, since spatio-temporal spline models often rely on spline-based spatial structures of risks, we are going to introduce them here. A good part of the spline literature on disease mapping has been developed from the frequentist point of view, although the Bayesian approach has allowed to include additional flexibility to the frequentist proposals (Lang and Brezger, 2004). We will pay particular attention to the Bayesian formulation of many of the frequentist proposals already made since they can be easily addressed with the current tools that we have already introduced throughout the book.

We have already introduced the use of bases of functions as a potential smoothing device, see Example 2.3 and Section 4.2 for two examples of their use in non-spatial and spatial problems, respectively. Spline are a particular case of smoothing devices relying on bases of functions. A *spline* is a piecewise polynomial function, of usually a variable, subject to continuity restrictions either on the own function or on its derivatives up to a specific order. These smooth functions can be used within regression models for reproducing smooth relationships between the mentioned variable and an outcome. *Cubic spline* are possibly the most popular family of spline since they are considered smooth enough and computationally convenient, we will focus on them from now on. Cubic spline are defined as the concatenation of a series of cubic polynomials, one for each pair of consecutive knots, on a given grid of knots. Continuity restrictions up to second-order derivatives are imposed on all the knots in the grid thus the resulting piece-wise function for cubic spline has second-order continuous derivatives everywhere.

Several families of piece-wise cubic functions accomplish these conditions. Cubic *B-spline* are surely the most popular due to their nice computational properties. In contrast to other popular basis of spline such as truncated power bases (Ruppert and Carroll, 2000), cubic B-spline have the particular feature of being non-zero for just a range of 5 consecutive knots (4 inter-knot intervals), thus they have compact support, which makes them particularly suited for modeling the local variability of a variable. Note that k-th order B-spline (cubic B-spline correspond to $k = 3$) on sets of equidistant knots tend to Normal probability density functions, up to a proportionality constant, when k grows (Brinks, 2008). Thus, B-spline in general can be viewed as compact support and finitely differentiable approximations of Gaussian bases. That is, B-spline are a kind of Gaussian-like functions whose location and dispersion is a function of the location of the knots used to define them. Specifically, a cubic B-spline defined on a set of equidistant knots $\{q_{i-2}, q_{i-1}, q_i, q_{i+1}, q_{i+2}\}$ will have its maximum at q_i and will have tails as long as the distance between q_i and q_{i+2}. Regular bases of cubic B-spline for univariate modeling are typically built by considering a set of sequentially ordered knots $\mathcal{Q} = \{q_i : i = 1, ..., Q\}$ and defining an ensemble of $Q - 4$ B-spline for each set of 5 consecutive knots in that set. The location of the knots in $\mathcal{Q}$ is typically chosen as equally spaced quantiles or as equidistant locations. For the knots in $\mathcal{Q}$, $[q_4, q_{Q-3}]$ usually span the range of values of the covariate modeled, while the rest of the knots in $\mathcal{Q}$ laying out of this range are outer knots intended to avoid edge effects on the fit. Being more precise, if we divided the range of a variable into K intervals (so $K + 1$ knots would be required), knots $q_1, q_2, q_3, q_{K+5}, q_{K+6}, q_{K+7}$ would be external to the range of values of the variable. In this case, if a cubic B-spline basis was considered, the i-th spline function will have as support $[q_i, q_{i+4}]$ and a total of $K + 3$ would be required in the spline basis for modeling the whole range of values considered. Note that the first three and the final three spline functions in the basis will also be positive for the outer intervals of the modeled variable. Thus, we will not have data contributing to estimate the corresponding coefficient for a good part of the support of those functions.

As mentioned above, we have already seen examples of the use of basis of functions for smoothing either time trends or spatial patterns. Those models are posed as generalized linear models, where the bases of functions act as covariates modeling the local performance of the pattern around the corresponding knot. Specifically, spline-based smoothing models are typically posed as generalized linear models with linear predictor of the form $\boldsymbol{X\beta} + \boldsymbol{B\gamma}$. In this expression, $\boldsymbol{X}$ is a matrix of covariates and $\boldsymbol{B}$ is an $I \times J$ matrix whose columns correspond to the $J(= Q - 4$ for the cubic case) spline functions in the basis considered, evaluated at each of the I areal units available. Since the number of spline in the corresponding basis, and therefore the length of $\boldsymbol{\gamma}$, is typically much lower than the number of available data, these models can be considered as low-rank smoothers. Specifically, they project the cloud of points into a low-dimensional space $\boldsymbol{B}$ fitting local features of the geographical distribution of risks. Inference should be made for both $\boldsymbol{\beta}$ and $\boldsymbol{\gamma}$ in the expression above so, under a Bayesian approach, prior distributions should be assigned to their components. Since $\boldsymbol{\beta}$ is intended to be a vector of fixed effects, its components will typically have vague prior distributions. Nevertheless, we showed (Example 2.3) that we could draw considerable advantage if $\boldsymbol{\gamma}$ had a random effect structure instead of a fixed effect one. Specifically, if $\boldsymbol{\gamma}$ is defined as a set of random effects, the final fit is much more robust. This robustness makes the influence of the knots used for spline models (one of the main drawbacks of this approach) much lower, making spline models in practice much less troublesome. A vast amount of literature exploits the use of random effects as coefficients for spline models, the resulting spline models are known as *P-spline* (Eilers and Marx, 1996), where the P in this term stands for penalized. The penalization in P-spline comes from the prior distribution of the vector $\boldsymbol{\gamma}$ which shrinks its values.

Under the frequentist point of view P-spline are just spline regression models whose coefficients are penalized in some way. They usually minimize an objective function of the kind $l(\boldsymbol{\beta}, \boldsymbol{\gamma}) - \boldsymbol{\gamma}' \boldsymbol{P} \boldsymbol{\gamma}$, where $l()$ stands for the log-likelihood function corresponding to a GLM with coefficients in the linear term given by $\boldsymbol{\beta}$ (as fixed effects) and $\boldsymbol{\gamma}$. The matrix $\boldsymbol{P}$ stands for a penalty matrix that may depend on one or more parameters (Lee and Durban, 2009). If we exponentiate the objective function above, we get the product of the likelihood function of the corresponding generalized linear model and $\exp(-\boldsymbol{\gamma}' \boldsymbol{P} \boldsymbol{\gamma})$. This expression is proportional to the posterior distribution of that GLM where the prior distribution of $\boldsymbol{\gamma}$ is multivariate Normal of mean $\boldsymbol{0}$ and precision matrix proportional to $\boldsymbol{P}$. If inference is made on the variance or correlation parameters of $\boldsymbol{P}$, this is equivalent to assuming a random effects structure for $\boldsymbol{\gamma}$ under a Bayesian point of view. Thus, the relationship between the penalizing term in frequentist spline models and assuming $\boldsymbol{\gamma}$ to be random effects in Bayesian spline models becomes clear.

In Example 2.3 and Section 4.2 the corresponding random effects were assumed to be independent, i.e., $\boldsymbol{P} = \sigma^{-2} \boldsymbol{I}_J$, but obviously the geometrical arrangement of the spatial units could induce some dependence that $\boldsymbol{P}$ would be convenient to take into account. Thus, setting $\boldsymbol{P} = \sigma^{-2}(\boldsymbol{D} - \boldsymbol{W})$ is quite usual for the univariate modeling of the effect of covariates by means of spline, where $\boldsymbol{D}$ and $\boldsymbol{W}$ are the typical diagonal and adjacency matrices used for ICAR distributions. In this case the $\boldsymbol{W}$ matrix would reflect adjacency for consecutive knots, i.e., $W_{j(j+1)} = W_{(j+1)j} = 1$ for consecutive knots for $j = 1, ..., J-1$. For the univariate modeling of covariates, this is known as a *difference penalty*. This would define a first-order random walk (RW1) on the components of $\boldsymbol{\gamma}$, taking into account the expected similarity between consecutive parameters of the spline regression model.

Higher order random walks could be also used as dependence structures for $\boldsymbol{\gamma}$. This could be achieved by setting $\boldsymbol{P} = \sigma^{-2}(\boldsymbol{D} - \boldsymbol{W})$ for another particular choices of $\boldsymbol{D}$ and $\boldsymbol{W}$ (see Section 3.4.1 of Rue and Held (2005) for a full description of $\boldsymbol{P}$ for the second-order random walk (RW2)). For the RW2 model $\boldsymbol{W}$ cells will be also non-zero for $W_{j(j+2)}$ and $W_{(j+2)j}$, $j = 1, ..., J-2$ as a consequence of the longer dependence on time in this process. The use of a first- or second-order random walk for modeling γ may have important consequences on the final fit of the corresponding spline regression model. Thus, the second-order random walk generally defines much smoother changes in the components of γ than the first-order counterpart (see for example Chapter 3 of Rue and Held (2005)). Thus, the election of a good dependence structure may not be as trivial as it could seem at a first glance. Nevertheless, it is important to mention that if P is rank-deficient for one dimension in the RW1 case, the rank-deficiency for the RW2 would be of two dimensions. Thus, besides the sum-to-zero restriction typically used for RW1 models, γ should be further constrained with the restriction $\gamma \cdot t = 0$, where $t = (1, ..., J)$ in order to fix the posterior impropriety problems of the RW2 model. In that case, an intercept and an additional linear term depending on t should be included in the model in order to fit the data along the space where γ has been restricted.

For spline-based disease mapping models, we will need a bidimensional basis of functions and a bidimensional grid of knots instead of a linear set, as for now. These knots are typically chosen as equidistant in both directions (latitude and longitude) and some additional knots are also used beyond the region of study in order to avoid edge effects on the final fit. Grids of knots will be in general of the kind $\mathcal{Q}_2 = \{q_{ij} : i = 1, ..., Q_1, j = 1, ..., Q_2\}$ and a bidimensional B-spline basis, for example, B would be intended to be built on this set of knots. Each column of B would be referred to a different basis function, centered at a different knot of $\mathcal{Q}_2$, whereas each row will contain the evaluations of the spline functions for a particular areal unit. Regarding the bidimensional basis to be used for disease mapping studies, let us assume $\{B_i^1(x) : i = 1, ..., J_1\}$ and $\{B_j^2(y) : j = 1, ..., J_2\}$ to be two basis of functions spanning the range of longitudes and latitudes of the region of study. Remind that for a cubic basis of spline $J_1 = Q_1 - 4$ and $J_2 = Q_2 - 4$. Therefore, the bidimensional basis $\{B_{(i-1)Q_2+j}(x, y) = B_i^1(x)B_j^2(y) : i = 1, ..., J_1, j = 1, ..., J_2\}$, which is the product of the two unidimensional bases mentioned, would be a suitable basis to be used for smoothing risks in disease mapping studies. If cubic B-spline were used in B^1 and B^2, the elements in B will be bidimensional piecewise cubic functions, mimicking Gaussian functions, and centered at different knots of $\mathcal{Q}_2$. Thus the B matrix will have $J_1 J_2$ columns, one per element in the bivariate spline basis, and I rows. Each row will correspond to the different elements of the basis of spline evaluated at a point-wise summary (usually the centroid) of a different areal unit.

Penalty differences are usually defined for fitting this model by considering knots $q_{i-1j}, q_{i+1j}, q_{ij-1}, q_{ij+1}$ as neighbours of q_{ij}. According to this adjacency relationship between knots, a precision matrix $P = \sigma^{-2}(D - W)$ for γ could be defined by setting $W_{ij} = 1$ if the central knots corresponding to the spline functions i and j are neighbours, and $W_{ij} = 0$ otherwise. In this manner we are imposing a kind of Markovian assumption on the bidimensional spline model. That is, given the parameters of the neighbouring spline, the parameter associated to any of the spline functions in the basis are assumed independent of the rest of the parameters modeling the spline surface. This model could be easily fitted within `WinBUGS` by defining the vector γ as a set of ICAR distributed random effects with the corresponding W matrix. This model could also be fitted in `INLA` by using a design matrix reproducing the basis of functions B by means of the "z" option for defining random effects. In this case the argument `Cmatrix` of the `f(,model="z")` function of `inla` should be used for setting the prior precision matrix for the random effects γ. Regretfully, the potential sparseness, for example, of `Cmatrix` will not be exploited here so this modeling is not particularly efficient. Nevertheless, as spline are low-dimensional smoothers, this should not be a huge problem for studies of moderate size.

From the frequentist point of view, the precision matrix P is used as a penalty difference matrix penalizing large differences between nearby knots. Lee and Durban (2009) propose penalty matrices of the form $P(\lambda_1, \lambda_2) = \lambda_1 P_1 \otimes I_{Q_2} + \lambda_2 I_{Q_1} \otimes P_2$ where P_1 and P_2 penalize differences between parameters of neighbouring knots along the longitude and latitude axes, respectively. An interesting feature of this matrix is that it includes different penalty terms λ_1 and λ_2 for each direction, northing and easting. This makes possible to reproduce anisotropic patterns with higher variability along one of these directions. The implementation of this model is not so straightforward with current Bayesian tools. That model would entail the use of a vector of random effects with precision matrix $P(\lambda_1, \lambda_2)$, where both λ_1 and λ_2 are in charge of controlling the spatial dependence of the pattern. This cannot be done with any of the prebuilt modeling tools neither in `WinBUGS` nor in `INLA`. Nevertheless, it could be implemented in `WinBUGS` by formulating the conditional distributions of the components of γ from their original joint distribution. This can be done by following standard results for the multivariate Normal distribution, yielding the following conditional distributions

$$\gamma_i | \gamma_{-i} \sim N \left(\frac{\lambda_1}{\lambda_1 n_i^1 + \lambda_2 n_i^2} \sum_{j \sim_1 i} \gamma_j + \frac{\lambda_2}{\lambda_1 n_i^1 + \lambda_2 n_i^2} \sum_{j \sim_2 i} \gamma_j, \frac{1}{\lambda_1 n_i^1 + \lambda_2 n_i^2} \right)$$

where n_i^1 and n_i^2 are the number of neighbours of knot i on the direction of each of the coordinate axis and $\cdot \sim_1 \cdot$ and $\cdot \sim_2 \cdot$ stand for neighbouring pairs of knots for each of those directions. The variance term of these conditional distributions shows that the λ_1 and λ_2 penalty parameters can be viewed as the factors controlling the decomposition of the conditional precisions into the two sources of variability of the spatial process, the X and Y axes. This consideration may be useful for putting prior distributions on these parameters, as they can be understood as precision terms.

Since regions of study are usually irregular, sometimes some of the knots in Q_2 will not have any nearby spatial unit. In fact, for B-spline, it could be that for some knot, none of the areal units fall within the compact region where the corresponding spline is positive. This could yield identification problems for the corresponding element in γ, that could be only weakly identified through their prior distribution and the information from other knots in the spline.

These identifiability problems could also entail additional convergence problems in MCMC-based Bayesian spline models. We have noticed these problems when fitting Bayesian spline models in `WinBUGS`, so we advise removing those problematic knots from Q_2 as they have no practical relevance on the fit of the risks in the areal units and can be troublesome in terms of convergence.

From our point of view, one potential problem of spline models in disease mapping studies could be oversmoothing. CAR-based random effects models have been described as prone to oversmoothing (Richardson et al., 2004). The case of spline models could be worse since they combine two different smoothing devices: spline and penalization. Spline themselves are smoothing devices since, as mentioned above, are low-rank smoothers projecting the set of risks on a lower dimensional space. Besides, under a Bayesian approach, penalization on γ is simply equivalent to treat their components as random effects, sometimes with CAR structure. Thus, the oversmoothing problems found in CAR-based random effects models in general could be exacerbated in spline models. Indeed, spline models have been said to smooth spatial patterns to a higher extent than CAR-based random effects models (Adín et al., 2017), although in terms of these authors this is not necessarily a drawback mainly for the modeling of very sparse data sets. In that case, the oversmoothing of spline models could make the transfer of information between neighbouring areas higher, robustifying the risk estimates drawn from these models. Nevertheless, the oversmoothing of spline models could obviously produce misfits in the geographical pattern fitted, which could introduce overdispersion into the model. In that case, additional random effects at the areal unit level could be introduced into the model in order to fit that overdispersion. Those random effects could be either independent, yielding a model called *PRIDE* 'Penalized Random Individual Dispersion effects' (Perperoglou and Eilers, 2010), or spatially structured with CAR structure, for example. Nevertheless, Lee and Durban (2009) recommend caution with the spatial structured case since confounding problems could arise between the spline term and the spatial random effect.

Example 6.1

We are going to fit now several non-CAR spatial structures to the oral cancer data set repeatedly studied in Chapter 4. Specifically, we have separately fitted: a geostatistical process, a spatial moving average process and P-spline for modeling the log-risks spatial pattern. Our goal is comparing the different fits of these non-CAR models with those obtained in Chapter 4 with CAR models, in particular for the BYM model that we will consider as a benchmark for this comparison. As always, you can find full details of the models fitted in the online supplementary material.

The size of the Valencian Region, with 540 municipalities, makes `WinBUGS` an inefficient tool for MCMC sampling in geostatistical models, which would need specific computational methods for efficiently sampling in this particular context. Thus, we have resorted to `INLA` for making inference on the geostatistical model proposed. Specifically, we have considered a point-based process, where the observed count for each municipality is assumed to be observed at the centroid of the corresponding areal unit. A Matérn covariance function, depending on the distance between centroids, is assumed for modeling the covariance function for the log-relative risks corresponding to those observed counts. The Matérn covariance function makes it feasible to use the SPDE approach for fitting the underlying geostatistical process in a computationally efficient manner (Lindgren et al., 2011).

The SMARS model has been the spatial moving average process chosen for this comparison. One of the most interesting features of this model is its capability for determining the spatial dependence range in the underlying process. However, this feature requires using trans-dimensional MCMC for the inference in this model. As a consequence, an ad-hoc coding of this model is necessary beyond `WinBUGS` and `INLA`. We have used the original `R` code made available by the authors of this proposal. A total of three chains have been sampled with these routines with 25,000 iterations per chain, whose first 5,000 iterations were discarded as burn-in period.

We have also fitted the P-spline model in this example with `INLA`. One-dimensional cubic B-spline bases of functions are considered for modeling the spatial variability for both coordinate axes. A bidimensional spatial basis is built as the product of those one-dimensional bases. These spline bases have 7 inner intervals for the longitude and 14 inner intervals for the latitude, since the Valencian Region is approximately twice longer than wider. This means that the knots are equally spaced, in practical terms, for both reference axes. The total number of bidimensional spline functions used as basis for this model is $170 = (7 + 3) * (14 + 3)$, where $7 + 3$ would be the total cubic spline needed to model the variability in the 7 inner horizontal intervals considered. The coefficients associated to these basis functions are considered as random effects in order to penalize its variability and avoid therefore overfitting. First-order penalty matrices are considered for the spline coefficients along both coordinate axes. This would be equivalent to assuming first-order random walk processes for those parameters along both coordinate axes. Anyway, different precision parameters are considered for both random walk processes, which would induce anisotropy if this was required by the data.

The geostatistical model took 101.6 seconds to run in `INLA` with the SPDE approach. The DIC for this geostatistical model was 1783.7, with 53.0 effective parameters. Remember that the BYM model attained a DIC of 1786.5 in Example 4.5, so the geostatistical model seems to yield a slight improvement over BYM. That improvement seems to come from the effective number of parameters of the geostatistical model, 53.0 vs. 83.3 of BYM. Thus, the geostatistical model seems to take more advantage of spatial dependence, which decreases the effective number of parameters in the model by making their coefficients more dependent. An interesting feature of geostatistical models is that they are defined in a continuous domain. As a consequence, they may predict the risk at every spatial location. Therefore, isopleth maps can be drawn with a continuous spatial prediction for the risk surface. The left-hand side of Figure 6.2 shows a risk isopleth map drawn from this geostatistical model. The shapefile with the municipalities of the Valencian Region has been overlaid to make easier the assessment of the results for this model but, as is evident, the underlying risk surface is continuous in contrast to the typical choropleth maps typically used in disease mapping. In this manner, the high visual influence of some particularly large areas in the choropleth maps is reduced. Note that this isopleth map entails the prediction of the continuous process at 7391 different points, which is a computationally demanding task. Thus, INLA took 669.9 seconds to run the model with all 7391 spatial predictions, instead of the 101.6 seconds of the model with no spatial prediction.

Regarding SMARS, it took 419 seconds to run the trans-dimensional MCMC algorithm. The DIC statistic for this model was of 1787.4, comparable to BYM, although a bit higher. The effective number of parameters for SMARS has been of 72.8, also similar to BYM, although evidently lower. One interesting feature of SMARS is that it may adapt itself to the spatial range of dependence of each data set. For our particular case, we have obtained the posterior mode for m, the order of the underlying spatial moving average model, to be equal to 3. Concretely, we have found a posterior probability of 49.7% for $m = 3$, 28.8% for $m = 4$ and 9.8% for $m = 5$. Thus, these three values sum nearly 90% of posterior probability for m. Bearing in mind that $m = 1$ stands for full independence between neighbouring spatial units, we can state that we have found spatial dependence in the oral cancer data set but of local extent. The ICAR distribution, for example, is not able to fit this feature for each data set. The risk for any spatial unit in SMARS will depend on the underlying pattern of at most 4, or maybe 5, neighbourhoods away. In contrast to BYM, every spatial unit placed further away will be independent instead of having negative correlation or some other counterintuitive relationship.

The P-spline model runs in 42.6 seconds with a full Laplace strategy. The DIC for this model was 1802.0 and the number of effective parameters was 26.6. According to this criterion, the fit of the P-spline model seems worse than the rest of the alternatives. Possibly the low effective number of parameters of this model makes it too rigid for explaining such a complex spatial pattern, with such large spatial variability. The right-hand side of Figure 6.2 shows a choropleth map with the posterior means of the municipal $sSMR$s for the P-spline model. This map shows less low-range spatial variability than the BYM model (Figure 4.4), which is able to depict more heterogeneous variability for some municipalities. One interesting feature of spline models is that they allow to fit anisotropic spatial patterns. Anisotropy is controlled by two separate hyperparameters of the precision matrix of the random effects used to fit the model, controlling the variability for both coordinate axes. Those parameters

Geostatistical model   **Spline model**

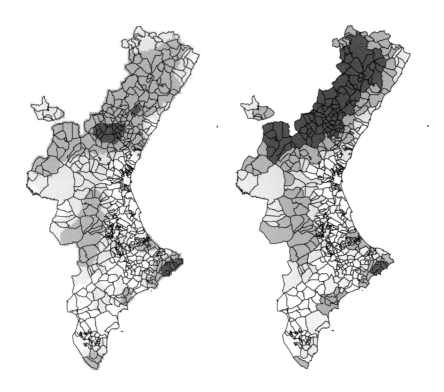

Figure 6.2
Left: isopleth $sSMR$s map for the geostatistical model. Right: choropleth $sSMR$s map for the P-spline model.

attained a posterior mean of 1.6 (95% credible interval of $[0.3, 5.0]$) and 2.2 (95% credible interval of $[0.4, 7.5]$), for both coordinates axes, so small evidence of anisotropy has been found for our data set. No evident sign of anisotropy can be noticed either in Figure 6.2.

Table 6.1 shows the correlations for the $sSMR$s of all possible pairs of models considered in this example. It can be noticed how all those correlations are rather high, so all 4 models yield similar $sSMR$ estimates. Although this could seem obvious, since all of them are smoothing the same process, the P-spline model seems to yield a more different spatial pattern than the rest of the options considered. All 3 random effects models in the comparison (geostatistics, SMARS and BYM) show correlations above 0.9, whereas the spline model shows such a high correlation only with the geostatistical model. This

	Geostatistics	SMARS	Spline	BYM
Geostatistics	1.00	0.93	0.91	0.93
SMARS	0.93	1.00	0.81	0.93
Spline	0.91	0.81	1.00	0.88
BYM	0.93	0.93	0.88	1.00

Table 6.1
Correlations for the $sSMRs$ (posterior means) for the different models considered.

could be due to the inability of spline for modeling spatial dependence of very low range, lower than the inter-knot distance. Maybe some modifications of the P-spline model fitted, such as PRIDE which considers additional heterogeneous variability or increasing the number of knots in the model, could improve the fit of the P-spline model in this comparison. According to the DICs of these models, this apparent lack of flexibility of the P-spline model has a negative impact on its final fit.

6.5 Modeling of specific features in disease mapping studies

This section introduces the specific modeling of two features shown by some data sets that have focussed considerable attention in the literature. These are the existence and modeling of geographical discontinuities in the underlying spatial pattern and the modeling of data sets with an excessive number of zeroes.

6.5.1 Modeling partitions and discontinuities

One of the main problems of most disease mapping models comes from the existence of discontinuities in the distribution of the risks along the region of study. Spatial smoothing models are based on sharing information between geographically nearby locations, according to the idea that the risk in those regions should be similar. Discontinuities or jumps in the geographical risks pattern are clear violations of that hypothesis, making disease mapping methods fail or produce inaccurate maps. Namely, disease mapping methods that do not specifically take this issue into account oversmooth those discontinuities since they consider spatial units placed in opposite sides of those discontinuities to be as similar as those which are on the same side. Thus, specific models are needed in case that we suspected that discontinuities were present in the geographical distribution of risks or if we had a particular interest in determining the existence and placement of those discontinuities if they really existed (Mollié, 1996).

Geographical discontinuities in risks distribution have focussed consider-able attention in the CAR-based disease mapping literature even from the earliest works in this field (Besag et al., 1991). As introduced in Section 4.3, geographical discontinuities could be taken into account within CAR distri-butions by changing the Gaussian assumptions for the conditional distribu-tions by Laplace distributions. This distribution can be easily implemented in WinBUGS, by means of the car.l1 built-in function, but not in INLA since the latter is conceived for specifically working with GMRF and the CAR-L1 distribution is no longer Gaussian. The CAR-L1 distribution would be partic-ularly suited if risk discontinuities were expected in the risk surface by allowing more abrupt risk differences between neighbouring units if these were really needed (Besag et al., 1991; Best et al., 1999). This is a consequence of the joint Laplace distribution underlying in this case instead of the more typical Gaussian alternative, which would penalize those large jumps more heavily. Nevertheless, CAR-L1 based models do not explicitly incorporate into the modeling the possibility of having discontinuities in the risk surface. Geo-graphical discontinuities are not explicitly acknowledged as a modeling issue in the CAR-L1 distribution and differences in risks between all neighbouring units are equally penalized. Regarding the performance of models with CAR-L1 random effects, Best et al. (1999) compare them with the traditional BYM model. As a result, they state that the BYM model achieves better results for modeling smooth risk surfaces, while the CAR-L1 distribution depicts better the rural-urban boundary in their example since this method is particularly suited for this kind of task. Interestingly, they also state that the choice of weights for the different neighbours in the map graph has a greater impact on the surface fitted than the choice between CAR-L1 or ICAR random effects.

Brezger et al. (2007) propose a CAR-based smoothing model for human brain mapping. They use the typical set of conditional Normal distributions for defining dependence:

$$\theta_i | \boldsymbol{\theta}_{-i} \sim N \left(\sum_{i \sim j} \frac{w_{ij}\theta_j}{w_{i+}}, \frac{\sigma^2}{w_{i+}} \right)$$

but they advise against the lack of adaptability of this proposal for a fixed vec-tor $\boldsymbol{w}$. They specifically warn against the excessive smoothing of this proposal for discontinuities of the risk surface that could be alleviated by modeling the vector of weights. Thus, they propose to model the components of $\boldsymbol{w}$ as independent variables with an informative $Gamma(1/2, 1/2)$ distribution. In this manner, this proposal could have an adaptive performance since edges corresponding to discontinuities in the risk function could have lower weights and therefore contribute to the smoothing to a lesser extent. The resulting joint posterior distribution of $\boldsymbol{\theta}$ will no longer be multivariate Normal (indeed it does not admit a simple analytic form) as in traditional CAR proposals with fixed weights, even though the conditional distributions $P(\theta_i|\boldsymbol{\theta}_{-i}, \boldsymbol{w})$ follow Normal distributions. According to several simulated data sets, the authors claim that the performance is better than that of typical Intrinsic CAR and CAR-L1 alternatives. Namely, their proposal separates better between spatial regions corresponding to signal and noise, depicting the borders delimiting those regions better.

The term *areal Wombling* (Lu and Carlin, 2005; Lu et al., 2007) has been coined after a foundational work by Womble (1951) trying to identify zones of abrupt changes (barriers or edges) in an underlying surface. Originally Womble's work referred to collections of points at some continuous space and that problem has been further developed in recent works, see for example Banerjee et al. (2003a) and Banerjee and Gelfand (2006). Areal Wombling consists of the identification of those abrupt changes in the context of geographical analysis of areal data, i.e., the identification of those borders that separate adjacent units with markedly different performance. The identification of those barriers associated with (more) independent risk estimates is additionally an issue of obvious epidemiological interest. More specifically, areal Wombling (Lu et al., 2007) can be seen as a variant of Brezger et al. (2007) but with a more explicit modeling of discontinuities between neighbouring units. Instead of assuming a continuous gamma distribution for the weights in the conditional distributions, Wombling proposals assume dichotomic 0/1 values for the adjacency matrix $\boldsymbol{W}$, modeled as:

$$w_{ij} \sim Bernoulli(p_{ij})$$

$$logit(p_{ij}) = \beta_0 + \beta_1 z_{ij}$$

for some covariate $\boldsymbol{Z}$ with information on the relationship between areal units. Lu et al. consider $\boldsymbol{Z}$ to be simply the adjacency matrix of the region of study, so all adjacent regions will have equal probabilities of being 'neighbours', while non-adjacent units will have another (supposedly lower) probability. Obviously, another different proposal for $\boldsymbol{Z}$ could also be used. In contrast to Brezger et al. (2007), which modeled the weights just for neighbouring units, this new proposal models the weights for all pairs (i, j) with $i \neq j$. This makes the number of variables in the model be of order $O(I^2)$ and therefore its use problematic for regions with a large number of units. Lu et al. use informative prior proposals for β and many of the parameters in the model and they warn of the use of non-informative priors. Moreover, although C routines are available at the author's website for doing inference in this model, its coding is in general not feasible in more friendly alternatives such as WinBUGS or INLA. This makes the modification of the routines (changing prior distributions, adding additional covariates, etc.) hard to do.

Another modeling proposal with even more explicit modeling of discontinuities in the risk surface is that in Knorr-Held and Raßer (2000). This proposal builds a risk surface by setting a discrete tessellation of the region of study, with constant risk for any of the tiles composing the whole partition. More specifically, they consider a set of k areal units $(\delta_1, ..., \delta_k) \subseteq \{1, ..., I\}$ as 'centroids' of those tiles and assign each areal unit to the tile with the closest centroid. Distance between two areas is defined as the number of regions that have to be crossed for going from one unit to the other since, as shown in the original paper, this yields tessellations with all the tiles being connected components. The number of components in the tessellation, k, is also considered an additional variable in the model. As a consequence the number of risks needed for defining the risk surface $(\lambda_1, ..., \lambda_k)$, depends also on this stochastic value and therefore a specific Reversible Jump trans-dimensional MCMC algorithm is needed for making inference in this model. A geometric prior distribution is set on k, i.e., $P(k) \propto (1-a)^k$. For $a = 0$ this is just a uniform prior distribution on the number of clusters that compose the risk surface. The authors suggest to fix a low value for a, such as 0.02 in order to put a 'close to uninformative' prior. Note that for low values of k, the model will yield spatial processes of high spatial dependence since the spatial units will be allocated to very few spatially connected clusters. On the contrary, for large values of k the variability in the risks will be mostly heterogeneous and full spatial independence is achieved for $k = I$. Given the number k of tiles in the tessellation, the locations $(\delta_1, ..., \delta_k)$ of the centroids of the tiles have a uniform prior distribution on the set of areal units of the region of study. Regarding the prior distribution of the risks for each of the tiles $(\lambda_1, ..., \lambda_k)$, a lognormal prior distribution of unknown mean and variance (which are assigned vague prior distributions) is used for them.

Interesting summaries such as the probability that two neighbouring units belong to the same connected component can be derived from this model. This would allow defining the most likely discontinuities in the risk surface as the borders between adjacent areas that most frequently belong to separate components of the tessellation. This kind of summaries could be of high epidemiologic interest and they are explored in detail, for example, in the Wombling literature but they could be also easily adapted to the Knorr-Held and Raßer's model. A second interesting feature of this model is that the prior variances for the risks are the same for all the units in the region of study. This is in contrast to many CAR distributions, where units with less neighbours have higher conditional variance and frequently show more variable estimates than those regions with a higher number of neighbours. As previously mentioned, MCMC simulation from this model requires the specific coding of the routines in nonconventional software since the Reversible Jump algorithm makes it unfeasible for `WinBUGS` or `INLA`. Fortunately, the authors have a compiled version of their code (`http://www.statistik.lmu.de/sfb386/software/bdcd/index.html`) ready to be run. Knorr-Held and Raßer's model is assessed and compared in Best et al. (2005) showing a good performance. This model attained the best fit in the comparison, in terms of DIC, for 2 out of the 5 data sets considered, so it seems to be a very competitive proposal.

Denison and Holmes (2001) propose a similar model to the Knorr-Held and Raßer proposal. The main difference between them is that Denison and Holmes's model uses a Voronoi tessellation so that each unit is allocated to the tile whose center is closer (in terms of Euclidean distance) to that unit's centroid. Risks for each tile in the tessellation are assumed to have gamma prior distributions so that their posterior distributions are conjugate. The authors state that this makes a great advantage from a computational point of view, but they do not make available any routine for potential users.

Mixture models are one of the obvious approaches for dividing the region of study into several disjoint sets. Mixture modeling proceeds as follows, the whole data set is considered to be composed of different subpopulations, each of them following a different distribution. Thus, in case of assuming a mixture model for modeling the observed cases we would have:

$$o_i | \boldsymbol{\omega}, \boldsymbol{\theta} \sim \sum_{k=1}^{K} \omega_k f_k(o_i | \boldsymbol{\theta}_k),$$

where $\boldsymbol{\omega} = (\omega_1, ..., \omega_K)$ is a vector of weights accounting for the proportion of observations corresponding to each subpopulation of the mixture. The components of this vector are all positive and are subject to the restriction $\sum_{k=1}^{K} \omega_k = 1$. This alternative formulation makes an explicit allocation of each observed count to a subpopulation by means of variables $\{\alpha_i : i = 1, ..., I\}$, where α_i takes values in $\{1, ..., K\}$ by following a multinomial distribution with probabilities $\boldsymbol{\omega}$. Conditioned to these auxiliary variables, the observed cases would be distributed as

$$o_i | \boldsymbol{\alpha}, \boldsymbol{\theta} \sim f_{\alpha_i}(o_i | \boldsymbol{\theta}_{\alpha_i}) \tag{6.5}$$

$$\alpha_i \sim Multinomial(\boldsymbol{\omega}).$$

The equivalence of both formulations is evident by just integrating out $\boldsymbol{\alpha}$ in the data-augmented formulation. This alternative formulation has lots of advantages from a computational point of view. Moreover, the explicit allocation of each observation to some of the components of the mixture brings additional opportunities for modeling that process.

For disease mapping models, a typical choice is to consider $f_1 = ... = f_K$ to be Poisson distributions, each of them having a different mean. That proposal has focussed considerable attention under the frequentist approach (Schlattmann and Böhning, 1993; Böhning and Schlattmann, 1999; Militino et al., 2001); and Ugarte et al. (2006). Namely, these proposals assume

$$o_i | \boldsymbol{\omega}, \boldsymbol{\theta} \sim \sum_{k=1}^{K} \omega_k Pois(o_i | e_i \theta_k).$$

Since these models are frequentist, no particular prior is assumed for either $\boldsymbol{\omega}$ or $\boldsymbol{\theta}$, the vector of expected risks for the components of the mixture. Inference on these models is done with EM algorithms. Software packages, such as C.A.MAN (Böhning et al., 1992), are available for carrying out inference on this model. The number of components in the mixture K is usually estimated by means of hypothesis testing, such as parametric bootstrap (Schlattmann and Böhning, 1993).

The main drawback of the mixture approach as introduced above is that it does not induce any spatial dependence on the data. The observed cases are i.i.d. given ω and θ, which does not take any advantage of the spatial arrangement of the data. Moreover, as also mentioned above, if the data-augmented version of this model was formulated, it would assume independent multinomial i.i.d. distributions on the vector of allocations α which would induce heterogeneous variability in the model. Thus, this proposal does not seem very appropriate for modeling patterns showing spatial dependence. Nevertheless, if the goal was identifying non-spatial subgroups in the units of the study, or those subgroups really exist, mixture modeling would be a good option (Militino et al., 2001). In any case, mixtures would do a reasonable work if there were geographic discontinuities in the risk surface, as they would not oversmooth by assuming spatial dependence.

Following a Bayesian approach, Green and Richardson (2002) propose an enhancement of the mixtures models above inducing spatial dependence on the data. This proposal makes an explicit division of the region of study into K disjoint regions, for K a variable to be estimated within the model. Knorr-Held and Raßer (2000) or Denison and Holmes (2001) make a hard-core division of the region of study given the centroids of the corresponding tessellations. In contrast, Green and Richardson make a soft division of the space where neighboring units could be perfectly assigned to different elements of the mixture and units placed very far apart can be assigned to the same component. As a consequence, this new model will use in general less components for dividing the region of study since a single component of the division may be used in separate regions placed very far apart. Green and Richardson propose a mixture modeling for the underlying risks, where the risk for each unit takes necessarily 1 out of K different possible values; therefore, the first layer of the data-augmented version of mixtures will also apply here. However, in contrast to traditional mixture models, spatial dependence is induced by rewarding nearby units to belong to the same component of the mixture, i.e., this model does not assume an i.i.d. multinomial process for the vector of allocations α. For achieving this goal, the authors propose a Potts model, an adaptation of hidden (discrete-state) Markov models for time series to irregular spatial domains, as those typically used in disease mapping studies. More specifically, Green and Richardson assume the observed counts to be distributed as in (6.5). The components in θ are assumed to have a $Gamma(a, b)$ prior distribution with $a = 1$ and $b = \sum_{i=1}^{I} e_i / \sum_{i=1}^{I} o_i$, which is often equal to 1 if internal standardization is used for calculating the expected cases e. The vector α is in charge of inducing spatial dependence in the process. Thus, its prior distribution is set as $P(\boldsymbol{\alpha}|\psi) \propto e^{\psi U(\boldsymbol{\alpha})}$, where $U(\boldsymbol{\alpha}) = \sum_{i \sim i'} I[\alpha_i = \alpha_{i'}]$ is the number of equally labelled neighbouring pairs. For $\psi = 0$ this is just a uniform distribution on $\boldsymbol{\alpha}$ but for $\psi > 0$ this favours neighboring units to be assigned to the same component of the mixture and so induces spatial dependence. Obviously, spatial dependence increases with ψ. The definition of the model by assuming a uniform prior on K between 1 and 10 (10 is assumed to be a high non-informative value) and another uniform prior on ψ between 0 and 1. The authors argue that 1 would induce enough spatial dependence in real terms. Although this model induces a partition of the space into K disjoint sets, the resulting risk surface does not show any striking discontinuity in general. The allocation of the areal units to the components of the mixture is not deterministic and its uncertainty makes those hypothetical discontinuities of the risk surface to be blurred, as in Knorr-Held and Raßer (2000), yielding in general smooth risk surfaces except for some few places.

Despite of the apparent simplicity of $P(\boldsymbol{\alpha}|\psi)$, its proportionality constant depends on all the I^K possible values of $\boldsymbol{\alpha}$, which introduces an important drawback from a computational perspective. Moreover, since the number of parameters in the model depends on K, the number of components in the mixture, Reversible jump trans-dimensional MCMC is needed in order to sample from the posterior distribution of this model. This makes the coding of this model to be unfeasible in `WinBUGS` or `INLA`. The authors state that the algorithm of this model has been programmed in `Fortran`, but no routines are made public for its use.

According to results on simulated data sets (Green and Richardson, 2002), the hidden Markov modeling of risks proposed yields in general lower mean squared errors than BYM. This proposal in terms of its authors depicts better spatial transitions when discontinuities are present in risk surfaces, avoiding oversmoothing. Additionally, it also provides good results, comparable to those of BYM, when the risk surface varies smoothly. In general, the hidden Markov-based model is less sensible to noise in the data as compared to BYM, which shows higher random variability when no pattern is present and higher uncertainty in general. In the model comparison performed in Best et al. (2005) this mixture model achieved very good results, being the best model in terms of DIC for 3 out of 5 data sets considered.

A second work inducing spatial dependence in mixture models would be that in Fernández and Green (2002). This model uses the original formulation of mixtures (non-data-augmented) with Poisson distributions as likelihood function, i.e.,

$$o_i|\boldsymbol{\omega}, \boldsymbol{\theta} \sim \sum_{k=1}^{K} \omega_{ik} Pois(o_i|e_i\theta_k),$$

but notice that now the weights ω_{ik} are different for each areal unit in contrast to the original formulation of mixture models. Informative gamma priors are assumed for the risks $\boldsymbol{\theta}$ for each component of the mixture.

Two different processes are proposed by Fernández and Green in order to induce spatial dependence in this model through the specific modeling of these weights. The basic underlying idea of both proposals is that observations that correspond to neighbouring locations should have similar vectors of weights. The first of these proposals considers K vectors of length I: $\{\varphi_1, ..., \varphi_K\}$ all of them following CAR processes. Then the vectors of weights are defined as:

$$\omega_{ik} = \frac{\exp((\varphi_k)_i)}{\sum_{j=1}^{K} \exp((\varphi_j)_i)}.$$

The spatial dependence on $\{\varphi_1, ..., \varphi_K\}$ induces spatial dependence on the set of weight vectors $\{\omega_1, ..., \omega_K\}$ making them similar to neighbouring sites. Alternatively, Fernández and Green consider a second process based on a single vector φ of length I which also follows a CAR process. Additionally, they consider a vector δ of length $K - 1$ and a distribution function Ψ (a logistic distribution function is considered in the paper) and they define the vector of weights for unit i as:

$$\omega_{ik} = \begin{cases} \Psi(\delta_1 - \varphi_i) & for\ k = 1, \\ \Psi(\delta_k - \varphi_i) - \Psi(\delta_{k-1} - \varphi_i) & for\ k = 1, ..., K - 1, \\ 1 - \Psi(\delta_{K-1} - \varphi_i) & for\ k = K. \end{cases}$$

Vector δ, which is essential for defining the vector of weights, is also estimated within the model and a prior distribution encouraging separation of their components is assumed. This prior distribution avoids having empty components within the mixture. The first of these modeling options for ω, which depends on a higher number of parameters, is more flexible. For example, it may give a high probability for one of the components of the mixture to just some areal neighbouring units, making the corresponding $(\varphi_k)_i$s high; this is not so easy to achieve with the second proposal.

Since the number of parameters in both modeling proposals of Fernández and Green depend on K, which is also a variable in the model, Reversible jump MCMC is required to sample from their posterior distribution. This makes its implementation infeasible for both `WinBUGS` and `INLA` and a specific coding of this model is done in `Fortran` in the original paper. Unfortunately, that code is not freely available for potential users. Simulation studies are carried out of these models in the original paper. In case of having a risk surface with discontinuities, these mixture models show an enhanced performance, as compared to BYM. Nevertheless, that performance is less satisfactory for modeling a smoothly changing gradient-like risk surface. For smooth patterns, BYM achieves lower mean squared errors than these correlated mixtures models. However, the sensitivity of these models to prior distributions is mostly unknown. Several of the prior distributions originally proposed are informative and their sensitivity should be further explored.

A final kind of partition models would be those where discontinuities may come from the own (known) data design. Sometimes the region of study is divided in different, usually nested, partitions with potential effect on the observed data. For example, countries may be divided into states and these could also be divided into counties, so nationwide municipal-level studies would show two sources of variation: counties within states and states within the whole country. This could mean that, for example, neighbouring counties belonging to different states were in general more different than any two counties belonging to the same state. Obviously this kind of data would require particular modeling. This case is different than the rest of the data and models introduced in this section since for this setting we know in advance which would be the main potential discontinuities in the risk surface. Several works have considered this setting in the spatial (see for example Langford et al. (1999); MacNab and Dean (2000)) and even in the spatio-temporal case (Schrödle et al., 2011; Ugarte et al., 2015).

Although spatio-temporal, the work of Ugarte et al. (2016) is in our opinion very enlightening of the modeling possibilities and issues of the spatial component for this kind of data. We will briefly reproduce their proposal. They consider a two-level model, counties and states, keeping on with the simile above, although this could be adapted to more general settings. Following Ugarte et al.'s terminology they call first-level areas (FLA) to the units in the finer division and second-level areas (SLA) to those in the coarse division. They assume the risk θ_i for each areal unit $i = 1, ..., I$ to be the sum of two components ξ_i and $\psi_{j(i)}$ corresponding, respectively, to the FLA and SLA of unit i. Note that j will vary from 1 to J, for $J << I$.

Both vectors $\boldsymbol{\xi}$ and $\boldsymbol{\psi}$ can be modeled in several different ways. Ugarte et al. propose 3 specific ways for $\boldsymbol{\xi}$. First, the whole vector $\boldsymbol{\xi}$ could be modeled by means of a joint spatial distribution (they use Leroux's proposal) considering as neighbours all those neighbouring FLAs, regardless of their SLAs. Alternatively, they consider as neighbours all those FLAs which are neighbours and belong to the same SLA. This second modeling proposal would be equivalent to consider a spatial distribution on that lattice, composed by several 'islands', one per SLA. Finally, as a third option, they propose a different spatial distribution (with different variance parameters) for each of the islands arising when considering each SLA separately. Obviously, additional sum-to-zero restrictions should be set for $\boldsymbol{\xi}$ in each SLA for the last two proposals, since for them these are considered as separate islands at the FLA level. Regarding the modeling of $\boldsymbol{\psi}$, Ugarte et al. propose to model it as either independent or spatially structured random effects, depending on the number of SLAs in the region of study. For very few SLAs, surely a heterogeneous random effect would be more appropriate, but if the number of SLAs was higher, a spatial random effect could be more convenient to reproduce the mid-range, in principle smooth, geographic variability of risks.

The differences in the modeling of FLAs, as for the three alternatives introduced in the previous paragraph, are substantial. As seen in the first section of this chapter the geometry of the regions of study plays an important role in the final fit and that geometry is very different for the three cases considered. According to the results in that section, Leroux's spatial structure considered in Ugarte et al. (2016), and used for the first scenario in that work, would describe a pattern with positive spatial correlations that would vanish to 0 for long distances. For the second of these modeling proposals, correlations would vanish to 0 for distant regions of each SLA and for units of different SLAs, yielding then much more local dependence patterns. Finally, the third modeling proposal would have different smoothing parameters for each SLA, yielding then local patterns with different smoothing features. This could be convenient mainly if the size of the SLAs is markedly different since then some values of the parameters could be very appropriate for some SLAs but not for others.

These models can be implemented in general in both WinBUGS and INLA, although both softwares find their own problems for some of the options introduced. Thus, the implementation of the second of the options above in WinBUGS is problematic since we have a single CAR distribution for all the FLAs corresponding to each SLA. Hence, a sum-to-zero restriction should be imposed for the FLAs in each SLA and the exponent of the precision in the corresponding GMRF should be also modified as a function of the number of SLAs (islands) in the region of study. According to our knowledge, there is no straightforward manner to do this in WinBUGS. On the contrary, regarding the third of the options above, although its implementation in INLA is feasible, that implementation is computationally problematic. In this case we would have as many different random effects as islands in the region of study. If the number of SLAs in that region is high, INLA would have a lot of parameters (precisions) to numerically integrate out. That integration is quite demanding for INLA when the number of parameters to integrate is high. Thus, Marí-Dell'Olmo and Martínez-Beneito (2015) opted for WinBUGS instead of INLA since the first was a faster alternative in a similar two-level ecological regression study. In their study they deal with census tracts corresponding to a set of 31 separate cities that would play the same role as SLAs in Ugarte et al. (2016).

6.5.2   Models for fitting zero excesses

One issue that disease mapping data sets could show and that deserves particular attention is the presence of an excessive number of zeroes in the observed counts. Having an excessive number of zeroes should not be confounded with having a lot of zeroes since the latter could be just a consequence of having a disease with low mortality or simply small units of analysis, but this should not mean necessarily there is a problem. The problem could come, for example, if we had a disease where the observed counts were distributed as a Poisson distribution with a common mean $\theta = 1$ (we will not consider different expected counts, i.e., $e_1 = e_2 = ... = e_I = 1$). In that case the probability of any observation to be equal to zero would be $P(O = 0|\theta = 1) = \exp(-1) \approx 0.37$, so we would expect a percentage of zero counts in our data set of around 37%. If two-thirds, for example, of the observed counts for this model were equal to 0, the number of zero counts would be then excessive according to those really expected under that model. This is what is known as a zero excess, which is just a particular misfit of the model assumed to the observed data with regard to the number of zero counts. Although the previous example considers a much more naive model than those we typically use for disease mapping, zero excesses could be also a problem for these studies as long as the fitted model is not able to reproduce as many zeroes as those contained in the data set.

Specific tests have been proposed in the frequentist setting for assessing the presence of zero excess problems such as Van Der Broek (1995), which has been later adapted for disease mapping problems (Ugarte et al., 2004). Other procedures have been also proposed for assessing zero excesses from a Bayesian setting (Bayarri et al., 2008), although predictive checkings are also useful tools under this approach. Basically, predictive checking samples from the predictive distribution of the number of zeroes in the model and compares that sample with the real observed zeroes in the data set. If the predictive distribution has most of its mass below those observed zeroes, it should be taken as an evidence of zero excess in the data set (with respect to the fitted model). This procedure can be easily integrated within MCMC algorithms by sampling a value of the predictive distribution of each observed count at every step of the MCMC and counting the number of zeroes among them. Corpas-Burgos et al. (2018) have shown that for the BYM model, for 46 geographical patterns studied in the Valencian Region, zero excess is present for about one-third of the data sets. Thus, the presence of this issue in regular mortality studies could be in general a prevalent problem that should deserve close attention.

Two main modifications of regular disease mapping models have been proposed for dealing with zero excess; these are *Zero Inflated Poisson* models (ZIP henceforth) and *hurdle* Poisson models (simply hurdle models henceforth). Both proposals make a specific treatment of zeroes by giving them a particular mass in the likelihood function, which both models assume to be a Poisson distribution (although this could be easily generalized to other families such as, for example, binomial). On one hand, ZIP models (originally introduced in Lambert (1992) outside of the disease mapping literature), assume the data likelihood to be a mixture of a Poisson distribution and a zero-specific component with all its mass at 0, instead of a simple Poisson distribution. More specifically, the observed cases are assumed to be distributed according to the following mixture:

$$o_i|\pi,\boldsymbol{\theta} \sim (1 - \pi)1_{\{0\}}(o_i) + \pi Pois(o_i|e_i\theta_i)$$

where $1_\Omega(o_i)$ is equal to 1 if $o_i \in \Omega$ or 0 otherwise, as defined in Chapter 1, and π, the probability of the Poisson component, takes values between 0 and 1.

For $\boldsymbol{\theta}$ modeled as in BYM, this proposal would be a ZIP version of that model for disease mapping. Nevertheless, some other spatial distributions could be alternatively used for inducing dependence in the risks. For ZIP models, the zero-specific term puts additional mass in 0 inflating the probability of zeroes corresponding to the Poisson distribution. Smoothed $sSMRs$ for ZIP models would be simply estimated as $\pi\theta_i$.

On the other hand, hurdle models (Mullahy, 1986) assume a mixture of a zero-specific component and a truncated Poisson distribution (taking just positive values), instead of a regular Poisson distribution as for ZIP. That is,

$$P(o_i|\pi,\boldsymbol{\theta}) = (1-\pi)^{1_{\{0\}}(o_i)} \left(\pi \left(\frac{\exp(-e_i\theta_i)\theta_i^{o_i}(o_i!)^{-1}}{1-\exp(-e_i\theta_i)} \right) \right)^{1_{]0,\infty[}(o_i)}, \quad (6.6)$$

so, the probability of observing a 0 is separately modeled with the zero-specific component, as the Poisson component only takes an effect for positive counts. For hurdle models π takes also values between 0 and 1 and $\boldsymbol{\theta}$ is typically modeled, with a BYM model for example, so that it induces spatial dependence on the risks. The smoothed SMR for the i-th spatial unit for hurdle models would be estimated as $((e_i\lambda_i)/(1-\exp(-e_i\lambda_i)))\cdot\pi/e_i$ (Neelon et al., 2013). This expression corresponds to the mean of the truncated Poisson component corrected by its probability and the number of expected cases, since we want to estimate the risk instead of the expected cases of the observed counts.

As stated above, both ZIP (Gschlößl and Czado, 2008; Musenge et al., 2013; Arab, 2015; MacNab, 2016b) and hurdle (Arab, 2015; Neyens et al., 2017) versions of regular spatial models could be posed by simply putting a prior distribution on π and using the corresponding spatial distribution for modeling $\boldsymbol{\theta}$. A uniform prior distribution between 0 and 1 is the most typical choice for π. Nevertheless, Corpas-Burgos et al. (2018) argue that using naive models with a common π for all areal units could yield inappropriate $sSMRs$ estimates. On one hand, for the ZIP case, those $sSMRs$ could be closely similar to those drawn from the spatial base model within the ZIP formulation. Thus, the zero-specific component would be basically ignored since otherwise it would put non-negligible probabilities of zeroes to all spatial units, even those with large populations where zeroes are impossible to be observed in practical terms. Thus, the zero-specific component is ignored due to its harmful effect on the most populated units, at least if the spatial units have very different populations. On the other hand, for hurdle models, using a common probability π for all units yields misleading risk estimates since that term takes the same effect on all the $sSMRs$, regardless of the size of each spatial unit. As a consequence, the $sSMRs$ estimates corresponding to more populated units are reduced, producing an infraestimation in these areas. Thus, more elaborated models considering different probabilities of the zero-specific component: $\boldsymbol{\pi} = \{\pi_i : i = 1, ..., I\}$ seem to be a convenient alternative.

The modularity of Bayesian hierarchical models allows to model the vector $\boldsymbol{\pi}$, instead of a common π, easily within the models above. Although some alternative proposals have been formulated for modeling $\boldsymbol{\pi}$ (Song et al., 2011), the most common choice is setting

$$logit(\boldsymbol{\pi}) = \boldsymbol{X\beta} + \boldsymbol{\varphi}$$

for $\boldsymbol{X}$ a matrix of covariates, $\boldsymbol{\beta}$ a vector of parameters to be estimated and $\boldsymbol{\varphi}$ a vector of (possibly spatial) random effects. Proposals of this kind have been repeatedly used in the literature for both ZIP (Nieto-Barajas and Bandy-opadhyay, 2013; MacNab, 2014) and hurdle models (Neelon et al., 2013, 2014; Arab, 2015). Nevertheless, this apparently innocuous modeling of the zero-specific probabilities hides unexpected dangers (Corpas-Burgos et al., 2018). Namely, the use of improper prior distributions for the dispersion parameter of $\boldsymbol{\varphi}$ makes also improper the posterior distribution. Moreover, the use of vague proper priors for this same parameter, trying to mimic improper non-informative priors does not seem to be an advisable procedure in this case. Thus, the use of random effects for modeling $logit(\boldsymbol{\pi})$ should be discouraged unless an informative prior distribution was used for its dispersion parameter, as proposed by Agarwal et al. (2002).

Regarding $\boldsymbol{\beta}$, important differences arise between ZIP and hurdle models, yielding ZIP models improper posterior distributions much more easily than hurdle models. Thus, it can be shown (Corpas-Burgos et al., 2018) that for ZIP, an improper prior distribution on $\boldsymbol{\beta}$ yields also an improper posterior distribution if any of the variables in $\boldsymbol{X}$ takes only positive (or negative) values. This is in general easily accomplished since including just an intercept into the model would fulfill this condition. In this case a vague prior distribution is not a reasonable option either since it would yield a very sensitive posterior distribution, identified only by that (arbitrary) prior distribution. For hurdle models, the condition for posterior impropriety is much milder: one of the variables should be positive (or negative) for those i with $o_i > 0$ and negative otherwise. So the use of fixed effects in hurdle models is much less troublesome than for ZIP models.

Those restrictions stated in the previous paragraph discard many of the modeling proposals already made in the literature. According to these restrictions, Corpas-Burgos et al. (2018) formulate several 'valid' modeling proposals. We put valid in quotation marks since the impropriety conditions in the previous paragraph are sufficient but not necessary, so we cannot really guarantee the posterior propriety of these proposals, but at least we know that they do not fall in the conditions for posterior impropriety mentioned above. We describe here one of them as an example. They propose a hurdle model with BYM modeling of the Poisson mean, as above, with

$$logit(\pi_i) = logit(1 - \exp(-e_i\theta_i)) + \gamma.$$

That is, they model $\boldsymbol{\pi}$ by means of a logistic regression with an offset depending on $P(o_i = 0)$ for the Poisson term in the model. This offset is leveraged with γ, which is supposed to control the zero excess in the data. Thus, for

$\gamma = 0$ this model is completely equivalent to a regular (uninflated) BYM model, whereas for $\gamma < 0$ the probabilities of zeroes $(1 - \pi)$ would be higher than that in the BYM model, producing then the pursued zero inflation. As shown in Corpas-Burgos et al. (2018), this proposal fixes the zero excess problems arising in regular mortality data sets that naive (without π's specific modeling) ZIP and hurdle models were not able to fix.

ZIP and hurdle models may be implemented in both `WinBUGS` and `INLA`. The implementation of ZIP models in `WinBUGS` is quite straightforward by coding that model as a mixture of two Poisson distributions, one of mean zero (zero-specific component) and a second one with positive mean (the spatial process). The `WinBUGS` code of the hurdle model is not so straightforward. In this case the mixture to be coded contains a truncated Poisson distribution which is not one of the prebuilt distributions in `WinBUGS` (the truncation device for `WinBUGS` is not valid in this case). As a consequence, the likelihood function of this model (Expression (6.6)) has to be specifically coded in `WinBUGS` with the 'zeros trick' (see pages 204–206 in Lunn et al. (2013)). Several ZIP and hurdle `WinBUGS` codes (with and without modeling of π) can be found as supplementary material in Corpas-Burgos et al. (2018).

`INLA` has also several prebuilt likelihood functions implementing ZIP and hurdle models. These functions implement hurdle (`zeroinflatedpoisson0` likelihood for `INLA`) and ZIP (`zeroinflatedpoisson1` likelihood for `INLA`) models with a common probability π for all spatial units. Additionally, a ZIP model with

$$\pi = 1 - \left(\frac{\exp(e\boldsymbol{\theta})}{1 + \exp(e\boldsymbol{\theta})} \right)^{\alpha}$$

where α is estimated by the model is also available (`zeroinflatedpoisson2` likelihood for `INLA`). Anyway, non-vague proper prior distributions are set by default on the ZIP and hurdle parameters of these models, so we would advise their users to perform tough sensitivity analyses for them.

Exercises

1. Alternatively to the CAR-based models repeatedly fitted in this book, fit now:

   - A geostatistical model
   - A moving average model (we suggest you fit SMARS)
   - A P-spline model

   to the COPD data also studied in the exercises of the previous chapters. Additionally, perform the following tasks:

- Determine the model which shows a better fit in terms of DIC.

- Do you find higher or lower differences for the $sSMR$s of these models than those corresponding to the CAR-based models in Chapter 4 exercises?

- Draw choropleth maps for all the models run and compare them. Additionally, draw an isopleth map for the COPD mortality risk for the geostatistical model.

- For the SMARS model, how many neighbours away do you find that the underlying risk in this model has an effect on?

- For the P-spline model fitted, do you find evidence of anisotropy in the estimated risk pattern?

- Fit several different P-spline models with different prior structures for the random effects, different number of knots, etc. and assess the sensitivity of the results in the model to these choices.

2. The `COPDFirst4.Rdata` file contains the COPD observed (and expected) death counts for the Valencia city census tracts, but just for the period 1996–1999. This data set, as the rest of data sets in the exercises, has been slightly modified for preserving the confidentiality of the original data set. These data contain 123 census tracts with no observed COPD death, a 23.3% of the whole census tracts in the data set. Maybe this may seem like a lot of zeroes at a first glance but, as discussed in this chapter, it does not necessarily mean the presence of a zero excess for this data set. Using the predictive distribution for the observed counts, assess the presence of a zero excess, with respect to the fit of a BYM model, for this data set.

7

Spatio-temporal disease mapping

So far, temporal variability in the geographical distribution of risks has been ignored in this book. Observed counts often corresponded to long time periods and geographical changes that could have happened during that time interval have been missed by such a long temporal aggregation. As a consequence, one could be missing important information on the evolution of the distribution of diseases that could be very relevant under an epidemiologic point of view. The main goal of this chapter is to include the temporal dimension into disease mapping studies so that we will be able to obtain a dynamic view of the geographical distribution of risks instead of a fixed picture for, sometimes long, periods of study.

Spatio-temporal analyses make the statistical small area problems arising in regular disease mapping studies even more serious. Using long periods of study in spatial analyses could apparently seem to be a solution for those problems, as these increase the number of observed counts of the corresponding disease per areal unit. Nevertheless, if spatio-temporal interaction exists, the use of long periods of analysis for estimating the overall risks for the whole period of study yields biased estimates. This bias persists even in the absence of spatio-temporal interaction, but just with an overall temporal trend in the mean risk for the whole region of study (Ocaña Riola, 2007). As a consequence, the use of spatio-temporal models that take the temporal evolution of risks into account becomes almost compulsory when long periods of analysis are considered.

The general spatio-temporal disease mapping modeling framework, followed by most studies in this area, may be formulated as follows. Let O_{it} be the number of observed deaths for the i-th areal unit ($i = 1, ..., I$) and t-th time period ($t = 1, ..., T$) for the corresponding cause of death. These observed counts are usually assumed to follow conditionally independent Poisson distributions

$$O_{it}|\Theta_{it} \sim Poisson(E_{it}\Theta_{it}). \tag{7.1}$$

Different spatio-temporal models arise for each different proposal for Θ, or to be more precise for $\log(\Theta)$ since a logarithmic link function will be typically used for modeling the log-risks. In contrast to pure spatial models, the spatio-temporal case will usually account for the spatial and temporal dependence of the risks. Thus, spatio-temporal models jointly induce dependence both across rows and columns of Θ. In contrast to spatial models, where there is just one source of dependence, the joint induction of two sources of dependence is the main challenge of spatio-temporal modeling that we will introduce in this chapter.

In this chapter, and until the end of this book, we start with the modeling of vectors (or even arrays at Chapter 9) of observations for each spatial unit, in contrast to all the previous chapters where we had just a single univariate observation for each of them. In addition, spatio-temporal modeling has the particularity that the elements in the vector of observations for each spatial unit follow a particular ordering that determines its dependence structure. This is in contrast to the rest of multivariate models developed in the next chapters where no particular order or structure is ever assumed for the dependence of the different outcomes within each spatial unit. Thus in this sense spatio-temporal models are a bit particular, although they have the advantage of a vast supporting literature devoted to the particular modeling of dependent data of this kind. Therefore, in some way, spatio-temporal models mostly fuse the methods developed for disease mapping, already introduced, and those used for the analysis of longitudinal data.

This chapter is structured as follows. First, we start with a general section discussing some general aspects of relevance in spatio-temporal studies. Later, Section 7.2 introduces spatio-temporal models whose time trends are defined as parametric functions of time. Spline modeling of time trends could also be seen as a particular case of parametric model (with a basis of spline used as parametric family for the time trends). Nevertheless, we devote Section 7.3 to spline-based spatio-temporal modeling due to the large literature developed on this issue. Finally, Section 7.4 introduces models inducing spatio-temporal dependence by means of correlated random effects, a less parametric alternative to the models developed in the previous sections.

7.1   Some general issues in spatio-temporal modeling

An important issue in the formulation of spatio-temporal models which usually gets hardly any attention is the calculation of the expected cases per spatio-temporal unit E_{it}. For spatial problems ignoring temporal variability, expected cases were calculated by considering a reference region and period and using the age-specific observed deaths along that region and period. This was previously explained in Section 4.1, but briefly: expected cases for spatial unit i were calculated as: $e_i = \sum_{j=1}^{J} p_{ij} r_j$ where j indexes the age groups considered, p_{ij} stands for the person-years at risk for the i-th spatial unit and j-th age group, and r_j is the observed risk for that age group in the reference population. The whole region and period of study corresponding to the set of observed deaths is usually taken as reference population, this was known as internal standardization in Section 4.1. Thus, SMRs above 1 are interpreted as risk excesses in comparison to the whole region and period of study considered.

For the spatio-temporal case, we do not have a single number of expected cases per spatial unit but a different number E_{it} per period considered. In this case, we will denote expected cases by an uppercase letter for stressing that they are elements of a general matrix $\boldsymbol{E}$ of dimension $I \times T$. The rows of $\boldsymbol{E} = (E_{it})$ intend to control temporal changes in the age composition of each spatial unit that could induce additional temporal changes in the observed deaths. If temporal variability in expected cases was not taken into account, these demographic changes would be absorbed by the risks and risk maps would reproduce changes in demography, instead of just changes in the risk distribution.

Mimicking the procedure for the spatial case, E_{it} could be naturally defined in at least two different manners for spatio-temporal studies. In practice, important differences could arise for these two different choices (López-Abente et al., 2014). Expected cases could be defined as either $E_{it} = \sum_{j=1}^{J} p_{ijt} r_{jt}$ or $E_{it} = \sum_{j=1}^{J} p_{ijt} r_j$. In the first case, period-specific rates would be used while, on the second, common age-specific rates will be used for all the periods considered, although exposed person-years will be updated for each period. The first of these cases has two important drawbacks. First, if internal standardization is carried out for each period and the time periods considered are short, this will make the r_{jt}s noisy and unreliable. As a consequence, noise in these age-specific rates is inherited also by the E_{it}s, making them also noisy and unreliable. Such a noisy behaviour of the expected cases could make spatial dependence, if present, hard to be captured and thus spatial patterns hard to be estimated since they are masked by the additional noise introduced in the model. Secondly, in the first of these options for computing E_{it}, a different reference population is used for each period considered, the population at risk during that specific period. Thus, SMRs for the different periods of analysis would be measuring risk excesses for each spatial unit in relation to different populations of comparison, thus they are not themselves comparable. As a consequence, we do recommend to define E_{it} as $\sum_{j=1}^{J} p_{ijt} r_j$ for age-specific rates r_j, which will be common to the whole period of analysis.

A second important issue in spatio-temporal modeling is related with the strengths of the different sources of variability underlying $\log(\boldsymbol{\Theta})$. In spatial studies there was a single source of variation, geographical variability, regardless of the degree of spatial dependence that it could show. Now $\log(\boldsymbol{\Theta})$ has three possible sources of variability: spatial, temporal and spatio-temporal variability. The predominance of any of these sources could make the spatio-temporal pattern of interest very different. For example, if spatial variability was the main source underlying $\log(\boldsymbol{\Theta})$, the maps for the different periods of analysis would mainly reproduce the same spatial pattern, with small variations between time periods. This would be the case of important and unmodifiable geographical risk factors that do not change either its strength or its geographical distribution along the whole period of analysis. An example of this would be diseases having radon as an important risk factor, whose geographical distribution mainly depends on the geology of the region of study. On the contrary, if the temporal component was the main source of variability in $\log(\Theta)$, all maps would be mostly flat for each time interval, changing the overall risk levels for each map as long as the period of analysis evolves. This would be the case, for example, of diseases with small geographical variability but with a strong temporal determinant that modifies its presence along the period of study, in the same manner for the whole region of analysis. Changes in clinical treatment of diseases, which are typically made available to all spatial units simultaneously, would be a typical cause for this. AIDS mortality studies starting in the nineties (the peak of the epidemic wave) until now would be a typical example of this setting since the temporal decrease of this cause of death has been very important. Finally, spatio-temporal variability shows its effect when the high(/low) risk areas for a cause of death move, change their strength (in different terms), appear or disappear throughout the period of study. In more statistical terms, we would be talking about the presence of interaction of the spatial and temporal terms instead of a simple (additive on the log-risks) combination of these factors. Spatio-temporal interaction would typically happen when substantial modifications of risk factors of local extent could have taken place. A typical example could be the progressive introduction of vaccination or screening programs for the incidence of a disease. As these programs are introduced, they modify the incidence in the areas covered by the program. If the introduction of the program is not simultaneous for the whole region of study, it could make different temporal trends for the different subregions under study.

Determining the relative weight of these three components in spatio-temporal studies is of high interest under an epidemiological point of view. Basically it tells us whether the risk factors determining a disease are mostly static in time, they are simultaneously modified in the same manner for the whole region of study or they show local changes that do not affect the whole region, at least simultaneously. This is very interesting information on the character and performance of the determinants of the corresponding disease. Thus, in general, we will be interested in measuring the contribution of all these three components to the overall variability in Θ. In this sense, the implementation of some ideas of Analysis of Variance (ANOVA) could be very useful in this context, since we really want to decompose the overall variability of the risks. We will perform that variance decomposition on $\log(\Theta)$ instead of on Θ. The reason for this is that many spatio-temporal models compound $\log(\Theta)$ as an additive combination of Gaussian terms (usually random effects), thus the ideas underlying ANOVA will work particularly well when applied to this Normal term.

Assuming that $\log(\boldsymbol{\Theta})$ is composed of spatial, temporal and spatio-temporal variability, we could decompose it as:

$$\log(\Theta_{it}) = \mu + \xi_i + \gamma_t + \Delta_{it} \tag{7.2}$$

where

$$\mu = (IT)^{-1} \sum_{i=1}^{I} \sum_{t=1}^{T} \log(\Theta_{it})$$

would be the overall (grand) mean of $\log(\boldsymbol{\Theta})$ for all spatial units and periods of study,

$$\xi_i = T^{-1} \sum_{t=1}^{T} \log(\Theta_{it}) - \mu$$

would be the overall spatial effect for unit i for the whole period of study

$$\gamma_t = I^{-1} \sum_{i=1}^{I} \log(\Theta_{it}) - \mu$$

would be the overall time effect for period t for the whole region of study, and

$$\Delta_{it} = \log(\Theta_{it}) - (\mu + \xi_i + \gamma_t)$$

would be the deviation of each cell in $\log(\boldsymbol{\Theta})$ from its expected value according to its spatial location and time period, considered as additive effects. Note that, as they are defined, all three $\boldsymbol{\xi}$, $\boldsymbol{\gamma}$ and $\boldsymbol{\Delta}$ are centered, in the sense that: $\sum_i \xi_i = 0$, $\sum_t \gamma_t = 0$ and $\sum_i \Delta_{it} = \sum_t \Delta_{it} = 0$. Thus, ξ_i stands for the overall deviation of the risks for the whole period of study in spatial unit i, in comparison to the overall risk for the whole region and period of study.

Bearing in mind that

$$\Theta_{it} = \exp(\mu) \exp(\xi_i) \exp(\gamma_t) \exp(\Delta_{it}), \tag{7.3}$$

then $\exp(\xi_i)$ could be understood as a kind of spatial $sSMR$ for the whole period of study. Since ξ_i has mean 0 for all i, these terms will take values around 1 and higher values will point out a higher risk excess for the corresponding site for the period of study as a whole. We will refer to $\exp(\boldsymbol{\xi})$, or to $\boldsymbol{\xi}$ when talking on a logarithmic scale, as the spatial component of the spatio-temporal pattern fitted. Likewise, $\exp(\boldsymbol{\gamma})$, or $\boldsymbol{\gamma}$ in logarithmic scale, will be also centred at 1 and will represent the overall risk excess for each period of study as compared to the overall time period analyzed. We will refer to these terms as the temporal component of the spatio-temporal pattern fitted. Finally, in a similar manner, we will refer to $\exp(\boldsymbol{\Delta})$, respectively $\boldsymbol{\Delta}$, as the spatio-temporal component which models the deviations of each spatio-temporal risk, in natural or logarithmic scale, from its expected value according to its corresponding location and period.

Expression (7.2) decomposes the matrix of log-risks as a sum of terms as in a balanced factorial two-way ANOVA. That expression allows decomposing the overall variance in the log-risks as follows:

$$(IT)^{-1} \sum_{i=1}^{I} \sum_{t=1}^{T} (\log(\Theta_{it}) - \mu)^2 = (IT)^{-1} \sum_{i=1}^{I} \sum_{t=1}^{T} (\xi_i + \gamma_t + \Delta_{it})^2.$$

With some algebra, it is direct to show that this last expression is equal to:

$$(IT)^{-1} \sum_{i=1}^{I} \sum_{t=1}^{T} \left((\xi_i)^2 + (\gamma_t)^2 + (\Delta_{it})^2 \right) =$$

$$I^{-1} \sum_{i=1}^{I} (\xi_i)^2 + T^{-1} \sum_{t=1}^{T} (\gamma_t)^2 + (IT)^{-1} \sum_{i=1}^{I} \sum_{t=1}^{T} (\Delta_{it})^2.$$

Therefore, according to this expression, we can decompose the overall variability in the log-risks as the sum of the corresponding spatial, temporal and spatio-temporal variability, i.e.:

$$\hat{\sigma}^2_{\log(\Theta)} = \hat{\sigma}^2_{\xi} + \hat{\sigma}^2_{\gamma} + \hat{\sigma}^2_{\Delta} \tag{7.4}$$

where $\hat{\sigma}^2_x$ stands for the biased sample variance estimator of the corresponding term in Expression (7.2). This last expression also allows to calculate the proportion of spatial, temporal and spatio-temporal variability in the whole variability of the log-risks as $\hat{\sigma}^2_x / (\hat{\sigma}^2_{\log(\Theta)})$ for $x = \xi$, γ or Δ, respectively, which are interesting indicators from an epidemiological perspective. Note that both decompositions in Expressions (7.2) and (7.4) can be done at every step of the MCMC, if inference was made by MCMC. This would allow deriving full posterior distributions of x and $\hat{\sigma}^2_x / (\hat{\sigma}^2_{\log(\Theta)})$ for $x = \xi$, γ or Δ instead of just point estimates. This would make it possible to map interesting statistics as, for example, $P(\xi > 0)$ for determining the spatial units with a high probability of risk excess for the overall period.

An interesting property of the variance decomposition proposed is that it is independent of the specific dependence structure assumed for $\log(\Theta)$. That is, that decomposition depends just on the values taken by the log-risks, so the particular structure used to model that matrix is irrelevant. This makes the variance decomposition above a very general tool, feasible for comparing the performance of different models, regardless of their dependence structure, which makes it particularly useful.

Although the variance decomposition of the log-risks is a nice consequence of Expression (7.2) allowing us to quantify the strength of each of the related components, Expression (7.3) has also an important practical use. As mentioned, spatio-temporal patterns could have predominant spatial, temporal or spatio-temporal components. Those predominant terms will make the rest of the features of the components very hard to be seen in naive maps plotting simply the different columns of $\boldsymbol{\Theta}$. Thus, it would be convenient to be able to filter out the different components in $\boldsymbol{\Theta}$ in our plots, in particular the main component, so that the rest of the terms could be explored in detail. Expression (7.3) allows us to do that. For example, plotting $\exp(\boldsymbol{\xi})$ would allow us to visualize the spatial component in the data set of study. In contrast, $\exp(\mu + \gamma_1 + \boldsymbol{\Delta}_{\cdot 1})$ would allow us to visualize the risk for the first period of study, removing the overall spatial pattern for the whole period of study. This will make it possible to visualize the geographic variability of risk in that precise period, beyond the overall spatial pattern which has been removed.

Example 7.1

We are going to illustrate in this example the variance decomposition introduced in this section. First we show the results obtained in the analysis of several simulated data sets and later we show the variance decompositions of some real data sets corresponding to some different mortality causes in the Valencian Region.

We start by the analysis of the simulated data sets. We have considered three different synthetic spatio-temporal patterns on the Valencian Region for a period of 10 years. We will analyze the data set as an ensemble of 10 annual separate periods. In the first data set, we assumed a risk pattern constant in time but showing substantial spatial variability. The spatial pattern considered shows a north-south gradient in risk, with a risk of 1.5 at the most northern point of the Valencian Region and a risk of 0.5 at the most southern point. The second data set shows no spatial variability at any time of the period of study but shows substantial temporal variability. Thus, the risk for all municipalities during the first year of study is 1.5, and this risk decreases steadily until 0.5 during the last year of study. The third data set shows neither temporal nor spatial variability for the risks of the Valencian Region; nevertheless, it shows substantial spatio-temporal interaction. Specifically, for the first year of study this data set reproduces the spatial gradient of the first data set. This gradient reverses steadily along the period of study showing, at the end of that period, an opposite gradient with higher risk in the south (1.5 vs. 0.5 at the northernmost point). These three data sets are supposed to reflect a different source of variability present at the variance decomposition introduced above. Expected cases for each of these data sets and year of study are set as the expected cases for oral cancer in the Valencian Region during 2011, which adds up a total of 215.1 expected cases for the whole Valencian Region. This low number of expected deaths (0.4 expected deaths per municipality and year) makes evident the need of spatio-temporal models, which share information also on time instead of just on space, in order to get reliable estimates.

We have run the auto-regressive spatio-temporal model of Martinez-Beneito et al. (2008) (to be introduced in Section 7.4) for all the previous data sets.

Expected cases/year	Setting	Spatial variability	Temporal variability	Spatio-temp. variability
oral 2011	1	83.4 [62.2,97.1]	3.9 [0,12.8]	12.6[1.6,33.6]
	2	1.8 [0,6.8]	92.2 [78.4,99.7]	6.0 [0.2,17.7]
	3	27.6 [9.7,51.5]	2.5 [0,12.4]	69.9 [45.6,88.3]
10·(oral 2011)	1	98.2 [95.3,99.7]	0.2 [0,0.8]	1.6 [0.2,4.7]
	2	0.2 [0,0.7]	98.0 [95.1,99.8]	1.8 [0.2,4.5]
	3	11.5 [5.8,19.8]	2.0 [0,7.1]	86.4 [76.9,93.0]

Table 7.1
Variance decomposition of the log-risks for all three simulated settings. Each cell shows the posterior mean and 95% credible interval for the percentage of variance explained by each component. The three last rows correspond to the same settings as for the upper rows with expected values multiplied by 10.

All simulations were run in WinBUGS. We have also performed the variance decomposition described above for the log-risks at each iteration of the MCMC, which yields posterior samples of $\hat{\sigma}_\xi^2$, $\hat{\sigma}_\gamma^2$ and $\hat{\sigma}_\delta^2$. Moreover, we have calculated the proportion of spatial variability in the patterns as $100\hat{\sigma}_\xi/(\hat{\sigma}_\xi^2+\hat{\sigma}_\gamma^2+\hat{\sigma}_\delta^2)$ and similar quantities have been also calculated for temporal and spatio-temporal variability. Columns 3 to 5 of Table 7.1 show the posterior means and 95% credible intervals for these proportions for each data set. Rows 2 to 4 at the right-hand side of Table 7.1 correspond to the settings mentioned and rows 5 to 7 correspond to the same settings, but observed cases are generated assuming 10 times more expected values per municipality and year than in the original simulated data sets.

Table 7.1 shows how the variance component with a more prominent contribution to each setting is found to have the most important contribution for each data set. Two additional conclusions can be drawn for that table. First, the spatio-temporal component is the one showing most confounding with the rest of the terms, particularly with the spatial component if spatio-temporal interaction do exist. Surely this could be avoided if more time intervals were available, instead of just 10 as in our example. Second, when the number of expected values per observation increases, the percentages in Table 7.1 are closer to their real values and show less variability, reducing also confounding between these components of variance. Although these estimates are necessarily biased since the real quantities are at the border of their domain, that bias is reduced as long as the expected values increase.

As a second illustration of the variance decomposition, we have run the auto-regressive spatio-temporal model mentioned above on several real mortality data sets of the Valencian Region. These data sets correspond to 28 causes of death and the period of study goes from 1988 to 2011. Some combination of causes of mortality and sex have been excluded either for lack of anatomical sense (such as prostate cancer in women) or too low mortality for that

Cause of death	Sex	Spatial variability	Temporal variability	Spatio-temp. variability
oral cancer	men	70.3	16.4	13.3
stomach cancer	men	39.6	52.8	7.6
stomach cancer	women	27.4	65.8	6.8
lung cancer	men	91.7	2.2	6.1
lung cancer	women	54.4	32.5	13.1
bladder cancer	men	83.9	0.5	15.6
cerebrovascular	men	22.3	69.8	7.8
cerebrovascular	women	21.0	67.7	11.3
pneumonia	men	56.6	17.0	26.4
pneumonia	women	46.4	17.2	36.4

Table 7.2
Variance decomposition of the log-risks for selected combinations of diseases and sexes in the Valencian Region. Each cell shows the posterior mean for the percentage of variance explained by each component.

combination (such as breast cancer in men), thus a total of 46 studies have been undertaken. For this spatio-temporal study, the whole period is divided into 12 biannual seasons. For these settings, we have performed a variance decomposition as that of Table 7.1.

Table 7.2 shows some of the results obtained for some particularly interesting cases in the Valencian mortality data set. Thus, Table 7.2 shows that the spatial pattern is in general the strongest component in variance decompositions, whereas the spatio-temporal pattern corresponds usually to the weaker component. This is a general fact for all 46 spatio-temporal patterns studied, where the spatial component explains on average a 52.4% of the variance, followed by the temporal component (28.2%) and finally the spatio-temporal component with a 19.4%. From this, we can conclude that a 24-year period has not produced big changes in the spatial distribution of death causes in the Valencian Region since spatial variability is, in general, substantially higher than that corresponding to changes in the spatio-temporal pattern (52.4% vs. 19.4%). Thus, although spatio-temporal variability is surely the most interesting variance component in epidemiological terms, it seems to be the rarest of these three components in real data. Spatio-temporal variability arises when temporal changes occur at different sites at different moments and our data show that this requirement does not take place so often in practice.

Table 7.2 shows the variance decomposition for oral cancer, the example that we have been mostly working on in this book. We can see that most of the variability for this disease (70.3%) comes from the spatial component followed by temporal and spatio-temporal variability to a similar extent. Thus we expect the maps for all 12 time intervals for this disease to reproduce basically similar spatial patterns with mild temporal changes. As in oral cancer, lung cancer for men and bladder cancer (which has been only studied for men) show also strong spatial patterns. Note that all three lung, bladder and oral cancers strongly depend on tobacco consumption, thus this result suggests that a marked geographical pattern on tobacco consumption could be behind the (supposedly common) spatial pattern(s) found for these diseases. Note also that the variance decomposition for lung cancer in women seems to be very different than that in men as were also the smoking habits for both sexes historically in the Valencian Region. This reinforces the idea that smoking habits could be highly influencing the spatio-temporal patterns found in lung, bladder and oral cancer mortality. In contrast, we find that stomach cancer and cerebrovascular disease, for both sexes, have a predominant temporal component. This points out that pharmacological/clinical changes in the treatment of those diseases could be having a higher impact than those coming from the distribution of risk factors for these diseases throughout the Valencian Region. Finally, pneumonia for both sexes are examples of spatio-temporal geographical patterns changing substantially the shape of the spatial pattern as long as the period of study evolves. Specifically, pneumonia in women is the case showing a more prominent spatio-temporal component. Note however that, even in this case, the spatial variability is higher than that of the spatio-temporal component. Finally note that all diseases in Table 7.2 show very similar variance decompositions for both sexes except lung cancer for the reasons already explained. This is a very general fact also for the rest of the diseases not included in that table. This points towards the common existence of risk factors, besides tobacco consumption, that have an influence on both sexes in a similar manner during the period of study.

In concluding this section, we find it convenient to introduce a concept that will be very useful from now on, *separability*. This concept is related to multivariate spatial processes in general, so it has also sense for spatio-temporal disease mapping studies in particular. Specifically, we say that a spatio-temporal process $\mathbf{\Phi} = \{\Phi_{it} = \Phi(S_i, P_t) : i = 1, ..., I; t = 1, ..., T\}$ observed at locations $\{S_i : i = 1, ..., I\}$ and periods $\{P_t : t = 1, ..., T\}$ is separable if $Cov_\Phi(\Phi_{it}, \Phi_{i't'}) = Cov_S(S_i, S_{i'})Cov_P(P_t, P_{t'})$ for $Cov_S(,)$ and $Cov_P(,)$ being covariance functions of the spatial and temporal underlying process, respectively. This means that a spatio-temporal process is said to be separable if there are two separate underlying sources of dependence, one inducing spatial dependence and another one inducing temporal dependence and the covariance for any two points of the original process is just the multiplication of the covariances for the two separate sources. Although the definition that we have just made of separability is referred to spatio-temporal processes, it also applies to multivariate models in Chapter 8 by simply considering the factor defining the columns in $\mathbf{\Phi}$ as the second source of dependence of the separable process, instead of time.

Separable processes are generally considered somewhat simple and restrictive. In particular, they implicitly assume that spatial covariance is exactly equal for all time periods considered and, similarly, temporal covariance is equal for all the areal units considered. These assumptions will be hard to accomplish, particularly in spatio-temporal problems with a large number of either areal units or temporal periods.

A second characterization of separability is by means of the covariance matrix of $vec(\mathbf{\Phi})$ (see Chapter 1 for the definition of the vec operator). Thus, the spatio-temporal process $\mathbf{\Phi}$ will be separable if and only if the covariance matrix of $vec(\mathbf{\Phi})$ is the Kronecker product (see also Chapter 1) of the covariance matrix between periods $\mathbf{\Sigma_P}$ and the spatial covariance matrix among areal units $\mathbf{\Sigma_S}$, that is: $\mathbf{\Sigma}_{vec(\mathbf{\Phi})} = \mathbf{\Sigma_P} \otimes \mathbf{\Sigma_S}$. The equivalence of both characterizations introduced of separability can be easily checked by developing the expression of the cells of $\mathbf{\Sigma}_{vec(\mathbf{\Phi})}$ as Kronecker product of the other two matrices. Moreover, separable processes combining valid processes (with symmetric and positive definite matrices) are also guaranteed to be valid. Thus, $\mathbf{\Sigma}_{vec(\mathbf{\Phi})}$ is clearly symmetric since

$$\mathbf{\Sigma}'_{vec(\mathbf{\Phi})} = (\mathbf{\Sigma_P} \otimes \mathbf{\Sigma_S})' = \mathbf{\Sigma}'_P \otimes \mathbf{\Sigma}'_S = \mathbf{\Sigma_P} \otimes \mathbf{\Sigma_S} = \mathbf{\Sigma}_{vec(\mathbf{\Phi})}.$$

In a similar manner, since the eigenvalues of $\mathbf{\Sigma}_{vec(\mathbf{\Phi})}$ are simply obtained as the product of the eigenvalues of $\mathbf{\Sigma_P}$ and $\mathbf{\Sigma_S}$, then $\mathbf{\Sigma}_{vec(\mathbf{\Phi})}$ will be evidently guaranteed to be also positive definite. Thus, although separable processes are usually treated as a restrictive class of spatio-temporal (or multivariate) processes, they are usually quite useful since they are guaranteed to lead to a valid process which can be easily generalized to more general non-separable processes. Hence, in some way, separable processes can be considered as linear models in statistical modeling, a kind of simple benchmark which can be later extended to more complex and tailor-made processes yielding enhanced fittings. This property of separable processes will be particularly useful in the multivariate context where guaranteeing the validity of some modeling proposals is a not so direct a task.

7.2 Parametric temporal modeling

Historically, the first modeling approach followed in spatio-temporal disease mapping relied on the parametric modeling of time trends for each spatial unit. This approach models each row of $\log(\mathbf{\Theta})$ as a parametric function of time with different regression coefficients for each spatial unit. These regression coefficients are usually modeled as spatially correlated random effects. Thus spatial dependence is induced in the coefficients of the linear regression model for each spatial unit, whereas temporal dependence is parametrically induced by regressing each temporal observation for each spatial unit as a function of time. These models are a particular case of the ecological regression models with spatially varying parameters introduced in Section 5.3, now with time being the covariate of interest. Note, however, that spatio-temporal studies will have several observations per spatial unit instead of one, as for typical spatially varying coefficient models. Bernardinelli et al. (1995b) and Sun et al. (2000) are two examples of this approach assuming a linear relationship between log-risks and time. Specifically, they assume

$$\log(\Theta_{it}) = (\alpha_0 + \alpha_i) + (\beta_0 + \beta_i) * (t - \bar{t}). \tag{7.5}$$

Note that the centered period $t - \bar{t}$ is used as a covariate instead of just t. This is usually made for two reasons: first, for interpreting the intercepts $\alpha_0 + \alpha_i$ as the log-risk at the middle of the period of study, and second, for diminishing the posterior covariance between the intercept and the slope of the regression lines. That posterior covariance could be particularly painful for MCMC (at least for WinBUGS) if t represented the year of observation, with values around two thousands. In that case, a slight increase in β_i, for example, for fitting a steeper time trend at some spatial unit would have a large impact on α_i (the value of the regression curve at $t = 0$), thus yielding a high negative posterior correlation between $\boldsymbol{\alpha}$ and $\boldsymbol{\beta}$. The centered version of time, shown above, avoids this. Nevertheless, Bernardinelli et al. (1995b) consider a proposal modeling the potential dependence between $\boldsymbol{\alpha}$ and $\boldsymbol{\beta}$, by defining $\beta_i \sim N(\rho\alpha_i, \sigma^2)$. Although $\boldsymbol{\alpha}$ is considered to follow some spatial distribution, this proposal does not implicitly induce spatial dependence on $\boldsymbol{\beta}$, thus the strength of the spatial dependence for $\boldsymbol{\beta}$ will be necessarily milder than for $\boldsymbol{\alpha}$. Moreover, this proposal puts necessarily related spatial patterns for both $\boldsymbol{\alpha}$ and $\boldsymbol{\beta}$ which will not necessarily hold in practice. A more elaborated dependence between $\boldsymbol{\alpha}$ and $\boldsymbol{\beta}$, explicitly considering spatial patterns for both vectors, could be done by using the multivariate spatial processes introduced in the next chapter.

Parameters α_0 and β_0 in the previous model are common for all spatial units. Specifically, α_0 models the overall log-risk for $t = \bar{t}$ for the whole region of study, so this term would be closely related to the overall intercept μ of the decomposition in the previous section. Similarly, β_0 models the overall time trend for the whole region of study so it will be referred to the temporal component/variability of the problem, γ in terms of the previous decomposition which is now assumed to be linear. Both α_0 and β_0 will be typically modeled as fixed effects with non-informative priors such as the usual improper uniform prior on the whole real line. As mentioned, $\boldsymbol{\alpha}$ and $\boldsymbol{\beta}$ are typically modeled as spatially correlated random effects following PCAR (Sun et al., 2000), BYM or any other suitable spatial distribution. The vector $\boldsymbol{\alpha}$ models the geographic differences in the log-risks at the middle of the period of study so, in some sense, it will be similar to the spatial component $\boldsymbol{\xi}$ of the spatio-temporal pattern, which depicts the overall risk for each spatial unit. Finally, $\boldsymbol{\beta}$ allows for different time trends for the different spatial units so it will introduce spatio-temporal interaction into the model, $\boldsymbol{\Delta}$ in Expression (7.2). Depending on the magnitudes/variabilities of these terms, the spatial, temporal or spatio-temporal components will play a more or less important role into the model.

Parametric spatio-temporal modeling proposals have a clear advantage over other alternatives, mainly their simplicity for both implementation and interpretation. In contrast, the main drawback of these models is their rigidity for modeling temporal trends. Since this restriction is tighter for simpler models, more elaborated parametric models have been proposed in the literature. For example, Assunção et al. (2001) and Earnest et al. (2007) proposed enhanced versions of the linear model above but with quadratic time trends for each spatial unit. These proposals also include spatial random effects for the coefficients of the model so that the risks fitted are able to reproduce spatio-temporal interactions. These quadratic models are a more flexible alternative for depicting time trends, which could be particularly advantageous for studying large periods where more intricate risk evolutions could have taken place. This will be particularly likely if the region of study has a large number of units and therefore very different time trends could have been followed for the different spatial units.

Although parametric models may seem somewhat simplistic proposals within the spatio-temporal literature, they are interesting tools that should be borne in mind. Namely, Torres-Avilés and Martinez-Beneito (2015) show that parametric models, as parameterized as their common non-parametric alternatives (to be introduced at Section 7.4), are also competitive proposals in terms of their fit. Moreover, parametric models have the advantage of relying on bases of functions (polynomial bases in the previous models) that, if wisely chosen, could yield important advantages. This is illustrated in that same work, which proposes *STANOVA* as an adaptation of a multivariate disease mapping tool, *Smoothed ANOVA* (Zhang et al., 2009), to the spatio-temporal case. Thus they propose to model $\log(\boldsymbol{\Theta}) = \boldsymbol{\beta H}$ for $\boldsymbol{H}$ a $J \times T$ matrix containing an orthogonal basis of J functions for modeling time trends and $\boldsymbol{\beta}$ an $I \times J$ matrix whose columns are mutually independent spatial structured random effects. Thus, temporal dependence is induced by the use of the temporal basis $\boldsymbol{H}$ and spatiality is induced by the dependence of the rows of $\boldsymbol{\beta}$, which contains the coefficients needed to model the different time trends for the whole set of spatial units.

Torres-Avilés and Martinez-Beneito (2015) consider a case study on monthly rheumatic heart disease mortality data in Spain. The period of study is 10 years, so 120 observations are available for each spatial unit. Mortality for this cause has a marked seasonal pattern, with higher mortality in the winter periods so, besides the main time trend for the whole period of analysis, a cyclic pattern within years should be fitted for achieving an appropriate fit. In that case, a Fourier polynomial basis, instead of a naive polynomial basis, makes possible to fit the seasonal yearly pattern of the data. This cyclic pattern may be difficult to be fitted without parametric time trend models, in particular without the used Fourier basis mentioned.

Parametric models have additional advantages. First, the use of parametric functions for modeling time trends does not require the observations to be equally spaced in time. Even time observations for the different spatial units could be misaligned and this should not be a problem, in contrast to spatio-temporal proposals relying on time series models, for example. On the other hand, as seen in the linear case above, few additional parameters are often needed for fitting the spatio-temporal variability in the data. In contrast, non-parametric alternatives, as we will see, are much more parameterized than most parametric proposals. This makes parametric models particularly competitive for spatio-temporal models with lots of temporal periods, let's say hundreds or thousands of observations. In those cases, non-parametric models which usually put at least one random effect per observation, are problematic and computationally hard to be fitted. The selection of a particularly wise basis of functions to be used for fitting the data could make a high reduction in the dimensionality of the problem, achieving a very reasonable fit with very few elements in the basis of functions. STANOVA, and SANOVA models in general, may be fitted with `WinBUGS` but can also be fitted with `INLA`. Nevertheless, for bases with lots of functions SANOVA models in `INLA` become very slow, slower than in `WinBUGS` (Torres-Avilés and Martinez-Beneito, 2015).

Another interesting result of the STANOVA seminal paper is the study of the joint covariance structure of these models made there. Specifically, that paper shows that if all the columns of β were assumed to have the same spatial prior distributions with common parameters, the corresponding STANOVA model would yield a temporally independent process. Basically, assuming the same variances on all the orthogonal components that compound time trends make them basically random and therefore independent. A second interesting case is when the covariance matrix of the columns of β, the different parameters of the parametric time trends, are assumed to be proportional: $\lambda_1 \Sigma, ..., \lambda_J \Sigma$. In this case the spatio-temporal covariance matrix would be separable and equal to $H' diag(\lambda_1, ...\lambda_J) H \otimes \Sigma$. That is, the overall spatial structure will be determined by Σ and $\lambda_1, ...\lambda_J$ will be the eigenvalues of the time structure, whose eigenvectors will be defined by the rows of H. Note that for $\lambda_1 = ... = \lambda_J$, the covariance matrix for the temporal component would be I_T which illustrates the performance of the case with common variances mentioned above. Finally, if the covariance matrices of β's columns were not proportional, the corresponding spatio-temporal structure would not be separable. As an illustrative example: (i) a temporally independent process would be defined if the columns of β were all assumed to follow a PCAR distribution of correlation parameter ρ and standard deviation σ, (ii) if $\sigma_1, ..., \sigma_J$ was assumed instead for the standard deviations we would have then a separable process, and (iii) if distinct correlation parameters $\rho_1, ..., \rho_J$ were considered, then we would reproduce a non-separable process. Similarly, if BYM models were assumed for modeling the regression parameters in a STANOVA, this would yield a non-separable process if each of these BYM processes had different standard deviations. Conversely, if all the BYM models had common standard deviations, the resulting process would be then temporally independent.

Example 7.2

We turn back once again to the oral cancer Valencian data, but we will consider now that data set disaggregated in 12 biannual periods, from 1988 to 2011. For this period, we have fitted two parametric spatio-temporal models, one assuming a different linear trend for each municipality and another one assuming quadratic trends. For both models, the parameters in charge of controlling the intercept and time trends for the set of municipalities are assumed to be spatially correlated random effects. Specifically, a BYM model is assumed for each of these vectors of parameters, each of them with different standard deviations. The first of the models fitted correspond to that in Expression (7.5), while the second model includes an additional term in that expression of the kind $(\gamma_0 + \gamma_i)(t - \bar{t})^2$ in order to model quadratic time trends. Note that both proposals correspond to particular cases of the model with $\log(\mathbf{\Theta}) = \boldsymbol{\beta}\mathbf{H}$ for $\mathbf{H}$ an orthogonal matrix, thus both are particular cases of STANOVA. As a consequence, the models proposed with BYM distributions of distinct standard deviations for the regression parameters will reproduce non-separable spatio-temporal patterns.

Both models have been fitted in `WinBUGS` although they could also be fitted with `INLA`. The annex material of the book contains the code used for fitting the model with both options. We have also calculated the DIC for both the linear and quadratic models yielding, respectively, 7340.8 and 7334.3, so quadratic time trends seem in principle a more satisfactory alternative. We have also decomposed the variance for both models in order to quantify their spatial, temporal and spatio-temporal components. For the linear model, that decomposition determines that a 82.7% of the variance in that model is of spatial character, a 14.2% corresponds to the temporal component and just a 3.0% corresponds to the spatio-temporal interaction. For the quadratic model, a 74.5% of the variance corresponds to the spatial component, a 17.3% of the variance belongs to the temporal component and a 8.2% of the variance corresponds to spatio-temporal interaction. Therefore, the additional flexibility induced by the quadratic term for modeling the time trends increases the amount of variance of the temporal and spatio-temporal terms, having an impact on the variance decomposition.

Figure 7.1 shows the municipal time trends fitted by both models. The left-hand side plot shows decreasing log-linear time trends for the period of study, whereas the right-hand side plot shows a peak for mortality, in general, around the 5th season of the period of study. This makes evident why the quadratic model is preferred in terms of DIC over its linear alternative. Specifically, the

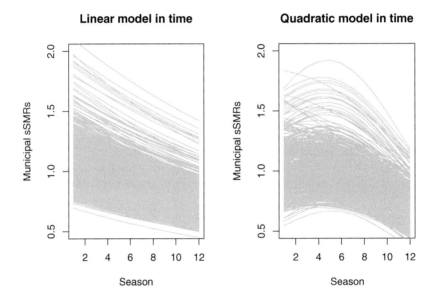

Figure 7.1
Time trends for the municipalities of the Valencian Region for the period of study. Left plot assumes linear time trends for the log-risks, and right plot assumes quadratic trends.

linear model is not able to reproduce the peak in mortality time trends in the nineties decade, which is also typical of other smoking-related diseases in men in the Valencian Region (Zurriaga et al., 2010). Although both models show substantial temporal variability in mortality, spatial variability is even more important, as evidenced in the variance decompositions above. Thus, Figure 7.1 shows how mortality for some municipalities, even at the end of the period of study, is way higher than that in other municipalities at the beginning of that period. This illustrates the important contribution of the spatial variability to the spatio-temporal pattern fitted. Finally, Figure 7.1 shows also the mild contribution of spatio-temporal interaction to the spatio-temporal pattern. This is evidenced by the mostly 'parallel' character of the municipal time trends in that figure, with few crossings between different municipal time trends. Note that, that lack of spatio-temporal interaction is more evident, with fewer crossings, for the time trends of the linear model, in accordance to the lower contribution of the spatio-temporal component found for that model. Finally, note that the spatio-temporal interaction of the quadratic model has allowed the time trends for the different municipalities to reproduce their mortality peaks at different seasons of the period of study. This could be the consequence of different temporal evolutions of tobacco consumption for the municipalities of the Valencian Region, which would be captured by the quadratic model but not by the lineal one.

The upper row of Figure 7.2 shows two choropleth maps for the $sSMR$s, these correspond to the 1st and 12th season of the period of study in the quadratic model, the preferred option in terms of DIC. Maps for the intermediate seasons show smooth constant transitions between these two images; therefore, we do not display them all. Since the overall time trend is decreasing during the period of study, the $sSMR$s for the first season show in general high risks, similarly the last season shows unanimously low risks. This effect makes evident that raw maps of the $sSMR$s, containing all the components in the spatio-temporal pattern, do not allow to explore the richness of the results generated with full detail. As a consequence, we would rather in some cases draw maps of the $sSMR$s filtering some of the components in the spatio-temporal component out. Thus the upper row of Figure 7.2 invites us to remove the temporal component of those maps in order to obtain more useful plots. If this was done (results not shown), we would see that the corresponding maps for the 1st and 12th season would be very similar, with few changes between them. This is a consequence of the high spatial variability of the patterns fitted, which is more than 10 times higher than that of the spatio-temporal interaction. Thus, it will be convenient to remove also the spatial component of the $sSMR$s in the upper row maps of Figure 7.2 since otherwise we would obtain two maps very similar to that in Figure 4.4, the spatial pattern for oral cancer during the whole period of study.

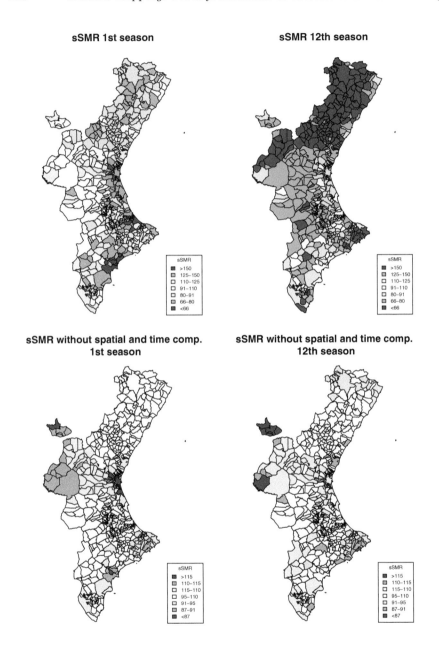

Figure 7.2
Upper row: choropleth maps for the $sSMR$s in the 1st and 12th season. Lower row: same maps as in the upper row but with the spatial and temporal components removed (pure spatio-temporal component).

The lower row of Figure 7.2 shows the same maps as in the upper row but with the temporal and spatial components removed, i.e., they represent $100 \cdot \exp(\mathbf{\Delta}_{\cdot 1})$ and $100 \cdot \exp(\mathbf{\Delta}_{\cdot 12})$, respectively. These maps do not show the unpleasant patterns shown in the upper row when the spatial and temporal components were present. These maps show how there are two regions in the central and south part of the Valencian Region with a particularly bad performance during the corresponding two seasons. Brown municipalities in these maps point out to those municipalities and seasons with worse performance than expected, according to the overall risks of that municipality (for all the period) and season (for all the Valencian Region). Thus, brown areas would correspond to municipalities having a particularly bad performance in that specific season, as compared to the average performance in that municipality in the whole period. Note that the scale of the lower two maps is different from that in the maps in the upper row since most of the variability in the upper maps has been removed with the spatial and temporal components.

Finally, regarding the maps in the lower row of Figure 7.2, we find it convenient to point out their strong similarities. High and low risk areas usually coincide for both seasons. This is a consequence of the rigidity of low-dimensional parametric models (the quadratic model in this case) for fitting time trends. If the quadratic component is required for increasing/decreasing a time trend at the beginning of the period, this quadratic trend will also produce an increase/decrease in the spatio-temporal interaction term at the end of the period. This is the reason why both maps are so similar and a clear example of the kind of problems of low-dimensional parametric models. If a wiser basis of functions was used for fitting time trends, a better low-dimensional parametric fit would be achieved. Nevertheless, if the basis of functions is not so appropriate, the corresponding fit may reproduce weird interactions at very distant time points, as evidenced.

7.3 Spline-based modeling

As stated in Section 6.4, spline are an alternative smoothing device to the use of correlated random effects. As compared to random effects models, spline models depend on a fewer number of parameters, which seems to be a considerable advantage. Nevertheless, spline models are usually far more parameterized than pure parametric models introduced in the previous section. Although spline models are frequently used as an alternative to random effects models, these two tools are frequently combined in spatio-temporal models in order to introduce the two sources of dependence existing in these types of studies. We are going to review now some modeling proposals following this approach.

Some spatio-temporal models propose the use of correlated random effects for modeling the spatial components and spline, with spatially correlated parameters over the temporal dimension. Specifically, this approach models the spatio-temporal log-risks as

$$\log(\Theta_{it}) = \mu + \alpha_i + S_0(t) + S_i(t)$$

where μ is an overall intercept modeling the mean log-risk for the whole period and region of study and $\boldsymbol{\alpha}$ is a vector of spatially structured random effects which induces spatial dependence on the mean log-risks for the set of areal units during the whole period of study. The term $S_0(t)$ models the overall temporal component of the spatio-temporal pattern, that is, the general time trend followed in average by the log-risks of all the areal units. This term is modeled as a linear combination of the elements of a spline basis

$$S_0(t) = \sum_{k=1}^{K} \gamma_{0j} B_k(t) = \boldsymbol{B}_{t\cdot} \boldsymbol{\gamma}_0$$

where $\{B_k(t) : k = 1, ..., K\}$ is a suitable time-dependent spline basis. The elements of this basis are combined as a function of the components of the vector $\boldsymbol{\gamma}_0$, which components are typically modeled as fixed effects, i.e., they take vague priors such as improper uniform distributions on the whole real line. Thus, $\boldsymbol{\alpha}$ and $S_0(t)$ (additively) model the spatial and temporal components of the spatio-temporal pattern fitted; therefore, $S_i(t)$ is the term in charge of modeling the spatio-temporal interaction. In a similar manner to $S_0(t)$, this term is a combination of spline, for each areal unit, of the form

$$S_i(t) = \sum_{k=1}^{K} \gamma_{ik} B_k(t) = \boldsymbol{B}_{t\cdot} \boldsymbol{\gamma}_i$$

where now the coefficients for these linear combinations are different for each spatial unit. These parameters, in contrast to those of $S_0(t)$, are modeled as spatially correlated random effects in order to induce spatial dependence on this spatio-temporal term. Namely, each vector $\{\boldsymbol{\gamma}_{\cdot k} : k = 1, ..., K\}$ is assumed to follow a spatially correlated distribution, such as BYM, Leroux, etc. Thus, under this approach, spatial smoothing is imposed by means of typical CAR distributions, temporal smoothing is imposed by means of spline, and spatio-temporal smoothing is imposed by fusing both tools into a single device: that is, a spline-based temporal model with spatially correlated components. Several works have followed different variants of this approach; see for example: MacNab and Dean (2001, 2002); Silva et al. (2008); Torabi and Rosychuk (2011); and Torabi (2013). Of particular interest are the works of MacNab and Gustafson (2007) and MacNab (2007) where the set of vectors $\{\boldsymbol{\gamma}_{\cdot k} : k = 1, ..., K\}$ have a joint multivariate CAR distribution (to be introduced in the next chapter) which assumes that these vectors, besides being spatially dependent, are also jointly correlated.

A second approach to spline-based spatio-temporal modeling relies on three-dimensional spline, where two dimensions are used for modeling the spatial variability and the third one for the temporal variability (Ugarte et al., 2010, 2012; Goicoa et al., 2016a). Specifically, let us assume $\boldsymbol{B}^X(x) = \{\boldsymbol{B}_i^X(x) : i = 1, ..., Q_X\}$ to be a one-dimensional spline basis defined on a set of knots $\mathcal{Q}^X = \{q_i^X : i = 1, ..., Q_X\}$ spanning the range of the longitudes of the geographic units of the region of study. Similarly, let $\boldsymbol{B}^Y(y)$ and $\boldsymbol{B}^T(t)$ be equivalent basis of functions for the latitudes and temporal components of lengths Q_Y and Q_T, respectively. This approach considers the following set of $Q_X \cdot Q_Y \cdot Q_T$ functions as a three-dimensional basis of spline:

$$\{\boldsymbol{B}_{(i-1)Q_Y Q_T + (j-1)Q_T + k}(x, y, t) = \boldsymbol{B}_i^X(x)\boldsymbol{B}_j^Y(y)\boldsymbol{B}_k^T(t)$$
$$:i = 1, ..., Q_X, j = 1, ..., Q_Y, k = 1, ..., Q_T\}.$$

The evaluation of these functions on the $I \cdot T$ spatio-temporal units yields a $\boldsymbol{B}$ matrix of dimensions $(I \cdot T) \times (Q_X \cdot Q_Y \cdot Q_T)$, whose rows correspond to each spatio-temporal available observation and each column to a function of the three-dimensional basis considered. If B-spline were considered for the univariate spline bases $\boldsymbol{B}^X(x), \boldsymbol{B}^Y(y)$ and $\boldsymbol{B}^T(t)$, the corresponding univariate functions would reproduce Gaussian-like functions on the different knots considered. Therefore, the functions in the three-dimensional basis $\boldsymbol{B}(x, y, t)$ will be positive for just a neighbourhood of some of the three-dimensional knots (q_i^X, q_j^Y, q_k^T) for some i, j and k. Thus, the functions in the three-dimensional spline basis will model the local performance of the spatio-temporal process on the surroundings of a set of locations of the spatio-temporal domain.

Under the three-dimensional spline approach, log-risks are modeled as a linear combination of the three-dimensional basis just introduced:

$$log(\boldsymbol{\Phi}) = \mu + \boldsymbol{B}\boldsymbol{\gamma}$$

where $\boldsymbol{\gamma}$ is modeled as a vector of random effects smoothing the spatio-temporal process and possibly inducing additional spatio-temporal structure. Under the frequentist literature (Ugarte et al., 2010; Lee and Durban, 2011), dependence between the components of $\boldsymbol{\gamma}$ is imposed by means of a penalty function of the kind $\boldsymbol{\gamma}'\boldsymbol{P}\boldsymbol{\gamma}$ where $\boldsymbol{P}$ usually takes the form

$$\boldsymbol{P} = \lambda_X \boldsymbol{P}_X \otimes \boldsymbol{I}_{Q_Y} \otimes \boldsymbol{I}_{Q_T} + \lambda_Y \boldsymbol{I}_{Q_X} \otimes \boldsymbol{P}_Y \otimes \boldsymbol{I}_{Q_T} + \lambda_T \boldsymbol{I}_{Q_X} \otimes \boldsymbol{I}_{Q_Y} \otimes \boldsymbol{P}_T$$

where $\boldsymbol{P}_X, \boldsymbol{P}_Y$ and $\boldsymbol{P}_T$ are penalty matrices that penalize differences between the components of $\boldsymbol{\gamma}$ corresponding to consecutive nodes in the longitudes, latitudes and temporal components, respectively. Those penalties impose additional smoothing in the spatial and temporal domains to that induced by the use of the spline. Moreover, the use of different penalty parameters λ_X, λ_Y and λ_T allows a different weighting of temporal and spatial neighbours and inducing spatial anisotropy. As mentioned in Section 6.4, the use of penalty functions in the frequentist literature can be translated into the Bayesian arena as the modeling of γ as a vector of structured random effects. Thus, in parallel to Section 6.4, if a random walk structure of first order was used for penalizing differences between consecutive nodes in the three dimensions of $B(x, y, t)$, this would mean that $\gamma_i | \gamma_{-i}$ would take as conditional distribution

$$N \left(\frac{\lambda_X \sum_{j \sim_X i} \gamma_j + \lambda_Y \sum_{j \sim_Y i} \gamma_j + \lambda_T \sum_{j \sim_T i} \gamma_j}{\lambda_X n_i^X + \lambda_Y n_i^Y + \lambda_T n_i^t}, \frac{1}{\lambda_X n_i^X + \lambda_Y n_i^Y + \lambda_t n_i^t} \right)$$

where n_i^X, n_i^Y, n_i^T denote the number of neighbours of the node corresponding to γ_i along each of the three dimensions of $B(x, y, t)$, and $\cdot \sim_X i, \cdot \sim_Y i, \cdot \sim_T i$ denote, respectively, the indexes of γ corresponding to those nodes which are neighbours of the node corresponding to γ_i along each of the mentioned directions. This set of conditional distributions for the components of γ can be coded in `WinBUGS` in order to implement this model under a Bayesian approach. The three-dimensional spline approach can be formulated without pure spatial and temporal terms, as just introduced, or it can also be accompanied with those terms so that the spatio-temporal component only has to reproduce the spatio-temporal interaction. The modeling proposal including specific spatial and temporal terms is usually known as *ANOVA-type interaction models* since variability is decomposed as in an ANOVA with main covariates effects and their interactions (Lee and Durban, 2011).

Finally, Bauer et al. (2016) propose to use spline smoothing but just for the spatial component. Specifically, they model the spatio-temporal component as

$$S_i(t) = \sum_{k=1}^{K} \gamma_{kt} B_k(x_i, y_i)$$

where the basis of functions B_k are the product of two univariate cubic B-spline functions, one for each spatial dimension. In this case, the rows of γ are modeled as a set of random effects with a value for each knot and time period, which can be either independent or temporal, spatial or spatio-temporally correlated. The last two cases induce additional spatial smoothing to that already induced by the spline spatial term. The modeling of the spline coefficients for the temporal and spatio-temporally correlated cases makes the $sSMR$s to be temporally dependent; otherwise, the spatio-temporal term will not induce temporal dependence at all. This is in some way similar to the STANOVA approach mentioned previously, which induced spatial dependence on the regression coefficients, and temporal dependence was induced by the bases of functions. Now, in contrast, temporal dependence is induced by the modeling of the spline coefficients, and spatial dependence is induced by the spline basis used for spatial smoothing.

Spatio-temporal spline models may be implemented with both `WinBUGS` and `INLA`. As mentioned in Section 6.4, `INLA` seems a better suited tool for fitting spline models from a Bayesian point of view. `WinBUGS` finds some convergence problems for the components of γ with few nearby spatial units, which makes it advisable to prune the originally devised, regular, grid of knots in order to improve convergence. Nevertheless, this does not preclude spline models to be reasonably fitted in `WinBUGS`. Anyway, we have used `INLA` for fitting the models in the next example.

Example 7.3

In this example, we have fitted several spatio-temporal spline models to the oral cancer data set used throughout all this chapter. Our goal now is fitting more flexible spatio-temporal patterns than the parametric models fitted in the previous example. We have run all the models in this example with `INLA` as it seems to be a better suited option (substantially faster) than `WinBUGS` for spline models. The code used for this example has been adapted from that used in Ugarte et al. (2017), which has been kindly shared by its authors.

The spline models fitted have been grouped into the following classification:

- **No spatio-temporal interaction**: First, we have fitted a spatio-temporal model with main spatial and temporal terms but without any specific spatio-temporal interaction term. The spatial term has been assumed to follow a LCAR distribution and P-spline have been used to fit the overall temporal term for the spatial units as a whole. A cubic B-spline basis has been used to fit the P-spline model in time. The period of study has been divided into 3 inner intervals, which means that a basis of 6 cubic spline functions in time has been used to fit the temporal component. More specific details on this, and the following models, can be found in the supplementary online material of this example. Appropriate constraints were imposed on the different terms of this and the following models in order to ensure the identifiability of their terms.

- **1-dimensional spatio-temporal interaction**: As a second option, we have modified the previous model by adding a particular spatio-temporal interaction term. This new term has been modeled by means of P-spline, in particular, a 1-dimensional P-spline has been considered per municipality for fitting its time trend departure from the overall time trend for the whole region of study. As for the main time term, 3 inner intervals have been considered for modeling the time trend in the spatio-temporal component for each municipality and cubic B-spline bases are defined on the corresponding set of knots.

- **2-dimensional spatio-temporal interaction**: Third, we have considered once again a model with spatial, temporal and spatio-temporal terms. Nevertheless, in this case, a bidimensional P-spline model is considered for fitting the spatio-temporal component at each time interval of the period of study. A bidimensional B-spline basis, which is the product of two one-dimensional bases, is considered for the spatio-temporal term with 7 (longitudes) and 14 (latitudes) inner intervals, as in Example 6.1. This knot arrangement makes the contiguous knots in the grid equally spaced, regardless of its relative position.

- **3-dimensional spatio-temporal interaction**: In this case, we have considered a model with just an intercept and a spatio-temporal term accounting also for pure spatial and temporal variability. Now, the spatio-temporal term is modeled by means of a P-spline with a 3-dimensional spatio-temporal basis, built as the product of univariate bases for the longitude, latitude and time. These bases are exactly those already used for the two previous proposals. The spatio-temporal term used would be in charge of modeling the spatio-temporal variability around several spatio-temporal locations (the knots in the 3-dimensional grid) covering the region/period of study. As this model does not have specific spatial and temporal terms, the spatio-temporal term avoids some particular restrictions so that this term is able to reproduce also the pure spatial and temporal variability in the data.

- **ANOVA type 3-dimensional spatio-temporal interaction**: In this case we have considered an ANOVA type 3-dimensional spline model. That is, besides the 3-dimensional term modeling the spatio-temporal interaction in the previous model, we have additionally considered pure spatial and temporal terms for separately fitting these components of variance. Obviously, additional restrictions have been imposed for the spatio-temporal component for this new proposal in order to ensure the identifiability of its terms. Except for these restrictions, the 3-dimensional spline model considered for the spatio-temporal component of this model is exactly the same as that used in the previous model.

We have fitted 4 different models for each of the 1- and 2-dimensional spline groups mentioned. Each model assumes a different penalty on the coefficients of the corresponding spatio-temporal interaction. These penalties can be: (i) spatially and temporally independent, (ii) spatially dependent, (iii) temporally dependent, or (iv) spatio-temporally dependent. A first-order random walk penalty, in time and(/or) space (depending on the kind of interaction used), is considered for the coefficients of the spline. These penalties correspond to the 4 interaction types introduced in Knorr-Held (2000) and further described in the next section. Additionally, for 2- and 3-dimensional spline models, spatial anisotropy is induced by considering different penalty parameters for the different dimensions of the spline.

As mentioned, INLA has been used to fit all the models in this example. Nevertheless, all the models in this example have been run with the option strategy="gaussian" since the computing time for the rest of the, supposedly safer, strategy options becomes prohibitive. Interestingly, computing times vary substantially as a function of the 4 dependence penalties chosen. Thus, the fastest model to be fitted is the model without spatio-temporal interaction, which was fitted in 0.29 minutes. Nevertheless, for the 1-dimensional spline models, computing times vary from 1.00 minutes (type I interaction for the parameters of the spatio-temporal term) to 36.23 minutes (type II interaction). These computing time differences were lower for the 2-dimensional spline model, where the ratio between the fastest and the slowest computing times was 9.27.

Table 7.3 shows the DICs and their components for the best model (in terms of DIC) for each of the settings in the classification above. For the 1-dimensional setting, the best model has been that assuming spatial and temporal independence for the coefficients of the spline, closely followed by the model assuming spatial dependence (DIC=7338.8). For the 2-dimensional case, the model assuming temporal dependence for the spline coefficients has been the best option. However, there are no large differences in DIC terms for the different interaction types in Table 7.3. In contrast, the main differences have been noticed between the different settings considered. Thus, 2- and 3-dimensional spline models show a worse fit than the model without interaction or the 1-dimensional model. In other words, the models using spline for fitting the spatial component in the spatio-temporal interaction achieve a worse fit than those using an LCAR distribution. Indeed, substantial differences (result not shown) can be noticed between the choropleth maps of the spline-based models vs. those implementing an LCAR distribution for the spatial term. Spline-based spatial patterns yield more smoothed geographical patterns than those based on LCAR distributions. At the end, the extra-smoothing of spline for the spatial term does not seem to bring any overall benefit, although the number of effective parameters (pD in Table 7.3) is drastically reduced by using this modeling device. These results are in accordance with those shown in Example 6.1 for a more simple spatial setting.

The right-hand side of Table 7.3 shows the variance decomposition for all the models summarized in that table. In general all those variance decompositions have a tiny fraction of the whole variance in the spatio-temporal term. Thus, according to these models, there seems to be hardly any spatio-temporal interaction in the data, which explains the competitive results of the model without interaction in terms of DIC. This model is hardly constrained for this data set by ignoring spatio-temporal interaction and, in contrast, is far less complex in statistical/computational terms than the rest of options. As in Example 7.2, the main variance component found for this data set is the spatial term, also for spline models. Note, however, that important differences in the variance decomposition can be noticed once again between models using spline for the spatial term and those that use LCAR distributions. The models using spline for the spatial component find a stronger contribution of that component to the variance decomposition. This could be surely due to the smooth spatial pattern reproduced by those models, which are forced to modify the risks for a large spatial area in order to reproduce some local variation in the risks.

Model	DICs components			Variance decomposition		
	Dev.	pD	DIC	% Spat.	% Temp.	% S.T.
No interaction	7248.0	90.6	7338.6	60.8	39.2	0.0
1 dim.	7231.5	106.9	7338.4	61.9	38.0	0.1
2 dim.	7297.9	44.9	7342.8	77.1	22.3	0.6
3 dim.	7305.3	47.9	7353.2	82.0	12.3	5.7
ANOVA 3 dim.	7303.7	38.6	7342.3	78.5	20.8	0.7

Table 7.3
DIC (with its components) and variance decompositions for the best model of each setting.

Figure 7.3 shows the time trends fitted for each municipality (gray lines) for the period of study. These time trends correspond to the spline model with 1-dimensional spatio-temporal interaction and no dependence on the penalty function of the parameters in the spline model (type I interaction), that is the model achieving the lowest DIC in Table 7.3. Note that the DIC for this model is slightly higher than that of the parametric quadratic model fitted in the previous example, so this particular spline model does not seem to be a better alternative than that parametric proposal. Figure 7.3 shows almost quadratic time trends, which justifies the practical equivalence of both models in DIC terms. Nevertheless, most of the time trends in Figure 7.3 become flat at the end of the period of study, in contrast to the quadratic parametric model. The quadratic model does not have enough flexibility for describing that stabilization, but the spline model, in contrast, is able to capture that particular feature in the time trends. In this sense, the additional flexibility of the spline model seems to bring some benefit, although not enough to outperform the quadratic models in terms of DIC. Finally, note the effect of the spatio-temporal interaction in Figure 7.3. That effect is particularly evident for the time trends corresponding to municipalities with higher risks. Concretely, we can see that the municipality with the highest risk reaches its maximum later, in general, than the rest of the municipalities. Moreover, we can also notice several municipal time trends crossing their trajectories. However, the effect of spatio-temporal interaction does not seem to be quite important, as also corroborated in Table 7.3.

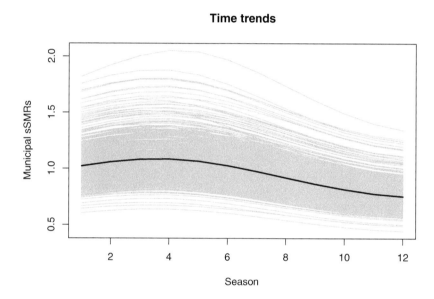

Figure 7.3
Time trends for the municipalities of the Valencian Region for the period of study. Black line corresponds to the overall time trend for the whole Valencian Region.

7.4   Non-parametric temporal modeling

Beyond temporal parametric models, either based on spline or on other alternative functions, we find also several proposals for non-parametric modeling in spatio-temporal problems. These models are a direct generalization of the (usually structured) random effects models used in pure spatial problems. As for the spatial case, spatio-temporal non-parametric models assume at least one random effect per spatio-temporal observation. Inducing a realistic and rich enough dependence structure on these random effects is the main challenge faced by this kind of models that avoid the use of additional smoothing devices, as for example bases of functions.

Within the non-parametric spatio-temporal literature, we find particularly enlightening the work by Knorr-Held (2000). This paper proposes to model the spatio-temporal log-risks as

$$\log(\Theta_{it}) = \mu + \alpha_i + \beta_t + \Delta_{ij} \tag{7.6}$$

where α and β are vectors of random effects modeling, respectively, the spatial and temporal components in the log-risks as in an ANOVA-type spline model. The term Δ, which will be also a matrix of random effects, will be in charge of modeling the spatio-temporal interaction in Θ. Knorr-Held (2000) proposes a classification of the models in this family as a function of the way how spatio-temporal dependence is structured in Δ. Knorr-held assumes two separate sources of variability in spatio-temporal problems, spatial and temporal variability. These two sources could either assume independence or dependence between observations and the classification proposed considers all four combinations of these two possibilities for the spatial and temporal components. The four combinations of these two sources of variation are made by considering the precision matrix of $vec(\Delta)$ as the Kronecker product of the corresponding spatial and temporal precision matrices. Therefore, the dependence structure in Δ will be a separable combination of the assumed spatial and temporal structures.

Specifically, the first of the spatio-temporal interactions in that classification (*type I interaction* according to the original paper) would be the combination of both independent spatial and temporal processes. This would yield a diagonal spatio-temporal precision matrix for Δ that would assume independence between all its cells. Thus, neither spatial nor temporal dependence would be induced with this interaction. Therefore, Δ in type I interaction induces further flexibility by allowing each specific cell in Θ to have a particular value which is not an additive combination of its spatial and temporal interactions. The interaction between cells of Θ takes independent values. Nevertheless, *Type II interaction* combines a structured temporal with an unstructured spatial term. This yields an interaction term Δ which is temporally correlated with each spatial unit, but these time trends are spatially independent. That is, Δ in this case will reproduce spatially independent time series or, in other words, Δ will show dependence within rows, but their rows will be mutually independent. On the contrary, *type III interaction* combines a spatially structured term with an independent temporal component. This yields an interaction term which is spatially correlated, but the corresponding period-specific spatial patterns are independent for each time period. That is, Δ shows dependence within columns but their columns are mutually independent. Finally, *type IV interaction* combines two structured effects for space and time, yielding an interaction term which is both spatially and temporally dependent. In principle, this would yield the more complex interaction since it would allow its components to share information for both spatial and temporal neighbours, yielding coherent estimates in these two aspects. Moreover, type IV interaction takes the maximum profit of the two sources of dependence in data, in contrast to the other three types, yielding in principle the most elaborated fit. In other words, for type IV interaction, both rows and columns of Δ will be dependent at a same time in contrast to the simpler interactions.

Note that the original paper of Knorr-Held (2000) assumes two particular spatial and temporal dependence structures. Specifically, spatial dependence, when considered, is assumed to follow an ICAR distribution and temporal dependence, when considered, is assumed to follow a Random Walk of first order, which is also an ICAR distribution considering as neighbours consecutive periods of time. This means that according to Knorr-Held (2000), type I to IV interactions have very specific and precise mathematical forms, with no parameter controlling the strength of spatial or temporal dependence, in the case that the cells of Δ were assumed to be dependent. We will understand Knorr-Held's classification of spatio-temporal interactions in a broader sense, assuming that a type I interaction is that which does not share information neither in space nor in time; type II interaction shares information just in time; type III interaction shares information just in space; and type IV interaction assumes dependence both in space and time. This makes in our opinion this classification even more useful and general as it contains also non-separable spatio-temporal processes, for example, whereas the original proposal only considered separable processes of specific spatial and temporal processes (their precision matrices were built as Kronecker products of these spatial and temporal precision matrices).

Knorr-Held's classification summarizes most of the spatio-temporal literature in non-parametric modeling. Thus, just to cite some examples, Waller et al. (1997), Knorr-Held (2000), and Ugarte et al. (2014) are three specific works that implement type I interaction models. Type II interaction has been used for example in Schmid and Held (2004), Schrödle et al. (2011), and Ugarte et al. (2016). Note that temporal structures such as Random Walks of second order are also used for modeling time trends for some of these works. Type III interaction has been used for example in Waller et al. (1997), Xia and Carlin (1998), and López-Abente et al. (2014) and type IV interaction in Schmid and Held (2004), and Dwyer-Lindgren et al. (2015). Additionally, some other works compare spatio-temporal models corresponding to these different types of interaction; thus Schmid and Held (2004) and Schrödle et al. (2011) compare type II and type IV interaction models, concluding both that type II interaction, ignoring spatial dependence in time trends, is the most advisable option for their respective data sets. Also, Ugarte et al. (2016) compare all four kinds of interaction in their work, concluding once again that type II interaction was the most advisable choice for their data set. Nevertheless, in our opinion, none of these types would be always the best choice for every setting, and this would depend on the particular data set at hand. The strength of spatial and temporal dependence for each data set would determine which of these interactions would be more appropriate for each particular case.

A second formulation of non-parametric spatio-temporal models could be done as a sequential concatenation of spatial processes instead of separable structures combining spatial and temporal processes. Specifically, Martinez-Beneito et al. (2008) propose to model spatio-temporal sets of risks as multi-variate first-order auto-regressive processes in time with spatially structured increments for each time interval. In more detail, they consider an $I \times T$ matrix $\mathbf{\Psi}$ with mutually independent columns which follow spatially correlated distributions such as ICAR, PCAR, BYM, etc. Given that matrix, the set of log-risks $\mathbf{\Theta}$ could be defined for each time interval, with $t > 1$, as

$$\mathbf{\Theta}_{\cdot t} = \rho\mathbf{\Theta}_{\cdot t-1} + \mathbf{\Psi}_{\cdot t}.$$

Temporal dependence in this model comes from the first-order auto-regressive structure imposed and spatial dependence is induced by the correlated character of the columns of $\mathbf{\Psi}$. Both sources of dependence induce the spatio-temporal structure of this proposal.

Typically all the columns of $\mathbf{\Psi}$, except $\mathbf{\Psi}_{\cdot 1}$ are assumed to have the same spatial distribution with the same hyperparameters. That is, all of them have a common covariance matrix $\sigma_{\mathbf{\Psi}}^2 \mathbf{\Sigma}_s$ where the structure matrix $\mathbf{\Sigma}_s$ could depend on additional parameters. In that case, it is commonly assumed $\mathbf{\Psi}_{\cdot 1}$ to have the same prior distribution than the rest of columns of $\mathbf{\Psi}$, but with variance equal to $(\sigma_{\mathbf{\Psi}}^2/(1-\rho^2))\mathbf{\Sigma}_s$. This gives higher variance to the risk pattern fitted for the first time period than for the subsequent differences in risks, which seems quite reasonable since inter-period variations would be expected to be small. That variance correction for the first time interval sets its variance to be equal to the stationary variance of the auto-regressive time series of each spatial unit. Additionally,

$$
\begin{aligned}
Var(\mathbf{\Theta}_{\cdot 2}) &= \rho^2 Var(\mathbf{\Theta}_{\cdot 1}) + \sigma_{\mathbf{\Psi}}^2 \mathbf{\Sigma}_s = (\rho^2/(1-\rho^2) + 1)\sigma_{\mathbf{\Psi}}^2 \mathbf{\Sigma}_s \\
&= (\sigma_{\mathbf{\Psi}}^2/(1-\rho^2))\mathbf{\Sigma}_s = Var(\mathbf{\Theta}_{\cdot 1})
\end{aligned}
$$

and in a similar manner we could show that $Var(\mathbf{\Theta}_{\cdot 1}) = Var(\mathbf{\Theta}_{\cdot 2}) = ... = Var(\mathbf{\Theta}_{\cdot T})$. Therefore, the variance correction in the first time interval makes the variances for the log-risks equal for all time periods.

A uniform prior distribution between -1 and 1 is usually set for ρ, which guarantees the positivity of the variance matrices above. It can be shown (Martinez-Beneito et al., 2008) that the variance-covariance matrix of the auto-regressive process is of the form

$$Var(vec(\boldsymbol{\Theta})) = \boldsymbol{\Sigma}(\rho) \otimes (\sigma_{\boldsymbol{\Psi}}^2 \boldsymbol{\Sigma}_s)$$

where

$$\boldsymbol{\Sigma}(\rho) = \frac{1}{1-\rho^2}\begin{pmatrix} 1 & \rho & \rho^2 & \cdots & \rho^{T-1} \\ \rho & 1 & \rho & \cdots & \rho^{T-2} \\ \rho^2 & \rho & 1 & \cdots & \rho^{T-3} \\ \vdots & \vdots & \vdots & \ddots & \vdots \\ \rho^{T-1} & \rho^{T-2} & \rho^{T-3} & \cdots & 1 \end{pmatrix}$$

is the covariance matrix of a first-order auto-regressive process of parameter ρ and of conditional variance fixed to 1. Therefore, the auto-regressive spatio-temporal process, as defined above, yields a spatio-temporal separable structure fusing the temporal and spatial structures used to build that process.

Note that all four types of Knorr-Held's interaction can be reproduced as particular cases of the auto-regressive process above with a BYM spatial structure for the columns of $\boldsymbol{\Theta}$. Specifically, type I interaction could be reproduced for $\rho = 0$ and σ_s^2 (the variance of the spatial term) equal to 0. Thus, neither temporal nor spatial dependence will be accounted for in this model. Similarly, type II interaction can be reproduced by setting $\sigma_s^2 = 0$ and $\rho \neq 0$. Specifically, for $\rho = 1$ we reproduce spatially independent first-order random walk structures, as originally proposed by Knorr-Held (2000). Type III interaction in general could be achieved by setting $\rho = 0$ and, in particular, for $\sigma_h = 0$ (the variance of the heterogeneous term in BYM) we would reproduce the original type III interaction proposal in Knorr-Held (2000). Finally, type IV interaction could be reproduced by setting $\rho \neq 0$ and $\sigma_s^2 \neq 0$, in particular if $\sigma_h^2 = 0$ we reproduce the original type IV interaction of Knorr-Held. Thus, in this manner we could reproduce all four interaction types in a single model without the need to specifically choose any of them, which seems to be a major advantage of this proposal. Moreover, the auto-regressive model is able to reproduce some models in between the four interaction types originally proposed, which constitutes an additional advantage.

Additionally, the auto-regressive spatio-temporal proposal can be easily modified to reproduce more general covariance structures that could be of use in some occasions. The auto-regressive process described is just an example of temporal concatenation of spatial processes. Nevertheless, there is no obligation to use specifically first-order auto-regressive process or BYM spatial processes in that process. Hence, this proposal could be easily modified by considering alternative spatial families (PCAR, LCAR, etc.) or alternative time series models (auto-regressive processes of higher order, random walks, etc.).

Moreover, although the original auto-regressive modeling proposal produces separable covariance structures, it is quite easy to reproduce non-separable covariances within that framework. For example, if spatial patterns of different hyperparameters (such as BYM models of different variances), or even of different spatial distributions, were allowed for each column of $\boldsymbol{\Psi}$ then $\boldsymbol{\Sigma_\Phi}$ would be no longer separable. In that case, we would not have a single correlation matrix for the spatial term, which makes unfeasible to represent the whole spatio-temporal covariance matrix as the Kronecker product of two temporal and spatial covariance matrices.

The implementation of the non-parametric models above requires some particular care. Specifically, Expression (7.6) decomposes the $I \times T$ matrix $\boldsymbol{\Theta}$ as the sum of μ, the I-vector $\boldsymbol{\alpha}$, the T-vector $\boldsymbol{\beta}$ and the $I \times T$ matrix $\boldsymbol{\Delta}$. Obviously, that decomposition of $\boldsymbol{\Theta}$ into $IT + I + T + 1$ parameters makes the corresponding models to be overparameterized if no additional restriction is imposed into the right-hand side variables of Expression (7.6). Regarding the auto-regressive process, this is solved by removing $\boldsymbol{\alpha}$, the overall spatial pattern for the whole period of study, from the log-risks decomposition. As a consequence, $\boldsymbol{\Delta}$ will be in charge of reproducing both the spatial and spatio-temporal terms of the log-risks. Therefore, the posterior distribution of ρ for this model often has most of its mass close to 1. This makes the columns of $\boldsymbol{\Phi}$ reproduce a single (overall) spatial pattern for the whole period of study with slight modifications for each particular time interval, that is, a strong spatial component, as a consequence of the removal of $\boldsymbol{\alpha}$. Moreover, $\boldsymbol{\beta}$ is assumed to follow a first-order random walk process, with a sum-to-zero restriction (ICAR distribution in time). This makes the number of free parameters in the spatio-temporal model to decrease to $IT + (T - 1) + 1 = IT + T$. If an ICAR spatial distribution, with the typical sum-to-zero restriction, was assumed for the columns of $\boldsymbol{\Psi}$ this would decrease the number of free parameters for each column in one unit and would make then the number of free parameters in this model to be equal to $(I - 1)T + T = IT$, solving the mentioned overparameterization. In contrast, a BYM distribution was originally assumed in Martinez-Beneito et al. (2008) for the columns of $\boldsymbol{\Psi}$. For that choice, the ICAR part of the BYM model would not be worrisome as we have already explained but the heterogeneous part will make the model to have $IT + T$ free parameters. As a consequence, a bit of confounding might exist between that heterogeneous part of $\boldsymbol{\Psi}$ and the overall time trend in the model. That confounding will come from the mean of those random effects that could compete with $\boldsymbol{\beta}$ for explaining the overall time trend. Nevertheless, the prior mean of the heterogeneous term of each column of $\boldsymbol{\Psi}$ will be distributed as a Normal of mean 0 and variance σ_h^2/I. Thus, for large lattices that confounding should be low. That confounding is also present in univariate BYM models between the heterogeneous random effect and the intercept and has not focussed particular attention in the literature. Beyond the auto-regressive model, for the decomposition of log-Risks in Expression (7.6), $\boldsymbol{\Delta}$ should be restricted with sum-to-zero restrictions for all their rows and columns, i.e., $\sum_{t=1}^{T} \Delta_{it} = 0$ and

$\sum_{i=1}^{I} \Delta_{it} = 0$ for all $i = 1, ..., I$ and $t = 1, ..., T$. In this manner confounding between $\boldsymbol{\alpha}$, $\boldsymbol{\beta}$ and $\boldsymbol{\Psi}$ would be completely avoided.

The four interaction types in Knorr-Held (2000) were coded in C++ in the original paper. Nevertheless, interaction types I-III can be also easily implemented in WinBUGS as independent random effects, a set of independent time series and a set of independent spatial patterns, respectively. Regretfully, the implementation of the type IV interaction in WinBUGS is not so straightforward. If pure spatial and temporal terms ($\boldsymbol{\alpha}$ and $\boldsymbol{\beta}$, respectively) were considered in the log-risks decomposition, $\boldsymbol{\Delta}$ should incorporate the previously mentioned sum-to-zero restrictions on their rows and columns. In principle, WinBUGS does not have any specific tool to implement restrictions of that kind. Anyway, type IV interaction could be implemented as a particular case of the auto-regressive model, which can be easily implemented in WinBUGS (see the online annex material for the next example).

All four spatio-temporal interaction types can be coded also within INLA. Section 7.1.2 of Blangiardo et al. (2013) shows the code needed to implement all four types of interaction in INLA. Additionally, Schrödle and Held (2011b) discusses the implementation of sum-to-zero restrictions in spatio-temporal models in INLA, and Ugarte et al. (2017) makes a similar discussion for spline-based spatio-temporal models with coefficients having a spatio-temporal interaction structure.

Example 7.4

We are going to retake our example of the spatio-temporal study of oral cancer in the Valencian Region. In this case, we are going to apply the auto-regressive model introduced in this section to the same data set used in the rest of the examples of this chapter. We have implemented the model in WinBUGS, whose code can be found in the online annex material to the book.

The variance decomposition for the auto-regressive model for the oral cancer data set yields a 73.1% of variance to the spatial term, a 16.1% of variance to the temporal term and a 10.8% for the spatio-temporal term. The high weight of the spatial component in that decomposition is a consequence of the posterior distribution of ρ, which has a posterior mean of 0.966. Therefore, the auto-regressive process reproduces spatial patterns with high temporal correlation, that is, similar spatial pattern with small variations per each time interval. Note that the contribution of the temporal and spatio-temporal terms increases for this model, in comparison to the models in the previous examples. This is surely as a consequence of the higher flexibility of auto-regressive time series to model the different temporal evolutions. The DIC for the auto-regressive model was 7332.8, slightly lower than that of the quadratic parametric model (7334.3) and the best spline model (7338.4), so the differences between these three models in terms of fit are modest.

Figure 7.4 shows several interesting features on the fit of the auto-regressive model. Specifically, the upper row of that figure shows the time trends for every municipality in the Valencian Region (gray lines). The plot on the left shows the evolution of the risks, whereas the plot on the right shows the evolution of the spatio-temporal components, where the spatial and temporal terms in the risks have been removed. The plot on the left shows, in addition, the overall time trend (black line) for the whole Valencian Region. For that overall time trend, the solid line stands for the posterior mean at each time interval and the dashed line stands for the corresponding 95% posterior credible interval. It can be noticed how the overall time trend has followed mostly a quadratic trend with a maximum peak around 1990-1997. According to the credible interval, a linear trend would seem discarded. This plot shows how all municipalities in the Valencian Region have followed a similar trend with small departures. Additionally, this plot makes evident why spatial variability is the main source of variation for this data set. Although all municipalities follow similar trends, the mean values for all of them are very different, pointing out different mean risk levels for each of them for the whole time period.

The particular features of the municipal trends can be better explored in the upper-right plot of Figure 7.4. Note first the different scales of the vertical axes for the two upper plots in that figure. The right plot shows a much narrower range making it clear that the interaction term controls a small part of the variability of the data set. The brown lines in this plot correspond to the municipalities with a spatial term for the risks above 1.5, that is, the municipalities with the highest overall risks. These municipalities correspond to those in the two clusters, around Alicante and Gandía, appearing in Figure 4.4. The few brown lines with a downwards trend for the whole period of study correspond to the southern cluster (Alicante), whereas the other brown lines, with a peak at the second half of the period of study, correspond to the northernmost cluster. This different interaction term for the two clusters points out a different temporal performance for both. The southern cluster has a worse performance at the beginning of the period of study making the peak of the disease appear before that for the rest of the Valencian Region. Interestingly, the region with the highest risk for 1988-89 (upper-left plot) belongs to this cluster. On the contrary, the municipalities in the northern cluster have a particularly bad performance once the overall trend has started to decline. As a consequence, the maximum risk peak for this cluster is reached later than for the overall Valencian Region. An example of municipality of this cluster is that with the second highest risk for 1998-99 (upper-left plot). Clear differences can be observed for the time trends of the two mentioned municipalities with diverging trajectories as the period of study evolves.

The lower row of Figure 7.4 shows two maps corresponding to the spatio-temporal interaction at the first and last intervals of study. We can see how the patterns for these two maps look uncorrelated, in contrast to those of the quadratic model in Figure 7.2 where those same maps showed closely similar patterns. This was a consequence of the parametric character of that

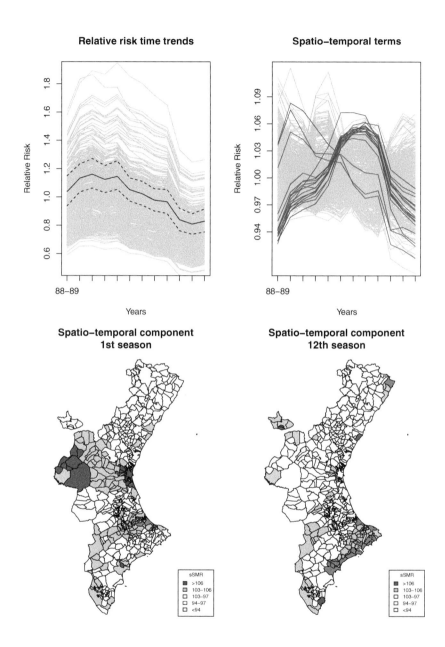

Figure 7.4
Upper row: Time trends for the risks and spatio-temporal interaction for each municipality in the Valencian Region. Lower row: Maps for the spatio-temporal interaction for the 1st and 12th seasons of study.

model. Now the higher flexibility of the auto-regressive model has made the correlation of these distant periods for the spatio-temporal term disappear. This performance of the auto-regressive model seems much more reasonable.

Finally, for concluding this section, we would like to point out that spatio-temporal disease mapping goes beyond the set of models described in the previous sections. Thus, besides CAR and spline models that have been by far the most popular tools for inducing spatial dependence in spatio-temporal studies, other tools such as Dirichlet processes have also been used for that goal (Kottas et al., 2007). Also, zero excesses could also occur in spatio-temporal disease mapping and they could be modeled with similar proposals, zero inflated and hurdle models, to those used in spatial studies (Balderama et al., 2016; Musenge et al., 2013; Neelon et al., 2014). Finally, we would also like to point out that longitudinal data have also focussed considerable attention on disease mapping studies. Longitudinal data are also a kind of temporal data, where people are observed for a period of time and the issue of interest is when they show a particular event, such as death. Thus, survival disease mapping studies have gotten, as mentioned, considerable attention (Osnes and Aalen, 1999; Li and Ryan, 2002; Banerjee and Carlin, 2003; Banerjee et al., 2003b; Carlin and Banerjee, 2003; Banerjee and Carlin, 2004); although other longitudinal data, such as general time to event data (Crook et al., 2003) or spatial age-period-cohort models (Lagazzio et al., 2003) have also received some attention.

Exercises

1. The `pop-ST.Rdata` file contains the age-specific populations for Valencia city census tracts for 10 biannual intervals covering the original period of study: 1996-2015. With this information and the age-specific observed counts for the whole period of study (see `COPD.Rdata` file), calculate the COPD expected deaths per census tract and time interval.

2. The `COPD-ST.Rdata` file contains the observed deaths counts per census tract corresponding to the 10 time intervals considered in the previous exercise. These data have been also slightly altered to preserve data confidentiality. Use the expected counts already calculated and pose the following models for estimating the corresponding spatio-temporal smoothed *SMR*s:

   • A parametric spatio-temporal model assuming spatially dependent quadratic time trends per census tract.

- One-, two- and three-dimensional (ANOVA type) P-spline models with specific spatial and temporal terms.

- A non-parametric spatio-temporal auto-regressive process.

Compare the fit for all the models proposed and describe the spatio-temporal changes that have occurred in the COPD mortality of Valencia city during the whole period of study. For the more convenient model in the previous comparison, report the variance decomposition of the spatio-temporal pattern fitted and separately describe the spatial, temporal and spatio-temporal components of the whole spatio-temporal pattern fitted.

8

Multivariate modeling

The main goal of spatio-temporal disease mapping studies, in the previous chapter, was generally to split the whole period of study into several smaller intervals while being able to draw reliable risk maps for any of them. As we showed, splitting the whole period of study into smaller parts produced a decrease in the amount of cases per observed unit, increasing the typical small area estimation problems of disease mapping studies. Being able to profit from the temporal dependence of risks in those time intervals, as well as spatial dependence between geographical units, was the key for obtaining reliable risk estimates.

In multivariate disease mapping studies, we have once again several outcomes per spatial unit, typically several different causes of death, instead of a single number of observed counts. In contrast to spatio-temporal modeling, those observations generally correspond to additional information sources instead of corresponding to a thinner temporal disaggregation of the original data. The goal now is taking advantage of those additional information sources in order to obtain improved risk estimates. Once again, sharing information between the variables in our models, by profiting from their dependence, is the key for improving their estimates. Therefore, as for spatio-temporal models, combining several sources of dependence in a sensible manner is the main methodological challenge that multivariate models pose.

Despite their different aims, multivariate and spatio-temporal modeling are in some way related methodological problems. Both settings consist of a set of spatial units with multivariate observations. From a mathematical point of view, the main issue that makes both problems different is that for spatio-temporal problems, those observations have an obvious ordering induced by time, while for multivariate studies there is no such order. Basically, for multivariate studies, the order followed by the causes of death is generally arbitrary and any alternative ordering could be equally good. This difference makes the tools used for inducing dependence between time periods (time series, spline, etc.) unfeasible for multivariate modeling, as all of them would depend on the ordering of the diseases in the study for inducing that dependence. For multivariate modeling, we would prefer modeling tools that could induce dependence between all the observations of each spatial unit regardless of their ordering. In this sense, multivariate modeling seeks to induce unstructured dependence between diseases in contrast to spatio-temporal models, which heavily rely on the ordering of the time sequence available.

In contrast to ecological regression, where we use also additional information sources (risk determinants) as covariates to improve risk estimates, multivariate models use other additional response variables as an additional information source. Specifically, ecological regression is devised for fitting some factor(s) that could be determining, or even causing, the geographical distribution of the disease. Nevertheless, covariates or proxies of specific desired determinants are not always available or so easy to obtain, so ecological regression may not be so feasible as a way for improving risk estimates. On the other hand, multivariate studies are generally performed on sets of related diseases or health events that could depend on common risk factors (regardless of whether we know that factor or not). Therefore, their geographical patterns should hypothetically show common features. Such association between those patterns will be used as a second source of dependence in order to improve risk estimates for all those diseases considered in the study. Thus, in this manner, multivariate models avoid the limitation of lacking a particular covariate by substituting the effect of that covariate for the dependence on some related diseases, that could possibly share the effect of the missing covariate or some other common risk factor.

A second important difference of multivariate modeling with respect to ecological regression is that, for the first, we would not be in general specially interested in the geographical pattern of one particular disease. We will be interested in retrieving reliable risk estimates for a set of diseases and all of them would be equally important, regardless of whether we could draw particular conclusions for any of them. For ecological regression, we would typically have a single outcome and therefore we will have a particular focus in explaining that particular disease. Thus, in summary, in contrast to ecological regression studies where there is one (or several) covariate(s) and a single geographical pattern to be studied, multivariate studies will not have in general covariate(s) to explain the corresponding geographical pattern, but they will have several response variables per spatial unit. Considering dependence among those response variables will be the main source of improvement of multivariate studies as compared to traditional univariate spatial studies.

According to the previous comments, the general formulation of multivariate problems would be very similar to that of spatio-temporal models and could be done as follows. Let O_{ij} be the number of observed deaths for the i-th areal unit ($i = 1, ..., I$) and j-th disease ($j = 1, ..., J$). We use now j instead of t to subindex the observations for any spatial unit, which will be typically different diseases or health events in contrast to the spatio-temporal setting. These observed counts are usually assumed to follow conditionally independent Poisson distributions

$$O_{ij}|\Theta_{ij} \sim Poisson(E_{ij}\Theta_{ij}) \tag{8.1}$$

$$\log(\Theta_{ij}) = \mu_j + \phi_{ij},$$

where μ_j denotes a disease-specific intercept. As for the spatial and spatio-temporal literature, different multivariate models arise for each different modeling proposal for $\boldsymbol{\Phi} = (\phi_{ij})$, the matrix of log-risks, which will typically account for the spatial and multivariate dependence of $\boldsymbol{\Theta}$. Thus, as for spatio-temporal models, multivariate models will have to jointly impose both sources of dependence, across rows and columns, in $\boldsymbol{\Phi}$. From now on, we will refer to spatial dependence for any of the diseases of study, dependence within columns of $\boldsymbol{\Phi}$, as dependence *within diseases*. In contrast, we will refer as dependence *between diseases* to that between columns of $\boldsymbol{\Phi}$, corresponding to the multivariate dependence of the components of the vector of observations for each spatial unit.

Similarly to univariate CAR models, $\boldsymbol{\Phi}$ will have to fulfill some conditions in order to be well defined, and not every definition of this matrix yields necessarily valid processes. For the univariate case, those conditions guaranteed the variance-covariance matrix of the corresponding vector to be symmetric and positive definite. Now $\boldsymbol{\Phi}$ is no longer a vector but a matrix. In this case the symmetry and positive definiteness conditions should be fulfilled by the covariance matrix of either $vec(\boldsymbol{\Phi})$ ($\boldsymbol{\Sigma}_{vec(\boldsymbol{\Phi})}$) or $vec(\boldsymbol{\Phi}')$ ($\boldsymbol{\Sigma}_{vec(\boldsymbol{\Phi}')}$). Note that, as mentioned in Section 1.1, $vec(\boldsymbol{\Phi}) = \boldsymbol{P}vec(\boldsymbol{\Phi}')$ for a permutation (and therefore orthogonal) full-rank matrix $\boldsymbol{P}$. Therefore,

$$\boldsymbol{\Sigma}_{vec(\boldsymbol{\Phi}')} = \boldsymbol{\Sigma}_{\boldsymbol{P}vec(\boldsymbol{\Phi})} = \boldsymbol{P}\boldsymbol{\Sigma}_{vec(\boldsymbol{\Phi})}\boldsymbol{P}'$$

and, as a direct consequence, $\boldsymbol{\Sigma}_{vec(\boldsymbol{\Phi})}$ is symmetric and positive definite if and only if $\boldsymbol{\Sigma}_{vec(\boldsymbol{\Phi}')}$ fulfills also both conditions. Note also that if $\boldsymbol{\Sigma}_{vec(\boldsymbol{\Phi}')} = \boldsymbol{A} \otimes \boldsymbol{B}$ for two square matrices $\boldsymbol{A}$ and $\boldsymbol{B}$, then $\boldsymbol{\Sigma}_{vec(\boldsymbol{\Phi})} = \boldsymbol{B} \otimes \boldsymbol{A}$, this can be easily shown, for example, as a direct consequence of expressions (12) and (13) of Henderson and Searle (1979). This property will allow us to put the covariance of many of the models to be introduced below in common terms since some works in the literature summarize their properties as a function of $\boldsymbol{\Sigma}_{vec(\boldsymbol{\Phi})}$ and others as a function of $\boldsymbol{\Sigma}_{vec(\boldsymbol{\Phi}')}$. This duality arises since some proposals model $vec(\boldsymbol{\Phi})$ and others $vec(\boldsymbol{\Phi}')$, so it will be convenient to derive the covariance matrix of all of them as a function of a single term. For all the models below, we will put all their covariance matrices as a function of $\boldsymbol{\Sigma}_{vec(\boldsymbol{\Phi})}$. The latter property will allow us to switch often between them, so we will use it extensively during this chapter. Thus, in summary, the main challenge of multivariate models is building sensible, computationally efficient models which yield valid covariance matrices including dependence both within and between diseases. This is not at all a straightforward task.

In contrast to univariate disease mapping, where most of the work done has been founded in the paper of Besag (1974), multivariate disease mapping models have been built following different approaches. Of these, we distinguish at least two main approaches in the literature. The first of these approaches corresponds to conditionally specified models, which would correspond to straightforward generalizations of the original work by Besag (1974) on spatial CAR distributions to the multivariate domain. We introduce this approach in Section 8.1 of this chapter. The second of these approaches corresponds to multivariate models inducing dependence by means of linear models of coregionalization. We introduce this approach in Section 8.2. Finally, we conclude this chapter with a final section on particular multivariate models that in our opinion deserve particular attention for some of their features or because of the interest that they have focussed on in the literature.

8.1 Conditionally specified models

Conditionally specified multivariate models are a natural generalization of the work done in univariate CAR models for sets of areal referenced vectors of observations. Based on MacNab (2018), we will classify the proposals in this approach into two big sets. Thus, for the multivariate CAR modeling of a matrix $\boldsymbol{\Phi}$ of log-risks, we introduce first a series of models formulated as a set of compatible conditional multivariate distributions for $\boldsymbol{\phi}_{i\cdot}|vec(\boldsymbol{\phi}_{-i\cdot})$, for $i = 1, ..., I$. On the other hand, we introduce later a second series of models formulated as a set of compatible univariate conditional distributions for $\phi_{ij}|vec(\boldsymbol{\phi}_{-(ij)})$ for $i = 1, ..., I$, $j = 1, ..., J$. We are going to review these two approaches in this section.

8.1.1 Multivariate models as sets of conditional multivariate distributions

Historically, this is the oldest formulation of multivariate CAR distributions (Mardia, 1988) and therefore the oldest approach to multivariate disease mapping. These models seek to generalize the conditional distributions in expressions (4.10) or (4.14) for the vectors $\boldsymbol{\phi}_{i\cdot}|vec(\boldsymbol{\phi}_{-i\cdot})$ for $i = 1, ..., I$. In more detail, Mardia proposes to set

$$\boldsymbol{\phi}_{i\cdot}|vec(\boldsymbol{\phi}_{-i\cdot}), \boldsymbol{\mu}, \boldsymbol{\beta}, \boldsymbol{\Sigma}_i \sim N_J\left(\boldsymbol{\mu}'_{i\cdot} + \sum_{i' \neq i} \boldsymbol{\beta}_{ii'}(\boldsymbol{\phi}_{i'\cdot} - \boldsymbol{\mu}_{i'\cdot})', \boldsymbol{\Sigma}_i\right) \quad (8.2)$$

for suitable J-dimensional square matrices $\{\boldsymbol{\beta}_{ii'} : i, i' = 1, ..., I\}$, for a collection of J-dimensional symmetric positive definite matrices $\{\boldsymbol{\Sigma}_i : i = 1, ..., I\}$ and for an $I \times J$ matrix $\boldsymbol{\mu} = (\mu_{ij})$. We will set from now $\boldsymbol{\mu} = \mathbf{0}_I$ since we will typically model the mean of any observation in the linear predictor of the corresponding hierarchical model, as usually done also for univariate models. The parameters in Expression (8.2) can be either fixed or unknown, possibly dependent on further model parameters, so we will denote them all by Greek letters, although some of them could be fixed.

   The set of conditional distributions in (8.2) are shown to be equivalent to a multivariate Normal distribution on $vec(\boldsymbol{\Phi}')$ of mean $vec(\boldsymbol{\mu}')$ and variance-covariance matrix $\boldsymbol{\Sigma}_{vec(\boldsymbol{\Phi}')} = (block(-\{\boldsymbol{\Sigma}_i^{-1}\boldsymbol{\beta}_{ii'}\}_{i,i'=1}^I))^{-1}$ (Mardia, 1988). As for univariate CARs, some constraints should be imposed on the previous conditional distributions so that they are compatible, i.e., so that they yield a symmetric and positive definite joint covariance matrix $\boldsymbol{\Sigma}_{vec(\boldsymbol{\Phi}')}$. Mardia states two conditions for this. First

$$\boldsymbol{\beta}_{ii'}\boldsymbol{\Sigma}_{i'} = \boldsymbol{\Sigma}_i\boldsymbol{\beta}'_{i'i}, \ i, i' = 1, ..., I \tag{8.3}$$

is a necessary and sufficient condition to guarantee the symmetry of $\boldsymbol{\Sigma}_{vec(\boldsymbol{\Phi}')}$. On the other hand, since

$$block(-\{\boldsymbol{\Sigma}_i^{-1}\boldsymbol{\beta}_{ii'}\}_{i,i'=1}^I) = Bdiag(\{\boldsymbol{\Sigma}_i^{-1}\}_{i=1}^I)block(-\{\boldsymbol{\beta}_{ii'}\}_{i,i'=1}^I)$$

and $\boldsymbol{\Sigma}_i$ is positive definite for $i = 1, ..., I$, the covariance matrix $\boldsymbol{\Sigma}_{vec(\boldsymbol{\Phi}')}$ will be definite positive if and only if $block(-\{\boldsymbol{\beta}_{ii'}\}_{i,i'=1}^I)$ is too. Note that for the two conditions above, and from now on, for convenience $\boldsymbol{\beta}_{ii}$ is assumed to be equal to $-\boldsymbol{I}_J$.

The multivariate setting above, as also stated by Mardia, is clearly overparameterized and too general to be applied as just formulated. Even in Sain and Cressie's opinion, one of the main contributors to this approach "the basic multivariate MRF model of Mardia (1988) is difficult to implement in practice without dramatic simplification of the matrices representing the spatial dependence parameters" (Sain et al., 2011). Hence, some simplifications of this general framework are often formulated yielding some of the different multivariate models in the literature. Specifically, an omnipresent assumption is assuming $\boldsymbol{\beta}_{ii'} = \boldsymbol{0}_{J\times J}$ for $i' \not\sim i$, since otherwise the proposed multivariate model would no longer be Markovian. We will consider this assumption henceforth.

Clearly, $\boldsymbol{\Sigma}_i$ in Expression (8.2) is in charge of modeling the covariance between diseases (for each spatial unit), while the modeling of spatial dependence will depend on the definition of $\boldsymbol{\beta}_{ii'}$. Specifically the diagonal terms of $\boldsymbol{\beta}_{ii'}$ will be in charge of modeling the dependence between neighbouring units for a single disease, whereas off-diagonal terms are in charge of modeling that same dependence but for different diseases. In this manner, if $\boldsymbol{\Sigma}_i = m_i^{-1}diag(\sigma_1^2, ..., \sigma_J^2)$ for all i and $\boldsymbol{\beta}_{ii'} = m_i^{-1}\boldsymbol{I}_J w_{ii'}$, where m_i stands for the number of neighbours for unit i and $w_{ii'} = 1$ for $i \sim i'$ and 0 otherwise, then Expression (8.2) would be equivalent to J independent ICAR distributions. On the contrary, for $\boldsymbol{\Sigma}_1 = ... = \boldsymbol{\Sigma}_I = \boldsymbol{\Omega}^{-1}$ and $\boldsymbol{\beta}_{ii'} = \boldsymbol{0}_J$ for $i, i' = 1, ..., I$, Expression (8.2) would define a set of I independent draws of a multivariate Normal distribution of covariance matrix $\boldsymbol{\Omega}^{-1}$.

A straightforward generalization of the ICAR distribution to the multivariate setting is achieved by assuming $\boldsymbol{\Sigma}_i = m_i^{-1}\boldsymbol{\Omega}^{-1}$, $\boldsymbol{\mu} = \boldsymbol{0}$ and $\boldsymbol{\beta}_{ii'} = m_i^{-1}\boldsymbol{I}_J w_{ii'}$. In this case, $\boldsymbol{\Omega}$ stands for a common, up to a constant, conditional precision matrix between diseases. This yields the following simplified version of Expression (8.2)

$$\boldsymbol{\Phi}_{i\cdot}|vec(\boldsymbol{\Phi}_{-i\cdot}), \boldsymbol{\Omega} \sim N_J\left(m_i^{-1}\sum_{i'\sim i}\boldsymbol{\Phi}'_{i'\cdot}, m_i^{-1}\boldsymbol{\Omega}^{-1}\right). \tag{8.4}$$

This collection of conditional distributions is known as the *Multivariate Intrinsic CAR* distribution (or just MCAR) for obvious reasons. For these conditional distributions, the symmetry condition (8.3) holds trivially. Moreover, the multivariate precision matrix $\Sigma^{-1}_{vec(\Phi')}$ for this model is a block matrix with blocks

$$-\Sigma^{-1}_i \beta_{ii'} = -(m_i\Omega)(m_i^{-1}I_J w_{ii'}) = -w_{ii'}\Omega,$$

for $i \neq i'$, and

$$-\Sigma^{-1}_i \beta_{ii} = -(m_i\Omega)(-I_J) = m_i\Omega,$$

for the diagonal blocks. Note that this makes the precision matrix of $vec(\Phi')$ separable, with $\Sigma^{-1}_{vec(\Phi')} = (D-W)\otimes\Omega$ or, equivalently, $\Sigma^{-1}_{vec(\Phi)} = \Omega\otimes(D-W)$ where D and W are the typical diagonal and sparse matrices, respectively, of the corresponding joint precision matrix of the ICAR distribution. That is, for the MCAR distribution $\Sigma^{-1}_{vec(\Phi')}$ is just the Kronecker product of the precision matrices within and between diseases, respectively. This implies that for the MCAR distribution there is a common spatial structure for all diseases, defined by the precision matrix $D-W$, and a common precision matrix between diseases Ω for all spatial units. Note that the typical scale term in the spatial precision matrix σ^{-2} no longer exists in the multivariate case. This term is now substituted by Ω, which controls the scale for all the diseases (diagonal terms of Ω) as well as their covariances (non-diagonal terms of Ω).

The precision matrix of the MCAR distribution is the Kronecker product of a positive semidefinite matrix, $D-W$, and a positive definite matrix Ω. This makes that joint precision matrix positive semidefinite, with its semidefiniteness arising from that same feature of the spatial precision matrix $D-W$. Moreover, the rank deficiency of the joint precision matrix will be $K\times J$ where K is the rank-deficiency of $D-W$. Thus, the MCAR distribution shows the same impropriety problems as the univariate ICAR distribution, multiplied by the number of dimensions in the multivariate study. These problems may (and should) be fixed by imposing similar sum-to-zero restrictions to those in the univariate case for each of the diseases in the corresponding multivariate study.

Similar generalizations of other spatial distributions can also be built by following this approach. Thus, if we set $\beta_{ii'} = m_i^{-1}\rho I_J w_{ii'}$ and $\Sigma_i = m_i^{-1}\Omega^{-1}$, as above, we would obtain an equivalent multivariate generalization of the univariate PCAR distribution with precision matrix $\Sigma^{-1}_{vec(\Phi)} = \Omega\otimes(D-\rho W)$ (Billheimer et al., 1997; Carlin and Banerjee, 2003). In this case, ρ would stand for a common parameter controlling the strength of spatial dependence, as for the PCAR distribution, so the same range of valid values for this parameter in the univariate PCAR distribution would also be feasible now (see Section 4.3). We will refer to this distribution as a *multivariate PCAR distribution* (although we will see more multivariate PCARs later) and will denote it as MPCAR(ρ). Once again this process is separable, with ρ being the common spatial parameter for all the diseases. In a similar manner, the LCAR distribution could be also generalized to the multivariate setting within the conditional multivariate approach by defining $\boldsymbol{\beta}_{ii'} = \lambda(1 - \lambda + \lambda m_i)^{-1}\boldsymbol{I}_p w_{ii'}$ and $\boldsymbol{\Sigma}_i = (1-\lambda+\lambda m_i)^{-1}\boldsymbol{\Omega}^{-1}$. It can be easily shown that these choices would yield a multivariate CAR distribution with separable precision matrix equal to $\boldsymbol{\Sigma}_{vec(\boldsymbol{\Phi})}^{-1} = \boldsymbol{\Omega} \otimes ((1 - \lambda)\boldsymbol{I}_I + \lambda(\boldsymbol{D} - \boldsymbol{W}))$. We will refer to this distribution as a *multivariate LCAR distribution* and we will denote it as MLCAR(λ).

All the models above have separable joint covariance matrices, which means a clear restriction in many cases. Separability assumes a common spatial structure for all the diseases and, in the same manner, a common covariance matrix between diseases for all the spatial units. Several attempts have been made to overcome this limitation and therefore go beyond separability. Gelfand and Vounatsou (2003) propose a model with marginal PCAR distributions, of different spatial parameters, for the set of diseases in the study. Although Gelfand and Vounatsou start following Mardia's conditional multivariate approach for building their most simple models, finally they resort to coregionalization (see Section 8.2) for building their non-separable proposals. This shows that, despite the generality of Mardia's conditional multivariate setting, that framework may find serious problems for generalizing even simple models. The underlying problem of the conditional multivariate setting is how to find sensible proposals, which are both analytically and computationally manageable while also fulfilling the symmetry and positive conditions above. As we see, these premises are not so easy to fulfill. We will turn back to Gelfand and Vounatsou's proposal in Section 8.2.

A second attempt for getting rid of separability under a conditional multivariate approach is that of Jin et al. (2005). This work also avoids Mardia's proposal in its attempt. Thus, it relies on the conditional distribution of the diseases instead of the conditional distributions for the spatial units (see Royle and Berliner (1999) for another example of this approach). Specifically, for $J = 2$ although this could be easily generalized to higher Js, they assume $\boldsymbol{\phi}_{\cdot 2} \sim N_I(\boldsymbol{0}_I, \sigma_2^{-2}(\boldsymbol{D} - \rho_2\boldsymbol{W})^{-1})$ and $\boldsymbol{\phi}_{\cdot 1}|\boldsymbol{\phi}_{\cdot 2} \sim N_I(\boldsymbol{A}\boldsymbol{\phi}_{\cdot 2}, \sigma_1^{-2}(\boldsymbol{D} - \rho_1\boldsymbol{W})^{-1})$ for an $I \times I$ matrix $\boldsymbol{A}$. Specifically, their model assumes $\boldsymbol{A}(\eta_0, \eta_1) = \eta_0\boldsymbol{I}_I + \eta_1\boldsymbol{W}$, which makes each element in $\boldsymbol{\phi}_1$ depend on the corresponding element of $\boldsymbol{\phi}_2$ and those of its neighbours. This choice yields the following covariance matrix $\boldsymbol{\Sigma}_vec(\boldsymbol{\Phi})$:

$$\begin{pmatrix} \boldsymbol{C}(\rho_1, \sigma_1) + \boldsymbol{A}(\eta_0, \eta_1)\boldsymbol{C}(\rho_2, \sigma_2)\boldsymbol{A}(\eta_0, \eta_1) & \boldsymbol{A}(\eta_0, \eta_1)\boldsymbol{C}(\rho_2, \sigma_2) \\ \boldsymbol{C}(\rho_2, \sigma_2)\boldsymbol{A}(\eta_0, \eta_1) & \boldsymbol{C}(\rho_2, \sigma_2) \end{pmatrix},$$

where $\boldsymbol{C}(\rho_j, \sigma_j) = \sigma_j^{-2}(\boldsymbol{D} - \rho_j\boldsymbol{W})^{-1}$, $j = 1, 2$. Jin et al. propose as sufficient conditions for the validity of this model to set ρ_1 and ρ_2 in the interval $]-1, 1[$. This covariance matrix allows us to directly control $Var(\boldsymbol{\phi}_{\cdot 2})$ and $Cov(\boldsymbol{\phi}_{\cdot 1}, \boldsymbol{\phi}_{\cdot 2})$, and sets $Var(\boldsymbol{\phi}_{\cdot 1})$ as a function of these. In any case this model generalizes the MCAR and the MPCAR(ρ) distributions which are just particular cases of this proposal. Despite getting rid of separability, this model shows two clear limitations, first the lack of direct control on $Var(\boldsymbol{\phi}_{\cdot 1})$ and second its order-dependent character. Specifically, Jin et al.'s proposal is formulated as a concatenation of spatial distributions as $p(\phi_{.1}|\phi_{.2})p(\phi_{.2})$. As a consequence $\phi_{.1}$ and $\phi_{.2}$ do not play a symmetric role in this formulation, which has evident consequences on $\Sigma_{vec(\Phi)}$. This makes the (usually arbitrary) ordering chosen for the diseases during the study play a non-negligible role on its results. This is a clear drawback of this proposal.

A third proposal for going beyond separability within the multivariate conditional framework is that of Sain and Cressie (2007), referred as *CAMCAR* (CAnonical Multivariate Conditional Auto-Regressive model) by these authors. Sain and Cressie propose a multivariate conditional model as Expression (8.2) with a generic μ typically modeled as a function of covariates. Regarding the rest of parameters, we are going to introduce a simplified version of CAMCAR assuming the typical adjacency relationship between spatial units, as for the rest of this book. Specifically, assuming that assumption CAMCAR sets:

$$\Sigma_i = m_i^{-1}\Gamma$$

for a joint covariance matrix Γ. That is, all the covariance matrices between diseases are proportional to a common matrix Γ and inversely proportional to the corresponding number of neighbours. On the other hand, CAMCAR assumes for $i < i'$

$$\beta_{ii'} = m_i^{-1/2}m_{i'}^{1/2}\Gamma^{1/2}\Lambda\Gamma^{-1/2}w_{ii'},$$

and for $i > i'$

$$\beta_{ii'} = m_i^{1/2}m_{i'}^{-1/2}\Gamma^{1/2}\Lambda'\Gamma^{-1/2}w_{ii'}$$

for an unknown $J \times J$ matrix Λ. Sain and Cressie further assume an informative inverse Wishart prior distribution on Γ and an informative Normal distribution for the cells of Λ. The use of 'restrictive' priors for these parameters is required in order to make feasible the fit of the model (Sain et al., 2011).

Sain and Cressie show how these choices for Σ_i and $\beta_{ii'}$, under some specific constraints, yield a symmetric and positive definite joint covariance matrix for $vec(\Phi')$. In particular $\Sigma_{vec(\Phi')} = \Gamma^* H^{-1}(\Gamma^*)'$, where $\Gamma^* = D^{-1/2} \otimes \Gamma^{1/2}$ with $D = diag(m)$ and

$$H = \begin{pmatrix} I_J & -\Lambda w_{12} & \cdots & -\Lambda w_{1I} \\ -\Lambda' w_{21} & I_J & \cdots & -\Lambda w_{2I} \\ \vdots & & \ddots & \vdots \\ -\Lambda' w_{I1} & -\Lambda' w_{I2} & \cdots & I_J \end{pmatrix}. \tag{8.5}$$

Obviously $\Sigma_{vec(\Phi')}$ is symmetric, moreover, since Γ is positive definite, the positive definiteness of $\Sigma_{vec(\Phi')}$ depends on that same condition on H. Sain and Cressie only provide a sufficient condition for the positive definiteness of H. This is a complex condition based on the diagonal dominance of H, which is shown to be restrictive (Greco and Trivisano, 2009). Regretfully all those feasible CAMCAR models not fulfilling that sufficient condition will be missed, which is an important drawback of this approach.

The CAMCAR model has an interesting interpretation when $\boldsymbol{\Lambda}$ is symmetric. In that case $\boldsymbol{H} = \boldsymbol{I}_{IJ} - \boldsymbol{W} \otimes \boldsymbol{\Lambda}$, for $\boldsymbol{W}$ being a typical adjacency matrix. Following the comment on the covariances of $vec(\boldsymbol{\Phi})$ and $vec(\boldsymbol{\Phi}')$ at the beginning of this chapter, this implies that the precision matrix for $vec(\boldsymbol{\Phi})$ would then be equal to

$$\begin{aligned} \boldsymbol{\Sigma}_{vec(\boldsymbol{\Phi})}^{-1} &= (\boldsymbol{\Gamma}^{-1/2} \otimes \boldsymbol{D}^{1/2})(\boldsymbol{I}_{IJ} - \boldsymbol{\Lambda} \otimes \boldsymbol{W})((\boldsymbol{\Gamma}^{-1/2})' \otimes \boldsymbol{D}^{1/2}) \\ &= (\boldsymbol{\Gamma}^{-1/2}(\boldsymbol{\Gamma}^{-1/2})' \otimes \boldsymbol{D}) - (\boldsymbol{\Gamma}^{-1/2}\boldsymbol{\Lambda}(\boldsymbol{\Gamma}^{-1/2})' \otimes \boldsymbol{D}^{1/2}\boldsymbol{W}\boldsymbol{D}^{1/2}). \end{aligned}$$

As a consequence, $\boldsymbol{\Sigma}_{vec(\boldsymbol{\Phi})}^{-1}$ is a block matrix with blocks equal to $\boldsymbol{D}^{1/2}(a_{jj'}\boldsymbol{I}_I - b_{jj'}\boldsymbol{W})\boldsymbol{D}^{1/2}$ for suitable values of $a_{jj'}$ and $b_{jj'}$. These blocks reproduce the covariance matrix of a Homogeneous CAR or HCAR distribution, of the form $(a\boldsymbol{I} - b\boldsymbol{W})$ (Expression (4.18) in this book), allowing for additional heteroscedasticity for the set of spatial units induced by the diagonal elements of $\boldsymbol{D}$. Hence, in this sense the CAMCAR model reproduces an enhanced multivariate HCAR spatial distribution. However, the CAMCAR model has different spatial covariance matrices for each disease (b_{jj} varies for all j) and different covariance matrices between diseases ($b_{jj'}$ varies for all j and j'). Thus, this model is much more flexible than the previous separable models in this section.

Nevertheless, the CAMCAR distribution allows $\boldsymbol{\Lambda}$ to be symmetric yielding, therefore, models beyond those mentioned in the last paragraph. For an asymmetric $\boldsymbol{\Lambda}$, $\boldsymbol{H}$ takes the general form mentioned in Expression (8.5). In that case $\boldsymbol{H}$ cannot be expressed as $\boldsymbol{I}_{IJ} - \boldsymbol{W} \otimes \boldsymbol{\Lambda}$, as for a symmetric $\boldsymbol{\Lambda}$, but as $\boldsymbol{H} = \boldsymbol{I}_{IJ} - \boldsymbol{W}_U \otimes \boldsymbol{\Lambda} - \boldsymbol{W}_U' \otimes \boldsymbol{\Lambda}'$ where now $\boldsymbol{W}_U$ denotes the upper triangle of $\boldsymbol{W}$. In this case

$$\boldsymbol{\Sigma}_{vec(\boldsymbol{\Phi})}^{-1} = (\boldsymbol{\Gamma}^{-1/2} \otimes \boldsymbol{D}^{1/2})(\boldsymbol{I}_{IJ} - \boldsymbol{\Lambda} \otimes \boldsymbol{W}_U - \boldsymbol{\Lambda}' \otimes \boldsymbol{W}_U')((\boldsymbol{\Gamma}^{-1/2})' \otimes \boldsymbol{D}^{1/2}).$$

This asymmetry of $\boldsymbol{\Lambda}$ induces an additional degree of freedom in the modeling since it allows $Cov(\Phi_{ij}, \Phi_{i'j'}) \neq Cov(\Phi_{ij'}, \Phi_{i'j})$, which is not possible when $\boldsymbol{\Lambda}$ is symmetric. Note also that $\boldsymbol{\Lambda}$ will be symmetric if and only if $\beta_{ii'} = \beta_{i'i}$ for all $i \neq i'$, therefore asymmetry in $\boldsymbol{\Lambda}$ induces dependence of the results on the ordering in which spatial units and diseases are considered. Thus, depending on whether $j < j'$ or not diseases j and j' will relate in one or another way. As a consequence, the fit of CAMCAR models depends on the (usually arbitrary) order chosen to tag the diseases in the study (MacNab, 2018). This arbitrary performance could be solved in principle, if J was low, by considering all or several permutations of the diseases and choosing the permutation yielding a better fit. Nevertheless, as mentioned, the effect of the asymmetry in $\boldsymbol{\Lambda}$ affects also the ordering of the spatial units, which is even more worrisome (MacNab, 2016b,a). Thus, covariances between diseases for two spatial units i and i' will be different depending on whether $i < i'$ or $i > i'$, when the labelling of spatial units is also usually arbitrary, frequently set according to an administrative criterion. In our opinion, this is a serious problem and without a reasonable solution so far since, in contrast to the case of diseases, the number of possible permutations of the spatial units is in general overwhelming. In our opinion, asymmetry in $\boldsymbol{\Lambda}$ induces a degree of freedom in the modeling that we are not sure that we would want to have. That asymmetry brings arbitrary results, making them order (diseases) and label (spatial units) dependent. Surely, more research is needed on asymmetric modeling of covariance matrices in order to assess the contribution in real terms of this particular modeling feature.

Greco and Trivisano (2009) formulate also a similar proposal to CAM-CAR. Specifically, for $i < i'$ they assume $\beta_{ii'} = m_i^{-1}\tilde{\boldsymbol{\Sigma}}\boldsymbol{\Lambda}\tilde{\boldsymbol{\Sigma}}^{-1}$ for $i \sim i'$ and 0 otherwise, where $\tilde{\boldsymbol{\Sigma}}$ is the lower-triangular Cholesky decomposition of $\boldsymbol{\Omega}^{-1}$, the conditional matrix for $\boldsymbol{\Phi}_{i\cdot}|\boldsymbol{\Phi}_{-i\cdot}$. In the same manner, they propose $\beta_{i'i} = m_{i'}^{-1}\tilde{\boldsymbol{\Sigma}}\boldsymbol{\Lambda}'\tilde{\boldsymbol{\Sigma}}^{-1}$. As a consequence of the different definitions of $\beta_{ii'}$ for $i < i'$ and for $i > i'$, this proposal yields also asymmetric covariances between diseases for different spatial units, which are usually known as *cross-covariances*. Specifically, for this proposal the covariance matrix $\boldsymbol{\Sigma}_{vec(\boldsymbol{\Phi})}$ will be equal to:

$$(\tilde{\boldsymbol{\Sigma}} \otimes \boldsymbol{I}_I)(\boldsymbol{I}_J \otimes \boldsymbol{D} - \boldsymbol{\Lambda} \otimes \boldsymbol{W}_U - \boldsymbol{\Lambda}' \otimes \boldsymbol{W}_U')^{-1}(\tilde{\boldsymbol{\Sigma}}' \otimes \boldsymbol{I}_I)$$
$$= \left(\boldsymbol{\Omega} \otimes \boldsymbol{D} - (\tilde{\boldsymbol{\Sigma}}')^{-1}\boldsymbol{\Lambda}\tilde{\boldsymbol{\Sigma}}^{-1} \otimes \boldsymbol{W}_U - (\tilde{\boldsymbol{\Sigma}}')^{-1}\boldsymbol{\Lambda}'\tilde{\boldsymbol{\Sigma}}^{-1} \otimes \boldsymbol{W}_U'\right)^{-1}.$$

Note that, for a symmetric $\boldsymbol{\Lambda}$, this expression results simply

$$\boldsymbol{\Sigma}_{vec(\boldsymbol{\Phi})} = (\boldsymbol{\Omega} \otimes \boldsymbol{D} - (\tilde{\boldsymbol{\Sigma}}')^{-1}\boldsymbol{\Lambda}\tilde{\boldsymbol{\Sigma}}^{-1} \otimes \boldsymbol{W})^{-1},$$

which is a straightforward generalization of the PCAR distribution to the multivariate domain. Specifically, all the covariance matrices for each disease $(Var(\boldsymbol{\Phi}_{\cdot j}|vec(\boldsymbol{\Phi}_{\cdot -j})))$ and covariance matrices between diseases $(Cov(\boldsymbol{\Phi}_{\cdot j}, \boldsymbol{\Phi}_{\cdot j'}|vec(\boldsymbol{\Phi}_{\cdot -(j,j')})))$ will follow PCAR distributions of different spatial parameters. Evidently, this proposal will not yield in general separable processes. Greco and Trivisano (2009) postulate as a sufficient condition for the validity of this model that the largest eigenvalue of $\boldsymbol{\Lambda}$ to be in the interval $]0,1[$. Although this condition is just sufficient, the authors show it to be less restrictive than that formulated by Sain and Cressie for the CAMCAR distribution.

Obviously, these distributions are used as tools within hierarchical models to induce multivariate spatial dependence on areal referenced vectors of observations. WinBUGS includes a specific function for developing multivariate models, the mv.car distribution, which corresponds to a built-in implementation of the intrinsic MCAR distribution. The syntax for this function is Phi[1:J,1:I]~mv.car(adj[],weights[],num[],omega[,]), where adj, weights and num have the same meaning than for the univariate intrinsic car.normal distribution. On the other hand, omega stands for the between diseases precision matrix of the MCAR distribution and has to necessarily follow a Wishart prior distribution, a multivariate generalization of the gamma distribution, so in this sense the `mv.car` is a bit restrictive. Note that, in contrast to the notation used in this chapter, `WinBUGS` assumes for the `mv.car` that the rows of $\boldsymbol{\Phi}$ correspond to the diseases and their columns to the different spatial units, so we will have to adapt our code accordingly. The Wishart restriction on the prior distribution of $\boldsymbol{\Omega}$ may be overcome, in principle, by coding the MCAR distribution in `WinBUGS` as a set of conditional multivariate distributions instead of using the `mv.car` function. Basically, we would just have to code into `WinBUGS` the set of conditional distributions in Expression (8.4) (see the code for the next example for more details on this). Nevertheless, this approach is computationally far less convenient as we will see in the next example. This conditional formulation would also make it possible to implement the MPCAR(ρ) or the MLCAR(λ) distributions in `WinBUGS`.

Regretfully, we are not aware of hardly any possible implementation in `INLA` of multivariate models, either posed as a set of conditional multivariate distributions or as any of the forms that we will introduce below. Some multivariate spatial models have been implemented with `INLA` by using the `copy` argument (Martins et al., 2013) of the `f()` function of this package (Blangiardo and Cameletti, 2015; Krainski et al., 2018). Although we do not have experience with the implementation in `INLA` of multivariate disease mapping models, we foresee a bad scalability of these models for a large number of diseases as they will depend on a large number of GMRFs. As a consequence, `INLA` will have a large number of parameters to integrate out, which makes this kind of model problematic to be fitted by `INLA`. In fact, Krainski et al. (2018) report some computational problems for fitting a trivariate geostatistical model. Therefore, we will just consider `WinBUGS` henceforth as an inference tool for multivariate (and multidimensional in Chapter 9) and multidimensional models.

Regarding the prior distribution for `omega` in the `mv.car` or for $\boldsymbol{\Sigma}_i^{-1}$ in general for conditional multivariate models, we have mentioned that a *Wishart distribution* is typically set for these variables. The Wishart distribution depends on two parameters, $\boldsymbol{R}$ and k, following the terminology in `WinBUGS`, where $\boldsymbol{R}$ is a $J \times J$ symmetric positive definite matrix and k is a positive number known as the degrees of freedom of the distribution. Take care if you search for further information on this distribution as the Wishart distribution may be defined in terms of either $\boldsymbol{R}$ or $\boldsymbol{R}^{-1}$ and its interpretation will depend on this. As defined in `WinBUGS`, if $\boldsymbol{\Omega} \sim Wishart(\boldsymbol{R}, k)$, then $\boldsymbol{\Omega}$ has as prior mean $k\boldsymbol{R}^{-1}$ and their cells are proportional to both k and inversely proportional to the scale of $\boldsymbol{R}$. The Wishart distribution is less informative as k is lower, so this parameter will be usually set to a low value. In practice k is usually set to J or $J+1$ when $\boldsymbol{\Omega}$ is a square J-dimensional matrix since for $k < J$ the Wishart distribution is improper and for $k \geq J + 1$ is finite everywhere. Regarding $\boldsymbol{R}$, it is commonly assumed to define it as $\lambda\boldsymbol{I}_J$ for a fixed value of λ, what will make the prior mean of $\boldsymbol{\Omega}$ to be equal to $(k/\lambda)\boldsymbol{I}_J$. Nevertheless, there is no clear agreement on the value of the proportionality constant λ. Thus, many authors (see for example, to cite just a few, Gelfand and Vounatsou (2003), Greco and Trivisano (2009), and Moraga and Lawson (2012)) fix λ

to 1 or a similar value. This makes the prior mean of Ω to be equal (or similar) to $k\boldsymbol{I}_J$, which could seem a reasonable choice for a precision matrix modeling random effects in a logarithmic scale. Nevertheless, some other authors (see for example Carlin and Banerjee (2003), Richardson et al. (2006), and Lawson et al. (2010)) fix it to a substantially lower value, such as 0.01 or 0.001, intended to be non-informative. These 'non-informative' prior proposals put more prior mass on higher values of the diagonal terms of the precision matrix; therefore, they shrink the multivariate random effects towards 0. In this regard, it would be surely wise to bear in mind that the Wishart distribution is a multivariate generalization of the gamma distribution to symmetric positive definite matrices. Therefore, the problems with vague gamma prior distributions for precisions mentioned in Chapter 4 that made us prefer uniform prior distributions on standard deviations could perfectly hold or even possibly be enhanced when using Wishart distributions. We will talk about this in the next example but, in general terms, we would advise to be cautious when setting vague Wishart prior distributions on precision matrices and to perform customary sensitivity analyses on the choice of its hyperparameter $\boldsymbol{R}$.

8.1.2   Multivariate models as sets of conditional univariate distributions

A second collection of formulations of multivariate CAR distributions relies on the definition of the univariate conditionals $\phi_{ij}|vec(\boldsymbol{\phi}_{-(ij)})$ for $i = 1, ..., I$ and $j = 1, ..., J$, where $vec(\boldsymbol{\phi}_{-(ij)})$ stands for the $IJ - 1$ vector $vec(\boldsymbol{\Phi}')$, removing the (i, j)th position of $\boldsymbol{\Phi}$. In this manner, the conditional distributions defining the multivariate ensemble are casted within the univariate CAR framework, where the univariate distribution of each observation in a vector is conditioned on the rest of its elements. The expression of these multivariate models as regular CAR processes makes all the available theory for these distributions apply also to them, which is a clear advantage.

Sain et al. (2011) formulated the most general proposal under this approach. The particular feature that distinguishes Sain et al.'s approach from regular univariate CAR distributions is that the former weighs each neighbour in $\boldsymbol{\phi}_{-(ij)}$ depending on its specific type of neighbour relationship (within diseases, between diseases, etc.). Specifically, Sain et al.'s proposal assumes $\phi_{ij}|vec(\boldsymbol{\phi}_{-(ij)})$ to follow a Normal distribution with

$$
\begin{aligned}
E(\phi_{ij}|vec(\boldsymbol{\phi}_{-(ij)})) = {} & \mu_{ij} + \sum_{i' \neq i} \beta_{iji'j}(\phi_{i'j} - \mu_{i'j}) + \\
& \sum_{j' \neq j} \beta_{ijij'}(\phi_{ij'} - \mu_{ij'}) + \sum_{i' \neq i}\sum_{j' \neq j} \beta_{iji'j'}(\phi_{i'j'} - \mu_{i'j'})
\end{aligned}
$$

and

$$Var(\phi_{ij}|vec(\boldsymbol{\phi}_{-(ij)})) = \sigma_{ij}^2.$$

In these expressions $\boldsymbol{\beta}$ stands for a 4-dimensional array, of dimensions $I \times J \times I \times J$, weighing the contribution of neighbours of each kind. Additionally, $\boldsymbol{\beta}$ is usually required to fulfill $\beta_{iji'j'} = 0$ for $i \nsim i'$ so that the model above is spatially Markovian. Sain et al.'s proposal distinguishes between three kinds of neighbouring (related) observations within the multivariate lattice:

- Observations corresponding to the same disease and a spatial neighbouring unit, with parameters $\beta_{iji'j}$ with $i \sim i'$. These observations, contained in the second term of $E(\phi_{ij}|vec(\boldsymbol{\phi}_{-(ij)}))$ are in charge of modeling (spatial) dependence within diseases.

- Observations corresponding to another disease in the same spatial unit, with parameters $\beta_{ijij'}$. These observations, contained in the third term of $E(\phi_{ij}|vec(\boldsymbol{\phi}_{-(ij)}))$ are in charge of modeling multivariate dependence between diseases.

- Observations corresponding to another disease in spatial neighbouring units, with parameters $\beta_{iji'j'}$ with $i \sim i'$. These observations, contained in the fourth term of $E(\phi_{ij}|vec(\boldsymbol{\phi}_{-(ij)}))$ are in charge of modeling multivariate dependence between different diseases for neighbouring sites. That is, this term would be in charge of modeling the strength of the cross-covariances mentioned above.

Sain et al.'s proposal yields a joint Normal distribution for $vec(\boldsymbol{\Phi}')$ with mean $vec(\boldsymbol{\mu}')$ and covariance matrix $\boldsymbol{\Sigma}_{vec(\boldsymbol{\Phi}')} = block(-\{\boldsymbol{\beta}_{i \cdot i'}\}_{i,i'=1}^I)^{-1} \cdot \boldsymbol{T}$, where $\boldsymbol{\beta}_{i \cdot i'} = (\beta_{iji'j'})_{j,j'=1}^J$, with $\boldsymbol{\beta}_{i \cdot i} = -\boldsymbol{I}_J$ and $\boldsymbol{\beta}_{i \cdot i'} = \boldsymbol{0}_{J \times J}$ for $i' \nsim i$. Finally $\boldsymbol{T}$ is a diagonal matrix equal to $diag(\sigma_{11}^2, ..., \sigma_{1J}^2, ..., \sigma_{I1}^2, ..., \sigma_{IJ}^2)$.

This modeling framework is once again quite large and contains lots of different potentially useful models as a consequence of its overparameterization. Nevertheless, the cells of $\boldsymbol{\beta}$ have to be chosen so that $\boldsymbol{\Sigma}_{vec(\boldsymbol{\Phi}')}$ yield a symmetric and positive definite matrix. Hence, this reduces the number of potential models that can be built. Thus, Sain et al.'s final proposal focusses in a less overparameterized version of the formulation above ensuring its validity. Specifically, they assume homogeneity of variances within diseases, i.e., $\sigma_{ij}^2 = \sigma_j^2$ for all i, so $\boldsymbol{T} = \boldsymbol{I}_n \otimes diag(\boldsymbol{\sigma}^2)$ for $\boldsymbol{\sigma}^2 = (\sigma_1^2, ..., \sigma_J^2)$. As a consequence, their model generalizes the HCAR univariate spatial distribution (see Section 4.3) to the multivariate setting, as for Sain and Cressie (2007). On the other hand, regarding dependence between diseases, which is controlled by the diagonal blocks of $\boldsymbol{\Sigma}_{vec(\boldsymbol{\Phi}')}$, they assume $\beta_{ijij'} = \rho_{jj'}\sigma_j/\sigma_{j'}$, with $\rho_{jj'} = \rho_{j'j}$. Therefore, $\boldsymbol{\Upsilon} = (\rho_{jj'})_{j,j'=1}^J$, with $\rho_{jj} = 1$ for all j, denotes a symmetric matrix controlling the covariances between diseases. Finally, for modeling within diseases and cross-spatial dependences they assume, for $i > i'$,

$\beta_{iji'j'} = \phi_{jj'}\sigma_j/\sigma_{j'}$ if $i \sim i'$ and 0 otherwise. In contrast to dependence between diseases, no symmetry is assumed now on $\boldsymbol{\Phi} = (\phi_{jj'})_{j,j'=1}^J$, as it does not affect the symmetry of $\boldsymbol{\Sigma}_{vec(\boldsymbol{\Phi}')}$. Nevertheless, for $i' > i$, $\beta_{iji'j'}$ has to be defined as $\phi_{j'j}\sigma_{j'}/\sigma_j$ in order to preserve that symmetry. Note that $\boldsymbol{\Phi}$ completely controls spatial dependence in this model. Specifically, the diagonal elements of $\boldsymbol{\Phi}$ control (spatial) dependence within diseases, while its non-diagonal terms control cross-spatial dependence.

For all the assumptions in the paragraph above, the joint covariance matrix $\boldsymbol{\Sigma}_{vec(\boldsymbol{\Phi}')}$ of Sain et al.'s proposal results:

$$\boldsymbol{\Sigma}_{vec(\boldsymbol{\Phi}')} = (\boldsymbol{I}_n \otimes diag(\boldsymbol{\sigma}))(\boldsymbol{I}_n \otimes \boldsymbol{\Upsilon} - \boldsymbol{W}_U \otimes \boldsymbol{\Phi} - \boldsymbol{W}_U' \otimes \boldsymbol{\Phi}')^{-1}(\boldsymbol{I}_n \otimes diag(\boldsymbol{\sigma}))$$

or, alternatively,

$$\boldsymbol{\Sigma}_{vec(\boldsymbol{\Phi})} = (diag(\boldsymbol{\sigma}) \otimes \boldsymbol{I}_n)(\boldsymbol{\Upsilon} \otimes \boldsymbol{I}_n - \boldsymbol{\Phi} \otimes \boldsymbol{W}_U - \boldsymbol{\Phi}' \otimes \boldsymbol{W}_U')^{-1}(diag(\boldsymbol{\sigma}) \otimes \boldsymbol{I}_n)$$

where $\boldsymbol{W}_U$ stands for the upper triangle of the adjacency matrix $\boldsymbol{W}$, as for the covariance matrix of Sain and Cressie (2007). Therefore, this proposal yields another example of asymmetric modeling of the cross-covariance matrices between diseases.

Note that the expression of $\boldsymbol{\Sigma}_{vec(\boldsymbol{\Phi}')}$ above yields a symmetric matrix, but its positive definiteness depends on that same feature of the central matrix in that expression. Sain et al. do not report any condition on the values of $\boldsymbol{\Upsilon}$ and $\boldsymbol{\Phi}$ leading to positive definite covariance matrices $\boldsymbol{\Sigma}_{vec(\boldsymbol{\Phi}')}$. Instead, they assume for these two matrices a uniform prior distribution over the set of values leading to a positive definite $\boldsymbol{\Sigma}_{vec(\boldsymbol{\Phi}')}$. This set is numerically determined in their example (with $J = 2$) in an empirical way, which may be problematic to be determined for higher values of J, where both matrices may have much more parameters.

For $J = 2$, Kim et al. (2001) formulates another modeling proposal that would fall into Sain et al.'s modeling framework. Specifically, they assume $\beta_{ijij'} = (\rho_0\sigma_j/\sigma_{j'})/(2m_i + 1)$ for modeling dependence between diseases and $\beta_{iji'j} = \rho_j/(2m_i + 1)$ for $i' \sim i$ (and 0 otherwise), for modeling dependence within diseases. For modeling cross-spatial dependence, they assume $\beta_{iji'j'} = (\rho_3\sigma_j/\sigma_{j'})/(2m_i + 1)$ for $j \neq j'$, $i \neq i'$ and $i' \sim i$ (and 0 otherwise). Thus, the vector $\boldsymbol{\rho} = (\rho_0, ..., \rho_3)$ controls the strength of the different kinds of dependence in the model. Regarding the conditional variances, Kim et al. assume $Var(\phi_{ij}|vec(\boldsymbol{\phi}_{-(ij)})) = \sigma_j^2/(2m_i + 1)$. For all these expressions $\rho_0, ..., \rho_3$ are assumed to take values in the interval $]-1, 1[$ (Kim et al. show that in that case the model is well defined) and $2m_i + 1$ denotes the number of neighbours (m_i within, 1 between and m_i cross-spatial) of unit (i, j). This model was named as *twofold CAR* model by its authors.

The original paper introducing the twofold CAR shows that this model yields the following covariance matrix

$$\boldsymbol{\Sigma}_{vec(\boldsymbol{\Phi})} = \begin{pmatrix} \sigma_1^{-2}(\boldsymbol{D} - \rho_1\boldsymbol{W}) & -(\sigma_1\sigma_2)^{-1}(\rho_0\boldsymbol{I}_I + \rho_3\boldsymbol{W}) \\ -(\sigma_1\sigma_2)^{-1}(\rho_0\boldsymbol{I}_I + \rho_3\boldsymbol{W}) & \sigma_2^{-2}(\boldsymbol{D} - \rho_2\boldsymbol{W}) \end{pmatrix}^{-1}$$

so this model yields a non-separable structure where $\phi_{\cdot j}|\phi_{\cdot j'}$, $j = 1, 2$, follow PCAR distributions of different parameters σ_j and ρ_j. Moreover, this model has two specific parameters ρ_0 and ρ_3 modeling the correlation between both diseases, so this model is more flexible than the typical PCAR or ICAR based multivariate models. Those parameters allow us to separately control dependence between diseases (ρ_0) and cross-spatial dependence (ρ_3). Specifically, if both parameters were equal to 0, the twofold CAR would be equivalent to setting independent PCAR distributions with different parameters per disease. Finally, note that, in contrast to Sain et al., the twofold CAR model has a symmetric cross-spatial covariance matrix. Nevertheless, two main drawbacks have been pointed out for the twofold CAR (Jin et al., 2005). First, conditions $|\rho_k| < 1; k = 0, ..., 3$ are only sufficient for $\Sigma_{vec(\Phi)}$ to be positive definite, so these conditions could be discarding some valid models that could be of interest. Second, and possibly most important, the generalization of this model to $J > 2$ does not seem to be straightforward which makes its use cumbersome for the study of several diseases.

Martinez-Beneito (2019) provides some insight on the relationship between the conditional multivariate and univariate approaches to multivariate GM-RFs. Specifically, this paper shows how any model following the multivariate approach in Mardia can be put as a univariate model as those formulated by Sain et al. (2011) and vice versa. Therefore, those two approaches can be seen as two different, but equivalent, ways of formulating a single model. In particular, Martinez-Beneito (2019) shows that any conditional multivariate model of the form

$$\phi_{i\cdot}|vec(\phi_{-i\cdot}) \sim N_J(\sum_{i' \sim i} \boldsymbol{\beta}_{ii'}\phi'_{i'\cdot}, \Sigma_i) \tag{8.6}$$

can be alternatively expressed as the conditional univariate model

$$\phi_{ij}|vec(\phi_{-(ij)}) \sim N\left(\sum_{i' \sim i}\beta^*_{iji'j}\phi_{i'j} + \sum_{j' \neq j}\beta^*_{ijij'}\phi_{ij'} + \sum_{i' \sim i}\sum_{j' \neq j}\beta^*_{iji'j'}\phi_{i'j'}, \sigma^2_{ij}\right) \tag{8.7}$$

with $\beta^*_{iji'j'} = (diag(\Sigma_i^{-1})^{-1}\Sigma_i^{-1}\boldsymbol{\beta}_{ii'})_{jj'}$ and $\sigma^2_{ij} = 1/(\Sigma_i^{-1})_{jj}$. Conversely, any conditional univariate model as that of (8.7) can be alternatively expressed as Expression (8.6) with $\boldsymbol{\beta}_{ii'} = (\beta^*_{ij'jj'})^J_{j,j'=1}$ and $\Sigma_i = diag(\boldsymbol{\sigma}^2_{i\cdot})$. Anyhow, beyond the equivalence of both conditional approaches, the reformulation of any conditional multivariate model as its univariate counterpart, and vice versa, may yield important advantages. Particularly, that reformulation could make it possible to profit from the theory of the models in its alternative formulation, which could make it easier, for example, to set conditions on the validity of that model. Moreover, that alternative reexpression could also bring additional computational advantages and make it possible to use previous code of one of these approaches for fitting models based on the other approach. Finally, the expression of univariate conditional models as multivariate conditional models could yield also some intuition on the proposal of valid univariate models. We have mentioned that the conditional univariate framework is quite flexible and allows to formulate lots of models, even invalid proposals. The multivariate counterpart is similar but, at least, has the guidance of restricting the Σ_is to be symmetric positive definite matrices, which makes it easier to formulate sensible proposals under this approach. The link above between both approaches could make the proposal of similar sensible models under the conditional univariate approach easier.

Regarding the implementation of the conditional univariate approach in WinBUGS, this is quite tricky since the conditional mean of each ϕ_{ij} depends on a sparse linear combination of elements in $vec(\phi_{-(ij)})$. That sparse linear combination has to be specifically coded within the model. The alternative formulation of any conditional univariate as a conditional multivariate model, according to the relationships pointed out at the previous paragraph, could make the coding of any of these models much easier.

Example 8.1

Tobacco and alcohol consumption are well-known risk factors for oral cancer, so it would be advisable to consider them in the study of the geographical distribution of this cause of mortality. Regretfully, there are not available covariates of alcohol and tobacco consumption at the municipal level for the Valencian Region, thus this goal in principle cannot be undertaken by means of ecological regression. Nevertheless, we could resort to additional causes of mortality, supposedly dependent on these risk factors, as a secondary information source. Dependence among the corresponding geographical patterns would be the statistical mechanism that would make it possible to use the common information on these risk factors underlying these causes of death. Thus, in order to improve the estimation of the geographical pattern in oral cancer mortality, we will perform a joint study of oral cancer with cirrhosis and lung cancer; all three causes referred to men. Cirrhosis depends heavily on alcohol consumption, so it should provide additional information on the unknown geographical distribution of this risk factor. On the other hand, lung cancer mortality depends heavily on tobacco consumption and its mortality is much higher than that of oral cancer, so it should be a very sensible surrogate of that risk factor.

We have run several models for the joint study of these three mortality causes. First, we have run independent BYM models for all three causes without considering dependence between their geographic patterns; we will refer to this model as *IND*. Second, we have run a second BYM model but, in this case, considering dependence between diseases. Specifically, we have included a multivariate MCAR spatial term in the corresponding WinBUGS model by using the mv.car function and have kept the spatial heterogeneous term also independent between diseases in order to reproduce completely random heterogeneity.

We have run this model twice, once with a Wishart distribution for the precision matrix between diseases with $\boldsymbol{R}$ equal to $\boldsymbol{I}_3$, and once equal to $0.01 \cdot \boldsymbol{I}_3$ in order to assess the sensitivity to these prior choices. We will refer to these two models as *MV1.1* and *MV1.01*, respectively. Additionally, we have also run a modification of these multivariate BYM models by assuming a correlated multivariate Normal distribution also for the heterogeneous term, allowing for dependence between diseases. For this model, we have assumed Wishart prior distributions for the precision matrices of both spatial and heterogeneous terms with $\boldsymbol{R} = 0.01 \cdot \boldsymbol{I}_3$. We will refer to this model as *MV2.01*.

Finally, we have also implemented an alternative version of model *MV2.01*. First, we have specifically coded the conditional multivariate approach for the MCAR distribution in `WinBUGS` instead of using the built-in `mv.car` function. This implementation makes use of Expression (8.4) for coding the conditional multivariate distributions conducing to a MCAR distribution. We have tried to implement also the conditional univariate approach for the MCAR distribution by making use of the conditional multivariate expression mentioned and its equivalence within the conditional univariate approach provided by Expression (8.7). Nevertheless, that implementation was far too complex and we desisted to implement it as a consequence of the results found (see comment below) for the conditional multivariate model, which is much simpler to code.

Figure 8.1 shows choropleth maps for the risks estimated with model *MV1.01* for all three causes of study. As can be appreciated, the geographic pattern for oral cancer shows a much more marked geographic pattern than that corresponding to the univariate BYM model (see left side of Figure 4.4). This new enhanced estimation of the oral cancer mortality pattern resembles that of both cirrhosis and lung cancer mortalities, as was expected, and takes profit of that resemblance to estimate its geographic pattern. Specifically, the risk for this disease in the northern and north-western parts of the Valencian Region is now substantially lower than for cirrhosis and lung cancer. Moreover, the risk for the cluster in the eastern side of the Valencian Region has also increased for the multivariate model, in particular, the region with the highest $sSMR$ for oral cancer in the univariate study (170.2) has now a $sSMR$ of 179.4 for the multivariate study. Moreover, the variability of the log-$sSMR$s is also higher for oral cancer in the multivariate study, pointing out more regions of higher or lower risk than for the univariate study. In particular, the standard deviation of the log-$sSMR$s (their posterior means) is 0.185 for the univariate study while it increases to 0.262 for the *MV1.01* model. This illustrates that multivariate modeling could be in part solving the oversmoothing on univariate $sSMR$s noted by some authors (Richardson et al., 2004). This fact has already been suggested by Best et al. (2005).

Besides the geographic distributions of risks, multivariate disease mapping provides also a second interesting outcome, the covariance matrix between diseases. That covariance matrix has only full sense for separable models, otherwise that matrix would change for each spatial unit and we could not strictly talk about a single covariance matrix between diseases. The intrinsic MCAR

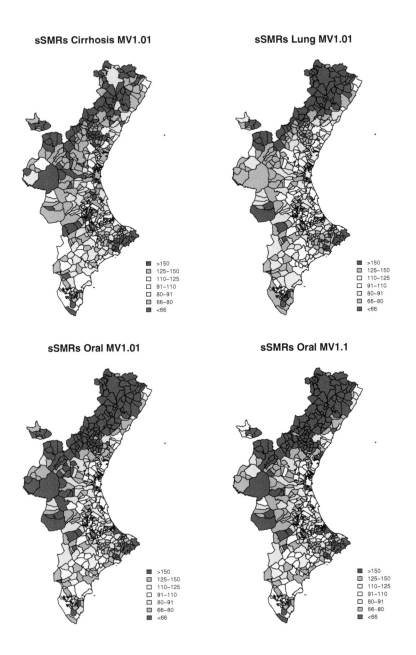

Figure 8.1
Choropleth maps for the $sSMRs$ estimated for cirrhosis, lung cancer and oral cancer for the $MV1.01$ multivariate model and oral cancer for $MV1.1$.

distribution used in our model has that separable structure so it is appropriate to talk about a covariance matrix between diseases for the spatial term. In our particular case, the posterior mean of the covariance and correlation matrices between diseases for the spatial term in model *MV1.01* are, respectively

$$
\begin{pmatrix} 0.08 & 0.10 & 0.12 \\ - & 0.14 & 0.17 \\ - & - & 0.22 \end{pmatrix}, \quad \begin{pmatrix} 1 & 0.92 & 0.95 \\ - & 1 & 0.93 \\ - & - & 1 \end{pmatrix}
$$

where the ordering for the diseases considered in those matrices is cirrhosis, lung cancer and oral cancer, respectively. Hence, on one hand, we see that oral cancer is the disease with higher variability, in the spatial term, of all three mortality causes considered. This explains the presence of a more marked spatial pattern for this disease. On the other hand, we see that all three mortality causes are highly positively correlated, as we initially expected. Particularly, although cirrhosis and lung cancer do not share known risk factors, they show a high correlation, even as high as the correlation of these diseases with oral cancer with whom they do share risk factors. Nevertheless, it is not surprising to check that the geographical patterns of those two mortality causes are tightly correlated, as it seems sensible to assume tobacco and alcohol consumption to be correlated as they reproduce similar lifestyles. Interestingly, for oral cancer, having such a high correlations with two mortality causes which have substantially higher mortality (12,342 deaths for cirrhosis, 39,420 for lung cancer and 4,005 for oral cancer) is a very important secondary information source for this disease. This is evidenced in the maps of the multivariate models as compared to the univariate oral cancer map.

Regarding the *MV1.1* model, the lower-right plot of Figure 8.1 shows also the map for oral cancer for this model. The differences between the oral cancer maps for the *MV1.01* and *MV1.1* models are quite mild. Nevertheless, strikingly, the differences in the correlation matrices between diseases in the spatial term for both models are not so mild. Thus, the posterior mean of that correlation matrix between diseases for the *MV1.1* model is

$$
\begin{pmatrix} 1 & 0.59 & 0.66 \\ - & 1 & 0.75 \\ - & - & 1 \end{pmatrix}.
$$

This makes evident that the choice of Wishart distributions for precision matrices of MCAR distributions should be done with extreme care. As shown, the two most widespread 'vague' choices for R yield very different estimates for the correlation matrix between diseases. Hence, we advise to perform customary sensitivity analyses when using these 'vague' Wishart prior distributions for precision matrices.

Table 8.1 shows the DIC for models *IND*, *MV1.01*, *MV1.1* and *MV2.01*. As can be appreciated, the model assuming independence between diseases is

Model	Dev.	n.eff	DIC
IND	6,977.3	463.6	7,440.9
MV1.01	6,963.9	396.3	7,360.1
MV1.1	6,927.5	443.2	7,370.7
MV2.01	6,961.2	397.3	7,358.5

Table 8.1
Posterior mean of the deviance, number of effective parameters and DIC for models *IND*, *MV1.01*, *MV1.1*, *MV2.01*.

clearly worse than the rest of multivariate models. Its number of effective parameters is higher than for the rest of the models as a consequence of assuming independence between diseases. These DICs also shed some light on the adequacy of the fit of the *MV1.01* model, as compared to model *MV1.1*. Thus the first has a substantial lower DIC, pointing out that choosing $R = I_3$ could be constraining the posterior distribution of the random effects and therefore providing a worse fit. *MV1.01* has a worse fit in terms of its deviance, but the corresponding reduction of the number of effective parameters, produced by a higher transference of information between diseases, compensates that loss.

Table 8.1 also illustrates that considering correlation between diseases for the heterogeneous term brings back a slight benefit in our case, at least in terms of DIC. Nevertheless, interestingly, the posterior mean of the correlation matrix for the spatial term for the *MV2.01* model

$$\begin{pmatrix} 1 & 0.89(0.78, 0.98) & 0.92(0.82, 0.99) \\ - & 1 & 0.92(0.83, 0.98) \\ - & - & 1 \end{pmatrix},$$

is quite similar to that of *MV1.01*. In the former correlation matrix, the values between brackets represent the 95% posterior credible interval for each cell. On the contrary, that same correlation matrix for the heterogeneous term:

$$\begin{pmatrix} 1 & 0.46(-0.28, 0.81) & 0.63(-0.30, 0.92) \\ - & 1 & 0.57(-0.27, 0.86) \\ - & - & 1 \end{pmatrix}$$

takes positive values but lower than those for the spatial component. Note that all the credible intervals for the correlations in this last matrix contain the value 0, which may explain why this model improves model *MV1.01*, although just slightly, in terms of DIC.

Regarding the implementation of the conditional multivariate approach, we have coded the conditional multivariate model in WinBUGS (available at the online supplementary material). Regretfully, the MCMC convergence of that implementation is substantitally worse than for the models using the mv.car distribution. Thus, the models using that distribution achieve a satisfactory convergence for 25,000 MCMC iterations, with 5,000 iterations used as burn-in period. The conditional multivariate implementation with 100,000 iterations, with 20,000 iterations used as burn-in, got substantially worse convergence statistics.

Finally, we find it convenient to mention that despite the convergence problems found in the implementation of the conditional multivariate approach, the implementation made corresponds to a relatively simple model. Specifically, this model corresponds to a separable MCAR distribution, which is surely the simplest multivariate spatial distribution. None of those models resorted to Cholesky or any other complex matrix decomposition as for many of the models described in the theory of this section. So the convergence problems found, with more complex models, could be substantially worse for those implementations. As a consequence, the implementation of more complex conditional multivariate models for moderate sized lattices would require for sure resorting to other programming tools beyond `WinBUGS`.

8.2 Coregionalization models

The second main approach to multivariate modeling relies on coregionalization, i.e., on linear combinations of sets of underlying spatial patterns, but we will refer to them for short as coregionalization models, in accordance to the literature. Coregionalization was originally proposed as a method for inducing multivariate dependence on continuous spatial Gaussian Random fields (Goulard and Voltz, 1992; Wackernagel, 1998, 2003; and Gelfand et al., 2004). Originally, coregionalization was proposed as a dimension reduction tool for building multivariate models as linear combinations of $J^* < J$ underlying spatial patterns. Later on, coregionalization has been applied to lattice data by means of linear combinations of underlying GMRFs in different manners.

The main idea of coregionalization models is defining the geographical patterns of the diseases considered as linear combinations of some common underlying geographic patterns. By doing this, those diseases having similar coefficients in their linear combinations induce high dependence on their respective spatial patterns. The link between correlated spatial patterns and linear combinations of spatial patterns can be easily illustrated for separable multivariate processes. Thus, let us consider an $I \times J$ matrix $\boldsymbol{\Phi}$ of zero mean Normal cells and covariance matrix $\boldsymbol{\Sigma}_{vec(\boldsymbol{\Phi})} = \boldsymbol{\Sigma}_b \otimes \boldsymbol{\Sigma}_w$, where $\boldsymbol{\Sigma}_b$ and $\boldsymbol{\Sigma}_w$ stand for covariance matrices between and within diseases. The multivariate process in

$vec(\mathbf{\Phi})$ can easily be built as

$$vec(\mathbf{\Phi}) = (\tilde{\mathbf{\Sigma}}_b \otimes \tilde{\mathbf{\Sigma}}_w)vec(\boldsymbol{\epsilon}) \qquad (8.8)$$

for an $I \times J$ matrix $\boldsymbol{\epsilon}$ with independent $N(0,1)$ cells and where $\tilde{\mathbf{\Sigma}}$ denotes the lower Cholesky triangle of a matrix $\mathbf{\Sigma}$. Standard linear algebra results (see for example page 74 of Gentle (2007)) establish that

$$vec(\mathbf{ABC}) = (\mathbf{C}' \otimes \mathbf{A})vec(\mathbf{B})$$

for any three matrices $\mathbf{A}, \mathbf{B}$ and $\mathbf{C}$ of suitable dimensions. Thus, if we applied this relationship to Expression (8.8), we would then have

$$\mathbf{\Phi} = \tilde{\mathbf{\Sigma}}_w \boldsymbol{\epsilon} \tilde{\mathbf{\Sigma}}_b'. \qquad (8.9)$$

Therefore, this expression shows how to obtain a separable multivariate spatial process as a result of simple matrix products on a matrix of independent Normal variables. The rows of $\boldsymbol{\epsilon}$ correspond to different spatial units and $\tilde{\mathbf{\Sigma}}_w$ gets in charge of combining the information of those rows and therefore sharing information between spatial units. How that information is combined depends on the specific form of the covariance matrix within diseases, in particular of its Cholesky decomposition. In a similar manner, postmultiplying by $\tilde{\mathbf{\Sigma}}_b'$ mixes up information on the different columns of $\boldsymbol{\epsilon}$, inducing therefore dependence on the columns of $\mathbf{\Phi}$, that is, inducing dependence between diseases. Thus, pre- and post-multiplication of a random matrix by suitable structured matrices can be considered a way of inducing dependence within and between diseases, respectively, in multivariate spatial models.

Note that Expression (8.9) entails the product of three matrices that could be carried out as either $(\tilde{\mathbf{\Sigma}}_w \boldsymbol{\epsilon})\tilde{\mathbf{\Sigma}}_b'$ or $\tilde{\mathbf{\Sigma}}_w(\boldsymbol{\epsilon}\tilde{\mathbf{\Sigma}}_b')$. As a consequence, for this separable model, the order in which spatial and multivariate dependence is induced is irrelevant; this could also be seen as a consequence of the following:

$$\begin{aligned} vec(\mathbf{\Phi}) &= (\tilde{\mathbf{\Sigma}}_b \otimes \tilde{\mathbf{\Sigma}}_w)vec(\boldsymbol{\epsilon}) \\ &= (\tilde{\mathbf{\Sigma}}_b \otimes \mathbf{I}_I)(\mathbf{I}_J \otimes \tilde{\mathbf{\Sigma}}_w)vec(\boldsymbol{\epsilon}) = (\mathbf{I}_J \otimes \tilde{\mathbf{\Sigma}}_w)(\tilde{\mathbf{\Sigma}}_b \otimes \mathbf{I}_I)vec(\boldsymbol{\epsilon}). \end{aligned}$$

As we will see below, this commutativity of the order of the spatial and multivariate dependence structure will not hold in general.

Note also that Expression (8.9) entails the product of two terms representing covariance matrices. If these matrices were not restricted in some manner, that expression would have two terms inducing scale on $\mathbf{\Phi}$. Obviously, these two terms could not be identified since the scale parameters in one of them could be increased by decreasing those same parameters in the other one in a similar quantity. A common solution to this ambiguity is to fix the scale of some of these matrices to some value. Thus, it is common to set the variance parameter of $\mathbf{\Sigma}_w$ to 1, i.e., for the particular case of an ICAR distribution we would consider $\mathbf{\Sigma}_w = (\mathbf{D} - \mathbf{W})^{-1}$ instead of the usual $\mathbf{\Sigma}_w = \sigma^2(\mathbf{D} - \mathbf{W})^{-1}$. Thus, broadly speaking, $\boldsymbol{\Sigma}_w$ would induce in some manner spatial correlation instead of spatial covariance. Alternatively, a similar restriction could be imposed on $\boldsymbol{\Sigma}_b$. Nevertheless, we will consider the restriction just mentioned on $\boldsymbol{\Sigma}_w$ for the models in this section.

Expression (8.9) yields important computational advantages as it allows us to implement multivariate processes with separable structures by avoiding specialized Kronecker products operations, which makes it feasible to run these models in `WinBUGS`, for example. This is not at all a negligible advantage. Nevertheless, Expression (8.9) has an even more convenient reexpression that we will use extensively in practice. Thus, the number of spatial units in multivariate studies is usually much larger than the number of diseases, as a consequence $\tilde{\boldsymbol{\Sigma}}_w$ will be generally much larger than $\tilde{\boldsymbol{\Sigma}}_b$. Moreover, although $\boldsymbol{\Sigma}_w^{-1}$ will be typically sparse for any GMRF, $\tilde{\boldsymbol{\Sigma}}_w$ will be no longer sparse so the computational benefits of dealing with GMRF are no longer present in Expression (8.9). Thus, it is quite advantageous to alternatively consider (8.9) as

$$\boldsymbol{\Phi} = \tilde{\boldsymbol{\Sigma}}_w \boldsymbol{\epsilon} \tilde{\boldsymbol{\Sigma}}_b' = (\tilde{\boldsymbol{\Sigma}}_w \boldsymbol{\epsilon}) \tilde{\boldsymbol{\Sigma}}_b' = \boldsymbol{\varphi} \tilde{\boldsymbol{\Sigma}}_b' \qquad (8.10)$$

where the columns of $\boldsymbol{\varphi} = \tilde{\boldsymbol{\Sigma}}_w \boldsymbol{\epsilon}$ have $\boldsymbol{\Sigma}_w$ as covariance matrix and therefore already show spatial dependence, so if we consider J spatial patterns, the J columns of $\boldsymbol{\varphi}$, we will avoid computing the costly operation $\tilde{\boldsymbol{\Sigma}}_w \boldsymbol{\epsilon}$ at every step of MCMC algorithms. Therefore, we can directly consider a set of spatially structured variables $\boldsymbol{\varphi}$, following ICAR, PCAR, etc. distributions, and induce dependence among them by means of $\tilde{\boldsymbol{\Sigma}}_b'$ instead of starting from a set of independent variables $\boldsymbol{\epsilon}$. Expression (8.10), which combines several underlying spatial patterns $\boldsymbol{\varphi}$ by means of a matrix product with a triangular matrix, is frequently known and referred to in the literature as a *coregionalization* model (Wackernagel, 2003; Gelfand et al., 2004; and MacNab, 2016b).

Expressions (8.9) and (8.10) allow us to express separable processes as simple matrix products. Thus, if we set the columns of $\boldsymbol{\varphi}$ to follow ICAR distributions, then $\boldsymbol{\Phi} = \boldsymbol{\varphi} \tilde{\boldsymbol{\Sigma}}_b'$ would follow a separable intrinsic MCAR distribution of covariance matrix between diseases $\boldsymbol{\Sigma}_b$. If those columns followed a PCAR distribution of common parameter ρ, then $\boldsymbol{\Phi}$ would follow a multivariate MPCAR(ρ) distribution with $\boldsymbol{\Sigma}_{vec(\boldsymbol{\Phi})} = \boldsymbol{\Sigma}_b \otimes (\boldsymbol{D} - \rho \boldsymbol{W})^{-1}$. In a similar manner, this procedure would allow posing separable multivariate processes with any underlying spatial distribution. Nevertheless, this procedure allows also proposing non-separable processes quite easily by simply setting the columns of $\boldsymbol{\varphi}$ as realizations of different spatial distributions. For example, let us assume those columns follow PCAR distributions of different spatial correlation parameters $\rho_1, ..., \rho_J$. In that case, $vec(\boldsymbol{\Phi}) = vec(\boldsymbol{\varphi} \tilde{\boldsymbol{\Sigma}}_b') = (\tilde{\boldsymbol{\Sigma}}_b \otimes \boldsymbol{I}_J) vec(\boldsymbol{\varphi})$ and therefore

$$
\begin{aligned}
\boldsymbol{\Sigma}_{vec(\boldsymbol{\Phi})} &= (\tilde{\boldsymbol{\Sigma}}_b \otimes \boldsymbol{I}_J) Bdiag(\{\boldsymbol{D} - \rho_j \boldsymbol{W}\}_{j=1}^J)^{-1} (\tilde{\boldsymbol{\Sigma}}_b' \otimes \boldsymbol{I}_J) \\
&= (\tilde{\boldsymbol{\Sigma}}_b \otimes \boldsymbol{I}_J)(\boldsymbol{I}_J \otimes \boldsymbol{D} - diag(\rho) \otimes \boldsymbol{W})^{-1} (\tilde{\boldsymbol{\Sigma}}_b' \otimes \boldsymbol{I}_J).
\end{aligned}
$$

This model was proposed as Case 2 in Jin et al. (2007) as a case of 'independent but not identical latent processes'. Note that

$$
\begin{aligned}
\Sigma_{vec(\Phi)}^{-1} &= ((\tilde{\Sigma}_b')^{-1} \otimes I_J)(I_J \otimes D - diag(\rho) \otimes W)(\tilde{\Sigma}_b^{-1} \otimes I_J) \\
&= ((\tilde{\Sigma}_b')^{-1}\tilde{\Sigma}_b^{-1} \otimes D) - (\tilde{\Sigma}_b')^{-1}diag(\rho)\tilde{\Sigma}_b^{-1} \otimes W) \\
&= (\Sigma_b^{-1} \otimes D) - (\tilde{\Sigma}_b diag(\rho^{-1})\tilde{\Sigma}_b')^{-1} \otimes W),
\end{aligned}
$$

so $\Sigma_{vec(\Phi)}^{-1}$ is a block matrix with blocks of the form $\sigma_{ij}^{-2}(D - \rho_{ij}W)$ where σ_{ij}^{-2} are the cells of the precision matrix between diseases Σ_b^{-1} and $\rho_{ij} = ((\tilde{\Sigma}_b diag(\rho^{-1})\tilde{\Sigma}_b')^{-1})_{ij}/(\Sigma_b^{-1})_{ij}$. Thus, for this model, both the covariances matrices of Φ columns and their cross-covariances follow PCAR distributions of different spatial parameters. Note that, as seen in the previous section, this goal was not so easy to achieve as a conditionally specified multivariate model but, as a coregionalization model, it is just a straightforward extension of the simplest (independent) modeling proposal under this approach.

Inseparable models might be easily derived within this approach by considering different spatial distributions (of different parameters) for each of the columns of φ. Specifically, in that case, φ can no longer be expressed as $\hat{\Sigma}_w \epsilon \tilde{\Sigma}_b'$ as there is not a single Σ_w for all the spatial patterns. Assuming different spatial patterns should be put instead as:

$$
\begin{aligned}
vec(\Phi) &= vec(\varphi\tilde{\Sigma}_b') = vec([(\tilde{\Sigma}_w)_1\epsilon_{.1} : ... : (\tilde{\Sigma}_w)_J\epsilon_{.J}]\tilde{\Sigma}_b') \\
&= (\tilde{\Sigma}_b \otimes I_I)vec([(\tilde{\Sigma}_w)_1\epsilon_{.1} : ... : (\tilde{\Sigma}_w)_J\epsilon_{.J}]) \\
&= (\tilde{\Sigma}_b \otimes I_I)Bdiag(\{(\tilde{\Sigma}_w)_j\}_{j=1}^J)vec(\epsilon).
\end{aligned}
$$

Thus, in contrast to the separable case, spatial dependence is now induced by premultiplying $vec(\epsilon)$ by $Bdiag(\{(\tilde{\Sigma}_w)_j\}_{j=1}^J)$ instead of $I_J \otimes \tilde{\Sigma}_w$. This change makes that, in contrast to separable models, the product of the matrices inducing spatial and multivariate dependence no longer commutes. As a consequence, the order in which dependences within and between diseases are induced in non-separable models does matter. We have just seen that inducing spatial dependence first in a non-separable multivariate PCAR model yields the Case 2 model of Jin et al. (2007). Interestingly, the model in Gelfand and Vounatsou (2003), already introduced in the previous section as a conditional multivariate model, can also be seen as a coregionalization model closely related to the Case 2 model of Jin et al. just mentioned. Specifically, that model corresponds to Jin et al.'s proposal but inducing multivariate dependence firstly and spatial dependence afterwards (Martinez-Beneito, 2013), i.e.,

$$
vec(\Phi) = Bdiag(\{(\tilde{\Sigma}_w)_j\}_{j=1}^J)(\tilde{\Sigma}_b \otimes I_I)vec(\epsilon),
$$

which yields a Gaussian process with the following covariance matrix

$$
\Sigma_{vec(\Phi)} = Bdiag(\{(\tilde{\Sigma}_w)_j\}_{j=1}^J)(\Sigma_b \otimes I_I)Bdiag(\{(\tilde{\Sigma}_w')_j\}_{j=1}^J)
$$

which no longer has a block-matrix structure of PCAR covariance matrices.

One drawback of the Case 2 non-separable model of Jin et al. (2007), introduced above, is its order dependence in relation to the set of diseases. Specifically, as $\hat{\boldsymbol{\Sigma}}_b$ is lower triangular, then the columns of $\boldsymbol{\Phi} = \boldsymbol{\varphi}\tilde{\boldsymbol{\Sigma}}_b'$ have increasing complexity for higher subindexes j. That is, $\boldsymbol{\Phi}_{.1}$ will be simply proportional to $\boldsymbol{\varphi}_{.1}$ while $\boldsymbol{\Phi}_{.2}$ will be a linear combination of $\boldsymbol{\varphi}_{.1}$ and $\boldsymbol{\varphi}_{.2}$ and so on. Thus, $\boldsymbol{\Phi}_{.2}$ is the combination of two different spatial families, making it possible to reproduce features of both families, while $\boldsymbol{\Phi}_{.1}$ is only able to reproduce features of the first of these families. As a consequence, for $j > j'$, $\boldsymbol{\Phi}_{.j}$ will be able to reproduce richer spatial structures than $\boldsymbol{\Phi}_{.j'}$. This asymmetry is worrisome since the order in which diseases are considered is usually arbitrary in multivariate studies. Note that this does not happen for separable models, since the linear combination of patterns with the same distribution produces always patterns following also that distribution. As a result, all the resulting patterns for all the diseases are equally complex.

This order dependence is closely related to the matrix decomposition used for $\boldsymbol{\Sigma}_b$. For all the previous models in this section, we have used the corresponding Cholesky lower triangle $\tilde{\boldsymbol{\Sigma}}_b$, when we just really needed a matrix $\hat{\boldsymbol{\Sigma}}_b$ accomplishing $\boldsymbol{\Sigma}_b = \hat{\boldsymbol{\Sigma}}_b\hat{\boldsymbol{\Sigma}}_b'$. Obviously, $\hat{\boldsymbol{\Sigma}}_b$ could be also obtained by resorting to the spectral decomposition of $\boldsymbol{\Sigma}_b$, for example, in fact Gelfand and Vounatsou base their proposal on that decomposition. Martinez-Beneito (2013) show that the set of matrices $\hat{\boldsymbol{\Sigma}}_b$ accomplishing $\boldsymbol{\Sigma}_b = \hat{\boldsymbol{\Sigma}}_b\hat{\boldsymbol{\Sigma}}_b'$ is precisely the set of right-orthogonal transformations of $\tilde{\boldsymbol{\Sigma}}_b$, i.e., $\{\tilde{\boldsymbol{\Sigma}}_b\boldsymbol{Q} : \boldsymbol{Q}\boldsymbol{Q}' = \boldsymbol{I}_J\}$. So, could we consider that whole set of matrices for any $\boldsymbol{\Sigma}_b$ instead of just its Cholesky decomposition for building multivariate models? In that case, for the separable case, we would have

$$\boldsymbol{\Phi} = \tilde{\boldsymbol{\Sigma}}_w \boldsymbol{\epsilon} \hat{\boldsymbol{\Sigma}}_b' = \tilde{\boldsymbol{\Sigma}}_w \boldsymbol{\epsilon} \boldsymbol{Q}' \tilde{\boldsymbol{\Sigma}}_b',$$

which yields the following covariance matrix

$$\boldsymbol{\Sigma}_{vec(\boldsymbol{\Phi})} = (\tilde{\boldsymbol{\Sigma}}_b\boldsymbol{Q} \otimes \tilde{\boldsymbol{\Sigma}}_w)(\boldsymbol{Q}'\tilde{\boldsymbol{\Sigma}}_b' \otimes \tilde{\boldsymbol{\Sigma}}_w') = \boldsymbol{\Sigma}_b \otimes \boldsymbol{\Sigma}_w.$$

Thus, for the separable case, considering all the suitable decompositions of $\boldsymbol{\Sigma}_b$ fulfilling $\boldsymbol{\Sigma}_b = \hat{\boldsymbol{\Sigma}}_b\hat{\boldsymbol{\Sigma}}_b'$ does not have any effect on the multivariate covariance structure. Nevertheless, for the PCAR based non-separable Case 2 of Jin et al. we would have

$$vec(\boldsymbol{\Phi}) = vec([(\tilde{\boldsymbol{\Sigma}}_w)_1\boldsymbol{\epsilon}_{.1} : ... : (\tilde{\boldsymbol{\Sigma}}_w)_J\boldsymbol{\epsilon}_{.J}]\boldsymbol{Q}'\tilde{\boldsymbol{\Sigma}}_b'),$$

which would yield the following covariance matrix

$$\begin{aligned}
\boldsymbol{\Sigma}_{vec(\boldsymbol{\Phi})} &= (\tilde{\boldsymbol{\Sigma}}_b\boldsymbol{Q} \otimes \boldsymbol{I}_I)Bdiag(\{\boldsymbol{D} - \rho_j\boldsymbol{W}\}_{j=1}^J)^{-1}(\boldsymbol{Q}'\tilde{\boldsymbol{\Sigma}}_b' \otimes \boldsymbol{I}_I) \\
&= (((\tilde{\boldsymbol{\Sigma}}_b')^{-1}\boldsymbol{Q} \otimes \boldsymbol{I}_I)(\boldsymbol{I}_J \otimes \boldsymbol{D} - diag(\boldsymbol{\rho}) \otimes \boldsymbol{W})(\boldsymbol{Q}'\tilde{\boldsymbol{\Sigma}}_b^{-1} \otimes \boldsymbol{I}_I))^{-1} \\
&= (\boldsymbol{\Sigma}_b^{-1} \otimes \boldsymbol{D} - (\tilde{\boldsymbol{\Sigma}}_b\boldsymbol{Q}diag(\boldsymbol{\rho}^{-1})\boldsymbol{Q}'\tilde{\boldsymbol{\Sigma}}_b')^{-1} \otimes \boldsymbol{W})^{-1}. \qquad (8.11)
\end{aligned}$$

Thus, for non-separable models, considering all the decompositions of $\mathbf{\Sigma}_b$ turns back a more general form of $\mathbf{\Sigma}_{vec(\mathbf{\Phi})}$, which depends on $\mathbf{Q}$. Thus, considering a single (and surely arbitrary) decomposition of $\mathbf{\Sigma}_b$ will (arbitrarily) restrict the set of processes that coregionalization models are able to fit. Moreover, permutation matrices are a particular subset of the set of orthogonal matrices. So, considering all orthogonal transformations of $\tilde{\mathbf{\Sigma}}_b$ solves the order dependence of the non-separable models mentioned above, as these models would implicitly consider any possible ordering of the set of diseases. As a consequence, any model defined as $\mathbf{\Phi} = \varphi \mathbf{Q}' \tilde{\mathbf{\Sigma}}_b'$ will be order-free as an effect of including the orthogonal matrix $\mathbf{Q}$ in its formulation. This order-free model is the most general multivariate proposal currently formulated as a coregionalization model. This model has been previously proposed for deriving multivariate generalizations of PCAR and BYM distributions (Martinez-Beneito, 2013). Jin et al. (2007) also formulated this process for PCAR distributions but following a mixed approach of conditionally specified and linear combinations of spatial patterns. We will refer henceforth to this model as the *QR-model* for reasons that we will see below.

One of the main disadvantages of the *QR*-model, and all the models introduced in this section, is that their formulations rely on a matrix decomposition $\tilde{\mathbf{\Sigma}}_b$. That matrix decomposition can be hard to compute in packages such as WinBUGS with such a limited collection of mathematical tools. Moreover, the modeling of the orthogonal matrix $\mathbf{Q}$ can be also very tricky as it is often built as a composition of $J(J-1)/2$ simpler orthogonal matrices, *Givens angles* (Jin et al., 2007), whose number grows quadratically as a function of J. This can be a particularly important problem when J is high since, in that case, these two problems may become prohibitive. Indeed, Botella-Rocamora et al. (2015) describe the implementation of the *QR*-model in WinBUGS for $J > 3$ as very problematic since it crashes, returning an error ('too complex' model), when trying to run that model. Fortunately, the *QR*-model can be reformulated in order to avoid the Cholesky decomposition of $\mathbf{\Sigma}_b$ or sampling from the orthogonal matrix $\mathbf{Q}$. That reformulation may be done by noticing that the product $\mathbf{Q}' \tilde{\mathbf{\Sigma}}_b'$ in the *QR*-model can be understood as the *QR decomposition* (see for example page 188 of Gentle (2007)) of a general $J \times J$ matrix $\mathbf{M}$. Note that, in general, we will be interested in making inference on $\mathbf{Q}$ and/or $\mathbf{M}$ so, in agreement with the rest of the book we should have noted those matrices with Greek letters. Nevertheless, for making sense of the *QR* and *M*-models (to be introduced just below) in the literature, which take their names from these matrices, we have preferred to denote them with Latin characters.

The *QR* factorization of a square matrix $\mathbf{M}$ decomposes that matrix as a product $\mathbf{QR}$ of an orthogonal matrix $\mathbf{Q}$ and an upper triangular matrix $\mathbf{R}$. Note that this decomposition exists, and is unique, for all square matrix $\mathbf{M}$. Note also that $\mathbf{M}'\mathbf{M} = \mathbf{R}'\mathbf{Q}'\mathbf{Q}\mathbf{R} = \mathbf{R}'\mathbf{R}$; therefore, $\mathbf{R}$ coincides with the upper Cholesky matrix of $\mathbf{M}'\mathbf{M}$. Since any square matrix can be expressed as $\mathbf{QR}$ for an orthogonal and an upper triangular matrix, we could substitute the term $\mathbf{Q}'\tilde{\mathbf{\Sigma}}_b'$ in the *QR*-model above by a general $J \times J$ matrix $\mathbf{M}$.

Therefore, $\boldsymbol{\Phi}$ could be equivalently modeled as simply $\boldsymbol{\varphi M}$ for a set of spatially correlated patterns $\boldsymbol{\varphi}$ and a general square matrix $\boldsymbol{M}$, which would yield an alternative reformulation of the QR-model but is much more manageable in computational terms. This model is known as the *M-model* in contrast to its original alternative, the QR-model, for obvious reasons (Botella-Rocamora et al., 2015). The computational advantage of the M-model has made it run multivariate studies with very complex multivariate covariance matrices, such as (8.11), and with up to 21 diseases in the Valencian Region (540 spatial units). Moreover, its mathematical simplicity has made that study be undertaken in WinBUGS.

QR and M-models solve the order dependence of the non-separable Case 2 model of Jin et al. (2005). Although this is a considerable improvement, it comes at a cost: many of the components of both models are no longer identifiable. Thus, if $\boldsymbol{\Phi} = \boldsymbol{\varphi Q}'\tilde{\boldsymbol{\Sigma}}_b'$ for suitable matrices $\boldsymbol{\varphi}$, $\boldsymbol{Q}$ and $\boldsymbol{\Sigma}_b$, then $\boldsymbol{\Phi} = \boldsymbol{\varphi}^*(\boldsymbol{Q}^*)'\tilde{\boldsymbol{\Sigma}}_b'$ also for $\boldsymbol{\varphi}^* = \boldsymbol{\varphi P}$ and $\boldsymbol{Q}^* = \boldsymbol{QP}$ for any permutation, and therefore orthogonal matrix $\boldsymbol{P}$. That is, we could change the order of the columns of $\boldsymbol{\varphi}$ by making a similar change in $\boldsymbol{Q}$, or $\boldsymbol{M}$ for the M-model, and get an exactly equivalent fit. This has important consequences on the convergence of the MCMC for these models, since these non-identifiable parameters often show weird performances. For example, for the vector $\boldsymbol{\rho}$ of spatial dependence parameters for a set of PCAR distributions, let us assume that we had just one column of $\boldsymbol{\varphi}$ with a high value for that parameter. We could perfectly find that such random effect is placed in the first column of $\boldsymbol{\varphi}$ for one chain, but it is placed in $\boldsymbol{\varphi}_{.2}$ for the second of the chains in the MCMC. This would make the convergence of ρ_1 seem faulty, as it will take in general high values for the first chain but not for the second, while the fit for all the chains could be perfectly equivalent. In principle, this could be fixed by setting a restriction in QR and M-models such as $\rho_1 > \rho_2 > ... > \rho_J$. Although this would fix the mentioned identifiability problems in theory, in our experience, this would introduce additional convergence problems for the chains, that could get trapped in constrained local maxima of the posterior distribution, making the convergence problems of these models even worse. So we would advise avoiding imposing any additional restriction on these models in order to favour their identifiability. In that case, we should consider the apparent convergence problems in the unconstrained QR and M-models as just a consequence of the multimodality of the posterior distribution (with $J!$ equivalent modes) and the fact that any of the chains run are exploring a different mode of this collection of equivalent modes. In some manner, this is similar to the MCMC convergence problems found in Bayesian fitting of mixtures models (Stephens, 2000a,b).

Fortunately, despite the convergence problems for the non-identifiable variables mentioned in the previous paragraph, the main quantities of interest of the QR and M-models can be perfectly identified. Thus, the log-risks $\boldsymbol{\Phi}$, and therefore the risks for each spatial unit, can be identified since the identifiability problems are related to the elements of the products $\boldsymbol{\varphi Q}'$ or $\boldsymbol{\varphi M}$, but not with the result of those products. In a similar manner, the covariance matrix between diseases can be also identified for the QR-model ($\boldsymbol{\Sigma}_b = \tilde{\boldsymbol{\Sigma}}_b \tilde{\boldsymbol{\Sigma}}'_b$) and the M-model in the following way:

$$\boldsymbol{\Sigma}_b = \boldsymbol{M}'\boldsymbol{M} = (\boldsymbol{Q}'\tilde{\boldsymbol{\Sigma}}'_b)'(\boldsymbol{Q}'\tilde{\boldsymbol{\Sigma}}'_b) = \tilde{\boldsymbol{\Sigma}}_b \boldsymbol{Q}\boldsymbol{Q}'\tilde{\boldsymbol{\Sigma}}'_b = \boldsymbol{\Sigma}_b.$$

Note that this is independent of whether any of the chains had a permuted version of the first chain, for example, since in that case:

$$\boldsymbol{\Sigma}_b = \boldsymbol{M}'\boldsymbol{M} = ((\boldsymbol{QP})'\tilde{\boldsymbol{\Sigma}}'_b)'((\boldsymbol{QP})'\tilde{\boldsymbol{\Sigma}}'_b) = \tilde{\boldsymbol{\Sigma}}_b \boldsymbol{Q}\boldsymbol{P}\boldsymbol{P}'\boldsymbol{Q}'\tilde{\boldsymbol{\Sigma}}'_b = \boldsymbol{\Sigma}_b.$$

Therefore, $\boldsymbol{M}'\boldsymbol{M}$ will return the covariance matrix between diseases, regardless of the ordering of the geographical patterns in $\boldsymbol{\varphi}$ for each of the chains run.

Regarding the prior distributions of the elements in the QR and M-models, several proposals have been made. As mentioned, there is no built-in function for modeling orthogonal matrices in `WinBUGS` so $\boldsymbol{Q}$ has been usually proposed in the literature to be modeled as a composition of Givens angles, which can be considered as a set of elemental orthogonal matrices. Given J and $1 \leq j < j' \leq J$, a set of $J(J-1)/2$ Givens matrices can be built by setting $\boldsymbol{G}_{jj'}$ as an $\boldsymbol{I}_J$ matrix with the jth and j'th diagonal elements replaced by $\cos(\varepsilon_{jj'})$ and the (j, j')-th and (j', j)-th elements replaced by $\sin(\varepsilon_{jj'})$ and $-\sin(\varepsilon_{jj'})$, respectively. For these matrices $\varepsilon_{12}, ..., \varepsilon_{(J-1)J}$ represent angles (Givens angles) for rotations around the main axis of a J-dimensional space. Thus, the orthogonal matrix $\boldsymbol{Q}$ is usually parameterized as a function of Givens angles as $\boldsymbol{Q} = \boldsymbol{G}_{12}\boldsymbol{G}_{13}...\boldsymbol{G}_{(J-1)J}$ where $\varepsilon_{jj'} \sim U(-\pi/2, \pi/2)$ for any j and j' (Daniels and Kass, 1999; Jin et al., 2007; Greco and Trivisano, 2009; MacNab, 2016b) or $\varepsilon_{jj'} \sim U(0, \pi/2)$ (Martinez-Beneito, 2013 and MacNab, 2016b). In our opinion, choosing $U(-\pi/2, \pi/2)$ has a disadvantage. Specifically, this prior choice could generate any possible orthogonal matrix $\boldsymbol{Q}$ so $\boldsymbol{\Phi}$ could be reproduced as either $\boldsymbol{\varphi}\boldsymbol{Q}\tilde{\boldsymbol{\Sigma}}_b$ or as $(-\boldsymbol{\varphi})(-\boldsymbol{Q})\tilde{\boldsymbol{\Sigma}}_b$, for example. This introduces an additional multimodality in the posterior distribution of $\boldsymbol{\varphi}$ and $\boldsymbol{Q}$. This may be responsible for the identification problems found for this prior choice in some works (MacNab, 2016a) and for MCMC convergence problems in general. Anyway, the use of Givens angles for parameterizing $\boldsymbol{Q}$ entails additional problems. First, choosing uniform prior distributions on the Givens angles $\boldsymbol{\varepsilon}$ does not yield a uniform prior distribution on the space of orthogonal matrices $\boldsymbol{Q}$ (Botella-Rocamora et al., 2015), as we would typically want. Daniels and Kass (1999) provide some insight on the induced prior distribution on $\boldsymbol{Q}$, concluding that such distribution favours low correlations between diseases, regardless of the real correlations underlying the data. Additionally, from a practical point of view, the composition of Givens angles for $J > 3$ could be a nightmare to be coded in `WinBUGS` and surely responsible for the excessive complexity of that code mentioned earlier.

Regarding the prior distribution of $\tilde{\boldsymbol{\Sigma}}_b$, two main proposals have been made. First, several authors (Gelfand and Vounatsou, 2003; Jin et al., 2007; and Greco and Trivisano, 2009) propose to set vague inverse Wishart prior distributions on $\boldsymbol{\Sigma}_b$. Although we discussed the prior sensitivity to this choice in the previous section, this is a common choice; surely because this is the conjugate prior distribution for this parameter, which could bring some computational advantage. Some other authors for Σ_b have proposed a uniform prior distribution on the set of symmetric, positive definite matrices of the corresponding dimension. Since that set is not so easy to determine, it could be previously determined by numerical procedures (Sain et al., 2011). Alternatively, we could separately model the elements of Σ_b setting a uniform prior distribution on the standard deviations and correlations between diseases for suitable ranges of values (Martinez-Beneito, 2013 and MacNab, 2016a). This would not guarantee the positive-definiteness of Σ_b, but an additional restriction could be imposed on the MCMC, checking this condition at every step and therefore guaranteeing it. See the online supplementary material for the next example for an example of implementation of this procedure in `WinBUGS`.

For the M-model, several prior distributions have been proposed for the cells of M. Originally, those cells were proposed to be modeled either as fixed effects, by setting an improper flat prior on the different $M_{jj'}$s, or as random effects by setting $M_{jj'} \sim N(0, \sigma^2)$ for $1 \leq j, j' \leq J$ and an unknown σ^2 also estimated within the model. These prior choices have been shown to be equivalent, in terms of the QR-model, to setting a Haar distribution on Q (a uniform prior distribution on the set of orthogonal matrices) and a Wishart prior distribution of $k = J$ degrees of freedom and $R = \sigma^2 I_J$ on Σ_b (Botella-Rocamora et al., 2015). Thus, these prior choices seem to solve the alleged problem of the uniform prior distributions on the Givens angles and its influence on the prior distribution of Q for the QR-model. Nevertheless, these prior choices have been found to yield sometimes unsatisfactory results (Corpas-Burgos et al., 2019). Thus, as shown by Corpas-Burgos et al., the fixed effects modeling of the M cells is, on one hand, prone to undersmooth the fitted $sSMRs$. This effect is more evident in studies with weak data, with low observed cases per spatial unit. On the other hand, the common variance term of the random effects modeling of M tends to give similar variabilities to the geographical patterns of all the diseases. This could be a problem in real terms if those diseases had spatial patterns of markedly different variability, since this model will shrink all of them towards a common value. As a solution to these problems, it has been proposed to model the cells $M_{jj'}$ as either $N(0, \sigma_j^2)$ or as $N(0, \sigma_{j'}^2)$, for both σ_j^2 or $\sigma_{j'}^2$ to be also estimated within the model. These two proposals are known as *Row Variance Adaptive (RVA)* and *Column Variance Adaptive (CVA)* models, respectively. The variance terms in RVA can be understood as the variances of the underlying spatial patterns, φ columns, while for CVA those terms are intended to model the specific variability of each separate disease. According to the fit, in terms of DIC, RVA seems to be superior to CVA, although the column adaptive proposal has also interesting interpretations in terms of the prior distribution that it induces on Σ_b, a scaled Wishart distribution (Corpas-Burgos et al., 2019). Nevertheless, the use of RVA and CVA models is just recommended for the analysis of a medium-high number of diseases, let's say $J > 5$, since the estimate of each σ_j

depends on J cells of $\boldsymbol{M}$. In this manner, we would have a reasonable number of values for estimating each of these variances.

One of the main advantages of coregionalization models is that they are in general valid by construction (Martinez-Beneito, 2013). Coregionalization models are built as the composition of simple matrix operations on a random matrix $\boldsymbol{\epsilon}$. These matrix operations can all be put as $vec(\boldsymbol{\Phi}) = \boldsymbol{A}vec(\boldsymbol{\varphi})$ for a positive definite matrix $\boldsymbol{A}$ and a random matrix $\boldsymbol{\varphi}$ with $\boldsymbol{\Sigma}_{vec(\boldsymbol{\varphi})} = \boldsymbol{\Sigma}$. This yields $\boldsymbol{\Sigma}_{vec(\boldsymbol{\Phi})} = \boldsymbol{A}\boldsymbol{\Sigma}\boldsymbol{A}'$, which is positive definite if $\boldsymbol{A}$ and $\boldsymbol{\Sigma}$ are too. Assuming $\boldsymbol{A}$ to be positive definite, this will be true if $\boldsymbol{\Sigma}$ is also positive definite, which will be generally true, except maybe if the columns of $\boldsymbol{\varphi}$ follow an ICAR distribution. In that case, $vec(\boldsymbol{\Phi})$ will be just positive semidefinite. Nevertheless, in that case the sum-to-zero restrictions of $\boldsymbol{\varphi}$'s columns will induce similar restrictions on the multivariate distribution of $\boldsymbol{\Phi}$, and we will just have to take care to include disease-specific intercepts so that everything works fine.

Although coregionalization and conditional models are two separate ways of formulating multivariate models, there are several works that have merged these two approaches (Jin et al., 2007; Greco and Trivisano, 2009; MacNab, 2016a). These proposals generally consider $\boldsymbol{\varphi}$ to be a conditionally defined multivariate model and induce afterwards additional multivariate dependence by making linear combinations of those, already correlated, underlying patterns. Martinez-Beneito (2019) explores in depth the relationship between 'pure' coregionalization models, those with column-independent $\boldsymbol{\varphi}$ matrices, and conditional multivariate models. That paper formulates a link between coregionalized and conditional models too. Thus, as shown there, any PCAR- or ICAR-based coregionalization model can be also reformulated as conditional multivariate and univariate models. Therefore, that set of coregionalized models can be seen as a subset of the class of multivariate conditional models. On the contrary, coregionalized models can be easily used to generalize other spatial families beyond GMRFs (see several examples in Chapter 6) to the multivariate case. Conditional models, since they build their multivariate ensemble in a similar manner to univariate GMRFs, are not able in principle to reproduce multivariate spatial structures beyond GMRFs so, in this sense, coregionalized models are however more general than conditional models. Finally, Martinez-Beneito (2019) proposes also a coregionalization model with asymmetric cross-spatial covariance matrices. Interestingly, this proposal does not show the label (spatial units) and order (diseases) dependence problems than previous asymmetric models showed (Greco and Trivisano, 2009; Sain et al., 2011). Currently this is the only asymmetric proposal formulated as a coregionalization model, although clearly the real potential of this model is to be explored.

Example 8.2

We are going to retake the three-dimensional study, already considered in Example 8.1, which jointly studied cirrhosis, lung cancer and oral cancer. We will consider now coregionalized models instead. We have coded and run several coregionalization models whose main results we illustrate just below. All models have been coded and run in WinBUGS.

First, we have coded a three variate M-model with underlying BYM models (Corpas-Burgos et al., 2019). This model considers a matrix $\boldsymbol{\varphi}$ of six columns, with the first three columns following an ICAR distribution and the final three columns following independent Normal distributions. Additionally, a 6×3 $\boldsymbol{M}$ matrix is considered. We have not considered a heteroscedastic version of this M-model due to the low number of diseases under study, as in that case we would have very few data to estimate each underlying variance of the elements in the $\boldsymbol{M}$ matrix. Note that the $\boldsymbol{M}$ matrix of this model can be expressed as $\boldsymbol{M} = [\boldsymbol{M}_1' : \boldsymbol{M}_2']' = [\tilde{\boldsymbol{\Sigma}}_1 \boldsymbol{Q}_1 : \tilde{\boldsymbol{\Sigma}}_2 \boldsymbol{Q}_2]'$ for suitable orthogonal ($\boldsymbol{Q}_1$ and $\boldsymbol{Q}_2$) and covariance ($\boldsymbol{\Sigma}_1$ and $\boldsymbol{\Sigma}_2$) matrices. Therefore, this M-model can be seen as the following decomposition of the log-risks:

$$\boldsymbol{\Phi} = \boldsymbol{\varphi}\boldsymbol{M} = \boldsymbol{\varphi}Bdiag(\{\boldsymbol{Q}_1', \boldsymbol{Q}_2'\})[\tilde{\boldsymbol{\Sigma}}_1 : \tilde{\boldsymbol{\Sigma}}_2]' = [\boldsymbol{\varphi}_1\boldsymbol{Q}_1' : \boldsymbol{\varphi}_2\boldsymbol{Q}_2'][\tilde{\boldsymbol{\Sigma}}_1 : \tilde{\boldsymbol{\Sigma}}_2]'$$

where $\boldsymbol{\varphi}_1$ and $\boldsymbol{\varphi}_2$ are the columns of $\boldsymbol{\varphi}$ having, respectively, ICAR and independent Normal distributions. As mentioned above, the orthogonal transformations $\boldsymbol{Q}_1$ and $\boldsymbol{Q}_2$ do not increase the scope of covariance structures generated by this model since the columns of $\boldsymbol{\varphi}_1^* = \boldsymbol{\varphi}_1\boldsymbol{Q}_1'$ follow once again ICAR distributions, in the same manner that the cells in the columns of $\boldsymbol{\varphi}_2^* = \boldsymbol{\varphi}_2\boldsymbol{Q}_2'$ follow independent Normal distributions. Therefore, the contribution of the orthogonal part of the $\boldsymbol{M}_1$ and $\boldsymbol{M}_2$ matrices is irrelevant for this model. Nevertheless, posing the model above as an M-model, with irrelevant orthogonal components, helps us avoid dealing with Cholesky matrices and makes it easier and more intuitive to assign prior distributions on the elements inducing the prior covariance structure of this model. Note that this M-model is equivalent to assuming a spatially correlated part $vec(\boldsymbol{\varphi}_1^*\tilde{\boldsymbol{\Sigma}}_1')$ which follows a multivariate Normal distribution of mean $\boldsymbol{0}_{3I}$ and variance-covariance matrix $\boldsymbol{\Sigma} \otimes (\boldsymbol{D} - \boldsymbol{W})$, i.e., an intrinsic MCAR distribution. Thus, in this manner, we are making a parallel implementation of the mv.car distribution in WinBUGS, but much more efficient than the implementation made as a conditional model in the previous section. Regarding the heterogeneous part of this model, $\boldsymbol{\varphi}_2^*\tilde{\boldsymbol{\Sigma}}_2'$ yields a multivariate Normal distribution of variance-covariance matrix $\boldsymbol{\Sigma}_2$. Thus, the M-model implemented here would be equivalent to the $MV2.01$ model in the previous example, with multivariate dependent spatial and heterogeneous terms, except for the differences coming from the prior assumptions on $\boldsymbol{M}$, $\boldsymbol{\Sigma}_1$ and $\boldsymbol{\Sigma}_2$, respectively. However, the prior assumptions on the M-model seem weaker than those for the mv.car-based alternatives since, for the first, the cells of M follow random effects; therefore, their scale is determined by the data. This is in contrast to the mv.car-based alternatives in the previous example where the prior scale of the covariance structure was set to some, supposedly vague, choice which at the end ended up being not so uninformative.

We implemented this M-model which attained a DIC of 7359.6. Regarding the covariance between diseases for the spatial and heterogeneous terms of this model these are the estimates (posterior means) for the corresponding correlations matrices of both components:

$$\begin{pmatrix} 1 & 0.86 & 0.89 \\ - & 1 & 0.89 \\ - & - & 1 \end{pmatrix}, \begin{pmatrix} 1 & 0.55 & 0.64 \\ - & 1 & 0.77 \\ - & - & 1 \end{pmatrix}.$$

Therefore, all three diseases have spatial patterns with similar correlations. Nevertheless, more marked differences are observed in the heterogeneous component with particularly high correlations between lung and oral cancer ((2,3)-th cell in the previous matrices). In consequence, municipalities with punctual risk excesses for any of these two diseases usually show also risk excesses for the other disease. Regarding the risk estimates for this model, the maps for all three diseases (not shown) hardly show differences with the maps of Figure 8.1. Nevertheless, the difference in computational terms with conditional models is evident since the coregionalized M-model has been able to run for the Valencian Region data without any convergence problem in a reasonable amount of time, 9.5 minutes or 10,000 iterations.

Alternatively, we have run the QR-model with underlying PCAR distributions on this same set of diseases. In principle, this would make it possible to fit a non-separable multivariate model instead of the sum of two (spatial and heterogeneous) separable processes as for the M-model above. The DIC for this model, 7384.0, is higher than for the previous M-model so in this case non-separability does not improve the model in terms of this criterion. The posterior mean for the correlation parameters of the PCAR distributions for this model were above 0.99 for two out of three of the underlying processes in φ and the third had a posterior mean of -0.23 with a posterior mode around 0. Therefore, it is not surprising that the DIC for the M-model was better since the columns of φ for this PCAR-based QR-model reproduce patterns resembling ICAR and heterogeneous Normal distributions, the components of the BYM model. The computing time for this model was far higher than for the M-model above (2.85 vs. 0.15 hours), even though the number of underlying patterns for the M-model doubled that of the QR-model. Nevertheless, the most important difference between both models in computational terms comes from their scalability in terms of the number of diseases under study. As we will see below, the M-model does not find any problem for fitting tens of diseases while the QR-model is unfeasible for jointly fitting even 4 diseases.

The QR-model is not separable, so we could not strictly talk about a covariance matrix between diseases, as that matrix would change for each spatial unit. Nevertheless, for comparative purposes, we could summarize the co-variance between diseases by calculating the posterior mean of the covariance matrix for the columns of $\log(\boldsymbol{\Phi})$. In that case, the correlation matrix between diseases for this model would be:

$$\begin{pmatrix} 1 & 0.59 & 0.63 \\ - & 1 & 0.88 \\ - & - & 1 \end{pmatrix}$$

This correlation matrix agrees with the correlation matrices for the spatial and heterogeneous terms of the M-model above, pointing out a closer association between lung and oral cancer than for cirrhosis.

Regarding the convergence of M-models, Figure 8.2 shows the history plot for four of the parameters of the QR-model. The first of the plots in Figure 8.2 corresponds to the $sSMR$ for the first municipality and cause of death of those considered. This variable can be perfectly identified in the model and no sign of worrisome convergence can be noticed in that history plot. The next three plots correspond to ρ_1, ρ_2 and ρ_3, the spatial dependence parameters of the underlying PCAR distributed vectors in the QR-model. Convergence for these three plots seems far different than that in the first plot. For all three plots, one of the chains moves in a different range of values (mostly negative) than the rest (close to 1). It is important to note that for each plot, the chain taking the negative values corresponds to a different chain of the MCMC. That is, for ρ_1, the first of the chains is that taking the low values, for ρ_2, the third simulated chain takes the low values, and for ρ_3 the second chain is that taking the low values. As a consequence, for each simulation, we find always two un-derlying random effects with substantial spatial dependence and a third factor without (or maybe negative) spatial dependence. Each simulation randomly puts the uncorrelated term in one of the underlying factors since we have not restricted the model in this sense. Nevertheless, all three models are finding the same performance for the random effects (two highly dependent patterns and another hardly dependent), although they are ordered in a different man-ner. If all three simulations had put the uncorrelated term in the first random effect, for example, we would not have found any worrisome sign in the history plots. Nevertheless, in terms of the $sSMRs$ fitted, the results of our model are not different than those that would apparently have an appropriate MCMC convergence for ρ_1, ρ_2 and ρ_3.

What happens for this model, and in general for M-models, is that it has $6(=3!)$ equivalent modes in the posterior mean, one for each possible per-mutation of the 3 underlying factors. Ideally, the MCMC chains should jump between these modes for every iteration as independently as possible but, as we introduced in Chapter 2, this is not so easy. Posterior modes are usually separated by large areas of low probability that are hard to be crossed by the MCMC chains. WinBUGS does not have any particular algorithm to make that task easier, so chains are usually trapped for non-identifiable quantities in one of the MCMC posterior modes for all (or a long part) of the iterations

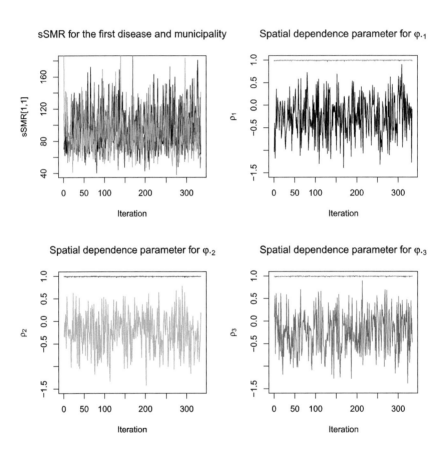

Figure 8.2
History plots for several parameters of the QR-model. Black corresponds to the first (out of three) chains simulated, and red, green correspond to the second and third chain, respectively.

of each chain. Nevertheless, having this consideration into account, we find several important quantities in the model that are not affected by this convergence problem, as for example the $sSMRs$, since they are independent of the mode visited by the non-identifiable elements of the model. If we restrict our attention to those identifiable quantities, we find the inference made valid. Moreover, for the non-identifiable quantities, inference has no sense since we should ideally see the chains jumping between the 6 modes of the posterior distribution, which would yield no sensible inference at all.

Additionally, we have run the heteroscedastic RVA M-model with underlying PCAR distributions for another two settings. First, we have run a four-dimensional M-model for the three causes of death above plus an additional synthetic pattern generated independently of the geographic patterns of those diseases. Specifically, this fourth 'cause of death' has been generated as a PCAR distribution of dependence parameter equal to 0.9 and independent of the other three diseases. We have repeated this process 10 times for 10 different underlying random patterns. With these analyses, we want to illustrate how the M-model appropriately fits an independent disease into the multivariate ensemble. Finally, we have also fitted a 21-dimensional version of the M-model containing the three original causes of death above and 18 additional causes. These 21 causes of death were those analyzed in Botella-Rocamora et al. (2015). This final study is intended to illustrate the analysis of a high-dimensional data set and the benefits that it yields in practical terms.

For the 4-dimensional study of cirrhosis, lung cancer, oral cancer and a synthetic simulated pattern we have considered 4 underlying PCAR distributions as for the QR-model. The mean correlation matrix for all 10 analyses carried out results:

$$\begin{pmatrix} 1 & 0.61 & 0.68 & -0.05 \\ - & 1 & 0.87 & -0.05 \\ - & - & 1 & -0.08 \\ - & - & - & 1 \end{pmatrix}.$$

As can be appreciated, the correlations of the three original diseases hardly change, in comparison to the QR-model, by the inclusion of the additional patterns. Additionally, the correlations of the new additional patterns with the 3 original diseases are all close to 0. Hence, this example illustrates how the M-model is able to appropriately fit the performance of diseases without relationship with the rest of the diseases if this was the case.

Regarding the analysis of the 21 diseases in Botella-Rocamora et al. (2015), the lower-right hand side of Figure 1.1 shows the geographical pattern fitted for oral cancer in that analysis. The geographical pattern of the risks in this map seems more evident than for any other plot for oral cancer in this book. Specifically, very few places are highlighted in that map as showing risk excesses in contrast to the original SMRs map. Furthermore, the standard deviation of the oral cancer log-risks (posterior means) for this analysis of 21 diseases is 0.30, in comparison to 0.21 in the previous analysis of 3 diseases.

This illustrates how taking into account more (hypothetically related) diseases makes it possible to depict more extreme smoothed risks by taking profit of that additional information. This could alleviate the oversmoothing that disease mapping models are usually blamed to produce.

Figure 8.3 shows the correlation matrix between diseases for all those 21 causes of death considered in this study. The first 12 rows (first 11 columns) correspond to tumoural causes of death, while the subsequent causes of death correspond to causes of death of another kind. That figure shows some interesting results. First, most of the correlations are clearly positive, except for atherosclerosis. This suggests that in general we find municipalities with high risk for all causes of death studied and, on the contrary, we find municipalities with low risks in general. We do not know the reasons for this, if this is caused by health services distribution, lifestyles, socioeconomic deprivation etc. It could seem a bit surprising that all the diseases go, in general terms, in the same direction; anyway, the previous example analyzing 4 spatial patterns showed that if one disease was independent of the rest, the M-model should be capable of fitting that performance. We find also interesting the correlations for atherosclerosis shown in Figure 8.3. Atherosclerosis is the cause of death showing the lowest correlations with the rest of diseases. We remind that the univariate map for atherosclerosis was already shown at Section 4.3 as an example of spatial independence. That map shows a completely unstructured spatial pattern, surely as a consequence of the bad quality of death notifications for this cause by health professionals. This makes the corresponding map show mainly noise, which hardly shows correlation with the rest of the diseases. Contrarily, we find that most of the highest correlation in Figure 8.3 corresponds to pairs of diseases that are well known to be related with tobacco consumption, such as lung, oral, bladder and larynx cancer. Most of the pairs of these diseases show correlations higher than 0.75. Additionally, liver cancer and cirrhosis show also a particularly high correlation (0.84). This is not surprising since both are hepatic diseases that could be clearly related. The M-model seems to capture that strong relationship.

8.3   Factor models, smoothed ANOVA and other approaches

In concluding this chapter, we are going to review in this section some approaches to multivariate modeling that do not fit within the previous conditional and coregionalized settings and that have attracted some attention in the literature. We will group these proposals into 3 sets: factor models, smooth ANOVA and a final miscellaneous group of proposals.

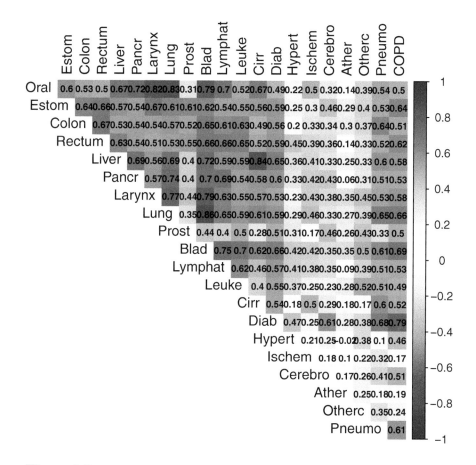

Figure 8.3
Correlation matrix between diseases for the joint analysis of 21 diseases by means of a RVA *M*-model.

8.3.1 Factor models

Multivariate spatial factor models reproduce the ideas of the popular statistical technique, with that same name, of multivariate analysis of regular (non-spatial) data. Factor models perform a low-dimensional approximation of the multivariate structure of the log-risks matrix. Specifically, they assume $\boldsymbol{\Phi} = \sum_{j=1}^{J^*} \boldsymbol{\lambda}_j \boldsymbol{\delta}_j' + \boldsymbol{\epsilon}$ where $\{\boldsymbol{\lambda}_1, ..., \boldsymbol{\lambda}_{J^*}\}$ is a set of I-vectors, the 'scores' of the spatial units, and $\{\boldsymbol{\delta}_1, ..., \boldsymbol{\delta}_{J^*}\}$ are J-vectors, with the weights of the factors for each variable. Usually J^* is much lower than J, so the number of common underlying factors assumed is far lower than the number of variables in the multivariate study. The underlying idea of these models is that there are a few underlying risk factors $\{\boldsymbol{\lambda}_1, ..., \boldsymbol{\lambda}_{J^*}\}$ in charge of inducing spatial dependence for all or many of the diseases considered. Leaving out the effect of these common factors, the remaining residual variability will be explained by J additional factors $\{\boldsymbol{\epsilon}_1, ..., \boldsymbol{\epsilon}_J\}$, uncorrelated between columns but possibly showing spatial dependence for each disease.

In contrast to traditional factor models, spatial factor models assume spatial dependence for the factor scores corresponding to the areal units. Since these scores correspond to geographical locations, it is reasonable to assume spatial dependence for them, thus $\boldsymbol{\lambda}_j, j = 1, ..., J^*$, are usually assumed to follow a spatial distribution such as PCAR, BYM, LCAR, etc. Similar spatial distributions could also be set for the columns of $\boldsymbol{\epsilon}$ if residual variability showed spatial dependence for some diseases. On the other hand, the vectors of weights $\boldsymbol{\delta}_j$, whose components could take both positive and negative values, modulate the contribution of the corresponding underlying factor to each disease. Those components are usually modeled as sets of independent zero-mean Normal variables.

Either the scale of the vectors of $\{\boldsymbol{\lambda}_1, ..., \boldsymbol{\lambda}_{J^*}\}$ or that of $\{\boldsymbol{\delta}_1, ..., \boldsymbol{\delta}_{J^*}\}$ should be fixed to a constant, normally 1, since otherwise the scales of these two groups would compensate between them and would not be identifiable in that case. Moreover, factor models show further identifiability problems since the vector of variables $(\boldsymbol{\delta}_1, ..., \boldsymbol{\delta}_{J^*}, \boldsymbol{\lambda}_1, ..., \boldsymbol{\lambda}_{J^*}, \boldsymbol{\epsilon})$ have the same likelihood as $(-\boldsymbol{\delta}_1, ..., -\boldsymbol{\delta}_{J^*}, -\boldsymbol{\lambda}_1, ..., -\boldsymbol{\lambda}_{J^*}, \boldsymbol{\epsilon})$ and usually have also the same prior probabilities. This effect makes the posterior distribution for these models multimodal, which induces problems for inference in general, and for MCMC convergence in particular. As a consequence, it may be advisable to restrict the parameter space in some way to avoid that multimodality and its associated problems. This could be done in several different ways, as for example restricting one of the components in each $\boldsymbol{\delta}_j$ to be positive. Nevertheless, in our experience, this procedure does not remove the MCMC convergence problems satisfactorily and the corresponding Markov chains for this component can easily get trapped in 0 for long runs of the simulation. In our experience, it is more satisfactory to change the orientation of $\boldsymbol{\lambda}_j$ and $\boldsymbol{\delta}_j$ accordingly at each step of the MCMC in order to fulfill the positivity condition on $\boldsymbol{\delta}_j$. In more detail, if we required $(\delta_j)_1$ to be positive, we would define

$$\hat{\boldsymbol{\delta}}_j = \left\{ \begin{array}{ll} \boldsymbol{\delta}_j & if \ (\delta_j)_1 > 0 \\ -\boldsymbol{\delta}_j & if \ (\delta_j)_1 \leq 0 \end{array} \right.$$

and

$$\hat{\boldsymbol{\lambda}}_j = \left\{ \begin{array}{ll} \boldsymbol{\lambda}_j & if \ (\delta_j)_1 > 0 \\ -\boldsymbol{\lambda}_j & if \ (\delta_j)_1 \leq 0 \end{array} \right.$$

and would define the linear predictor for the log-risks as a function of $\hat{\boldsymbol{\delta}}_j$ and $\hat{\boldsymbol{\lambda}}_j$, instead of $\boldsymbol{\delta}_j$ and $\boldsymbol{\lambda}_j$ (Marí-Dell'Olmo et al., 2011).

Interestingly, factor models can also be casted within the set of coregionalization models. Thus, let us assume a coregionalized M-model with the following particular structure for $\boldsymbol{M}' = [\boldsymbol{\delta}_1 : \ldots : \boldsymbol{\delta}_{J^*} : diag(\sigma_1, \ldots, \sigma_J)]$, i.e., $\boldsymbol{M}$ is matrix of dimensions $(J^* + J) \times J$. In a similar manner, let $\boldsymbol{\varphi} = [\boldsymbol{\lambda}_1 : \ldots : \boldsymbol{\lambda}_{J^*} : \epsilon_{.1} : \ldots : \epsilon_{.J}]$ be an $I \times (J^* + J)$ matrix, with the scales of its columns fixed, for example to 1. Then for these choices of $\boldsymbol{M}$ and $\boldsymbol{\varphi}$ it is easy to check that

$$\boldsymbol{\varphi}\boldsymbol{M} = \sum_{j=1}^{J^*} \boldsymbol{\lambda}_j \boldsymbol{\delta}_j' + \boldsymbol{\epsilon} \cdot diag(\boldsymbol{\sigma}).$$

The $diag(\boldsymbol{\sigma})$ term puts different scales to the residual variability of each disease as this seems to be a reasonable assumption. Then, any factor model can be expressed as a coregionalized M-model with the $\boldsymbol{M}$ and $\boldsymbol{\varphi}$ matrices as defined above.

Anyway, although closely related, factor models are usually posed with a different aim to general multivariate models. Factor models usually focus their interest on making inference on the common score vectors $\boldsymbol{\lambda}_j$, which could yield interesting information on the spatial distribution of risk factors or other quantities of interest. In particular, spatial factor analysis has been used on social data (Hogan and Tchernis, 2004; Abellán et al., 2007; Marí-Dell'Olmo et al., 2011) in order to build socioeconomic indicators which cannot be directly measured, such as material deprivation, but they have an effect on measurable observed variables coming from census or other surveys. The spatial distribution of those indicators is estimated as that of the common underlying pattern to all those related outcomes. On the other hand, Tzala and Best (2008) use spatial factor analysis for modeling the temporal evolution of the common factor underlying 6 diet-related cancers and Christensen and Amemiya (2002) apply it in an agricultural context in order to summarize the distribution of a set of soil properties.

Shared component models (Knorr-Held and Best, 2001) is a modeling proposal closely related to factor models which have attracted some attention in the literature. As originally formulated, for the study of $J = 2$ diseases, shared component models assume

$$O_{i1} \sim Pois(E_{i1} \cdot \varphi_i^{\delta} \cdot \varepsilon_{i1}) \ i = 1, \ldots, I$$

$$O_{i2} \sim Pois(E_{i2} \cdot \varphi_i^{1/\delta} \cdot \varepsilon_{i2}) \; i = 1, ..., I$$

where φ is a shared component for both diseases whose strength for each disease is modulated by δ, a positive parameter. The columns of ε model two disease-specific components that cannot be explained by the shared component. Taking logarithms of the relative risks in the expressions above, shared component models would be equivalent to assume

$$\boldsymbol{\Phi}_{\cdot 1} = \log(\varphi)\delta + \log(\varepsilon_{\cdot 1})$$

$$\boldsymbol{\Phi}_{\cdot 2} = \log(\varphi)/\delta + \log(\varepsilon_{\cdot 2}),$$

which clearly resembles a factor model of a single common factor with $\boldsymbol{\delta}_1 = (\delta, \delta^{-1})$, $\boldsymbol{\lambda}_1 = \log(\varphi)$ and $\boldsymbol{\epsilon} = \log(\varepsilon)$. In the original paper, a zero-centered Normal vague prior is assumed for δ and a spatial process, designed for detecting clusters (Knorr-Held and Raßer, 2000), is used for $\log(\varphi), \log(\varepsilon_{\cdot 1})$ and $\log(\varepsilon_{\cdot 2})$ instead of the omnipresent GMRFs typically used. Nevertheless, GMRFs are also frequently used for inducing spatial dependence on these vectors in shared component models (Richardson et al., 2006; Earnest et al., 2010; Ibañez Beroiz et al., 2011).

Extensions of shared component models to the study of more than 2 diseases have also been discussed in the literature (Held et al., 2005; MacNab, 2010). These attempts can also be understood as factor models with a particular restriction on the vector of weights $\boldsymbol{\delta}$. Specifically, a sum-to-zero restriction is assumed on the logarithms of those weights, i.e., $\sum_{j=1}^{J} \log(\delta_j) = 0$. Note that this restriction was also implicitly assumed for the case $J = 2$ as, in that case, $\boldsymbol{\delta} = (\delta, \delta^{-1})$; therefore, $\sum \log(\delta_j) = \log(\delta) + \log(\delta^{-1}) = 0$. This restriction fixes the geometric mean of the components of $\boldsymbol{\delta}$ (which are all positive); otherwise that mean would be confounded with the standard deviation of φ; that is; an increase in that mean could be compensated by a decrease in the mean of $\boldsymbol{\delta}$, and vice versa.

The main difference between factor and shared component models comes from the modeling of the weights of the common component $\boldsymbol{\delta}$ for these two approaches. For factor models, these weights can be either positive or negative, while for shared component models, those weights are necessarily positive. For the case of a factor model with a single underlying factor and $J = 2$ diseases, we would have

$$Cov(\boldsymbol{\Phi}_{\cdot 1}, \boldsymbol{\Phi}_{\cdot 2}) = Cov(\boldsymbol{\lambda}\delta_1 + \boldsymbol{\epsilon}_{\cdot 1}, \boldsymbol{\lambda}\delta_2 + \boldsymbol{\epsilon}_{\cdot 2}) = \delta_1\delta_2\sigma_\lambda^2.$$

This covariance can be either positive or negative, or even zero, depending on the signs of δ_1 and δ_2. However, for shared component models that covariance would be simply: $Cov(\boldsymbol{\Phi}_{\cdot 1}, \boldsymbol{\Phi}_{\cdot 2}) = \delta\delta^{-1}\sigma_\lambda^2 = \sigma_\lambda^2$, which is obviously positive. Therefore, shared component models always induce positive correlations on the geographical patterns modeled. Although this performance may be appropriate in some particular cases, it may not be so suitable in general settings with hypothetically possible negative correlations or simply no relationship between geographic patterns. In this sense, shared component models are more restrictive than general factor models.

8.3.2 Smoothed ANOVA

Another approach to multivariate modeling with considerable interest in our opinion is smoothed ANOVA, usually known as simply SANOVA. The main interest of this approach is the possibility that it offers to incorporate a specific design of a study into the analysis, if it existed, in order to model multivariate dependence. Most of the proposals in multivariate modeling are conceived for estimating, and therefore using, multivariate dependence between diseases, which is assumed, in principle, as fully unstructured. Nevertheless, in some cases, the design of a study could induce some specific structure on that dependence matrix. For example, let us assume that we wanted to perform a multivariate study comprising the joint analysis of 4 geographical patterns: chronic obstructive pulmonary disease (COPD) in men, COPD in women, lung cancer in men and lung cancer in women. Obviously, the mortality outcomes considered induce a particular dependence structure, making the correlation between the first and fourth patterns (or that between the second and third patterns) to be expectedly lower than that of the first and second or first and third patterns, for example. If possible, it would be convenient to incorporate that fact in the corresponding multivariate model. Moreover, in the previous setting it could be of particular interest to estimate the geographical pattern depicting the geographical differences between men and women, for these two causes as a whole. In a similar manner, we could be interested in determining the geographical pattern depicting the places with a higher COPD mortality, as compared to that of lung cancer and vice versa. All these are interesting questions that arise naturally as a consequence of the design assumed, which SANOVA seeks to answer.

SANOVA was originally proposed outside of the disease mapping context with different goals (Nobile and Green, 2000; Gelman, 2005a; Hodges et al., 2007). Zhang et al. (2009) originally proposed the use of SANOVA for multivariate disease mapping as an alternative to the use of the intrinsic MCAR distribution. This proposal structures the different sources of variability in multivariate studies as fixed and random effects in an ANOVA, incorporating spatial dependence structure for some of the terms in the model. This work was conceived as a simplified, lower dimensional approach to multivariate disease mapping studies where the eigenvectors of the covariance matrix between diseases are fixed by some specific statistical design or set by the modeler. As a consequence, the estimation of Σ_b reduces to the estimation of a set of eigenvalues, which is a parsimonious alternative to the use of the original MCAR distribution. Although this model was formulated as a simplified alternative to the MCAR distribution, its formulation relies heavily on the eigendecomposition of the covariance matrices between and within diseases. As a consequence, this proposal cannot be easily implemented in WinBUGS; indeed their authors coded it in R for the original paper.

In parallel, Marí Dell'Olmo et al. (2014) reformulated SANOVA with a very different aim, which makes it possible to incorporate easily the underlying design of the multivariate ensemble. As formulated by Marí-Dell'Olmo et al., SANOVA can be posed as a kind of factor model with given weights for each underlying factor. More in detail, SANOVA assumes a $J \times J$ orthogonal matrix $\boldsymbol{H}$ containing the coefficients of the 'contrasts' of interest that the modeler could be interested in. For example, for the COPD/lung cancer setting above $\boldsymbol{H}$ could be naturally defined as:

$$\boldsymbol{H} = \frac{1}{\sqrt{4}} \cdot \begin{pmatrix} 1 & 1 & 1 & 1 \\ 1 & 1 & -1 & -1 \\ 1 & -1 & 1 & -1 \\ 1 & -1 & -1 & 1 \end{pmatrix}$$

where the first column of $\boldsymbol{H}$ gives a common coefficient to all four patterns, so it corresponds to a common underlying component to all of them. The second component compares the COPD terms against those corresponding to lung cancer, so this component compares the different diseases considered. The third pattern compares the mortality causes corresponding to men against those corresponding to women and, finally, the fourth component would correspond to the interaction cause–sex for an ANOVA of the 4 groups considered. Note that the $1/\sqrt{4}$ term in $\boldsymbol{H}$ is needed to ensure the orthogonality of this matrix.

Given $\boldsymbol{H}$, SANOVA models the matrix of log-risks as $\boldsymbol{\Phi} = \sum_{j=1}^{J} \boldsymbol{\varphi}_{\cdot j}(\boldsymbol{H}_{\cdot j})' = \boldsymbol{\varphi}\boldsymbol{H}'$ for a matrix $\boldsymbol{\varphi}$ of spatially correlated random effects, where the relationship between SANOVA and factor models (with given vectors of weights) becomes clear. Note that SANOVA, as just formulated, do not have a specific unstructured error term $\boldsymbol{\epsilon}$ in contrast to factor models. This is because SANOVA models are often assumed to have as many underlying common factors (columns of $\boldsymbol{\varphi}$) as maps to be modeled (columns of $\boldsymbol{\Phi}$). In this sense factor models are typically considered to have just a limited number $J^*(< J)$ of factors, so the additional unstructured terms are required to model the remaining (univariate) variability in $\boldsymbol{\Phi}$. In contrast to factor models, SANOVA does not estimate the weights of each factor for each dimension but, on the contrary, it fixes them to some specific values given by the design of the study. Obviously, this is useful when the multivariate side of the study has a sensible design; otherwise, SANOVA does not seem to be the best modeling option.

The elements $\boldsymbol{\varphi}_{\cdot j}$ in the above formulation of SANOVA are I-vectors of spatial random effects. Interestingly, for the Marí-Dell'Olmo et al.'s reformulation these vectors could take any spatial distribution: ICAR, PCAR, BYM, etc. while for the original formulation this was not possible, they had to necessarily follow ICAR distributions. The reason for this limitation is that the original formulation depended on the eigenvectors of the covariance matrix of $\mathbf{\Sigma}_{vec(\mathbf{\Phi})}$. This matrix is fixed for ICAR distributions, which makes that eigendecomposition to be calculated just once, which yielded substantial computational benefit. For other spatial distributions, $\mathbf{\Sigma}_{vec(\mathbf{\Phi})}$ typically depends on one (or more) parameter(s), which forces that eigendecomposition to be computed at every step of the MCMC. Additionally, the coding of Marí-Dell'Olmo et al.'s reformulation of SANOVA in `WinBUGS`, or even in `INLA` (Marí Dell'Olmo et al., 2014), is fairly simple, which makes that proposal available to a more general community of users.

One of the more attractive features of SANOVA for multivariate modeling is that it allows us to take advantage of the ANOVA tools and concepts for studies of this kind. Specifically, SANOVA allows us to decompose the variance in the spatial patterns of $\mathbf{\Phi}$ as a function of the components considered in our model, which could be of even more interest than those patterns. More in detail, the total variance for the log-risks considered can be decomposed as

$$\sum_{j=1}^{J} Var(\mathbf{\Phi}_{\cdot j}) = \sum_{j=1}^{J} Var((\boldsymbol{\varphi}\boldsymbol{H}')_{\cdot j}) = \sum_{j=1}^{J} Var(\boldsymbol{\varphi}(\boldsymbol{H}_{j\cdot})')$$

$$= \sum_{j=1}^{J} \boldsymbol{H}_{j\cdot} Var(\boldsymbol{\varphi})(\boldsymbol{H}_{j\cdot})' = \sum_{j=1}^{J}\sum_{k=1}^{J} H_{jk}(\sigma_\varphi^2)_k H_{jk}$$

$$= \sum_{k=1}^{J} (\sigma_\varphi^2)_k (\sum_{j=1}^{J} H_{jk}^2) = \sum_{k=1}^{J}(\sigma_\varphi^2)_k,$$

where σ_φ^2 stands for the variances of the columns of matrix φ, the spatial underlying random effects. This expression makes clear how the variance of the set of log-risks is split into several components of particular meaning. Hence, the quantities $(\sigma_\varphi^2)_j / \sum_{k=1}^{J}(\sigma_\varphi^2)_k$ represent the proportion of variance of all the spatial patterns studied that is explained by the j-th column of φ. In a similar manner, we can also calculate the covariance between the spatial patterns in $\mathbf{\Phi}$ as

$$Cov(\mathbf{\Phi}_{\cdot j}, \mathbf{\Phi}_{\cdot j'}) = Cov(\boldsymbol{\varphi}(\boldsymbol{H}_{j\cdot})', \boldsymbol{\varphi}(\boldsymbol{H}_{j'\cdot})') = \boldsymbol{H}_{j\cdot} Cov(\boldsymbol{\varphi},\boldsymbol{\varphi})(\boldsymbol{H}_{j'\cdot})'$$

$$= \sum_{k=1}^{J} H_{jk} H_{j'k}(\sigma_\varphi^2)_k.$$

Thus, if the variances of the columns of φ were all equal, then $Cov(\mathbf{\Phi}_{\cdot j}, \mathbf{\Phi}_{\cdot j'}) \propto \sum_{k=1}^{J} H_{jk} H_{j'k}$ which would be 0 for $j \neq j'$. As a consequence, dependence between columns of $\mathbf{\Phi}$ arises as a product of the heteroscedasticity of φ's columns. Specifically, for the setting above, if $(\sigma_\varphi)_1$ was substantially higher than the rest of variances for φ's columns, a strong common underlying pattern will prevail for all 4 spatial patterns modeled. If, on the contrary, $\varphi_{\cdot 2}$

was the column with higher variance, geographical differences for the patterns corresponding to each of the two diseases will prevail regardless of the sex, and so on.

SANOVA has been also used in other contexts beyond multivariate disease mapping studies. For example, SANOVA-based spatio-temporal models have been also proposed by considering the columns of Φ as data corresponding to different periods of study and the columns of H as basis of functions for modeling the time trends for each spatial unit (Torres-Avilés and Martinez-Beneito, 2015). This approach makes it possible, by setting bases of functions of dimension much lower than J, to perform a low-dimensional fit of the spatio-temporal pattern, quite convenient for large spatio-temporal data sets. On the other hand SANOVA, as proposed by Marí-Dell'Olmo et al. and further developed in Marí-Dell'Olmo et al. (2014) or Martinez-Beneito et al. (2016), was devised as a method for performing multivariate ecological regression studies. Thus, for these studies, the columns of φ are modeled as a function of a covariate and a residual spatial component, which is assumed to be orthogonal to that covariate. This allows us to decompose the variance of the original log-risks into several components whose variance is further decomposed into a component associated with that covariate and a second component that cannot be explained by the covariate. This approach produces very rich results of high epidemiological interest.

Example 8.3

We are going to illustrate the use of SANOVA on a mortality study at the census tract level for Valencia city, as that in Example 5.2. In this case, we have studied two causes of death, lung cancer and chronic obstructive pulmonary disease (COPD) for both sexes, by separate, and the period of study has been split into two subperiods 1996-2001 and 2002-2007. These two causes of death are the two main respiratory causes of death; therefore, we would like to jointly study both causes in order to evidence any environmental potential risk factor that could increase respiratory deaths in general. We have the observed and expected death per census tract for each 2^3 combinations of these 3 factors; therefore, we have 8 maps to study altogether. In this case, it becomes clear that we have a particular design of the multivariate structure of the observations that we would like to take into account. In particular, we would like to know which is the common geographical pattern for all 8 maps, that is, which are the areas of Valencia city with an increased risk in general for all 8 combinations of the 3 factors considered. Additionally, we would like to know, which areas of Valencia have an increased risk for one of the causes of death in comparison to the mortality observed for the other cause, regardless of the sex or period. In the same manner, we would like to know if there is a region with particular high risk for one of the sexes and, finally, if there are regions

Pattern	Variance	% Variance explained
common	0.142	58.2%
Dif. diseases	0.056	23.0%
Dif. sexes	0.008	3.1%
Dif. periods	0.034	13.8%
Interaction 1	0.003	1.2%
Interaction 2	0.001	0.2%
Interaction 3	0.001	0.3%
Interaction 4	0.000	0.2%

Table 8.2
Variance decomposition for the terms considered in the SANOVA model.

with particularly increased risk for any of the periods of study. In addition, we will be interested in quantifying the contribution of all these factors to the whole variability of the 8 geographical patterns considered. A similar study for Barcelona city has also been undertaken in Martinez-Beneito et al. (2016).

We have considered 8 underlying patterns in our SANOVA model. The first one models the geographical variability for all 8 risk maps as a whole; the second pattern studies the geographical differences in risks between diseases; the third pattern compares the risk patterns between sexes; and the fourth pattern compares both periods of study. The four additional underlying risk patterns model several interaction terms between these main factors. Table 8.2 shows the variance accounted for each of these underlying patterns and the proportion of variance explained by each of them. This table shows how the common pattern is the factor taking the main effect on the set of risk patterns considered, which explains the 58.2% of the variance of the 8 original risk patterns. The second main factor explaining the geographical variability of all 8 maps is the common pattern to all of them, which explains a 23% of the whole variance, so all 8 maps show substantial differences between diseases despite the strong common component to all of them. Differences between periods and differences between sexes have a much milder contribution to the explanation of that whole variance. These main factors explain the 98.2% of the whole variance, while the remaining 1.8% is explained by interactions between those main factors.

Figure 8.4 shows the geographical patterns corresponding to the main factors in the SANOVA model. It is evident how the patterns explaining a higher proportion of variance have a more clear risk pattern than the rest. The upper left plot shows the common geographical risk pattern for the 8 combinations of factors analyzed. The brown areas in this plot correspond to regions showing in general an increased risk for all 8 factor combinations, while green areas correspond to regions with a lower risk. It can be seen that there are several isolated high-risk neighbourhoods scattered around Valencia. These

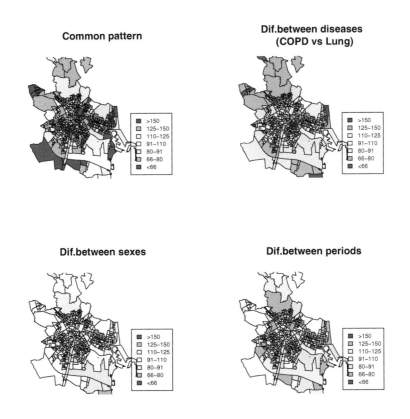

Figure 8.4
Geographical patterns for the main factors considered in the SANOVA model.

neighbourhoods correspond mainly to those locations with a high deprivation, as can be checked in Figure 5.1. Thus, the overall mortality for all 8 geographical patterns in this study is mainly associated with deprivation, being the regions with a higher deprivation those showing also a higher mortality. The upper-right figure corresponds to disease differences in mortality. Specifically, the brown areas correspond to those having a larger lung cancer mortality as compared to the COPD mortality found in those regions. Conversely, the green areas show larger COPD mortality as compared to the observed lung cancer mortality in those regions. We can see that the north-east side of Valencia has more lung cancer than COPD risk for all two sexes and periods. The lower-left map shows mortality differences between sexes. In this map, the brown areas correspond to those regions with higher mortality in men as compared to the female mortality observed there. This map shows hardly any noticeable pattern, as it could be anticipated by the variance decomposition above. Finally, the lower-right plot shows mortality differences between periods. In this map brown areas stand for regions with higher mortality at the first period of study, in comparison to the observed mortality for the second period. This map does not show any clear geographical pattern. In contrast, it shows a high heterogeneity, thus temporal changes in mortality have had a very local scope.

8.3.3 Other approaches

To conclude this chapter, we find it convenient to mention some multivariate modeling proposals that would not fall within the categories previously introduced. Although these works could be seen as more or less isolated efforts for building multivariate structures, their ideas may be of help for future developments in this field. Hence, it may be of interest to mention them here. Specifically, we introduce first some works that rely on non-GMRF spatial structures and conclude with some proposals that estimate the multivariate dependence structure between diseases but also estimate the spatial dependence structure according to the set of spatial patterns considered.

Meligkotsidou (2007) proposes a multivariate disease mapping model based on mixtures of multivariate Poisson distributions (Karlis and Meligkotsidou, 2007). In contrast to multivariate Poisson models, mixtures of these processes are able to reproduce negative correlations between diseases or overdispersion. Anyway, this mixture model does not explicitly induce any prior spatial structure on the risks so they are spatially independent. Thus, although applied to a multivariate disease mapping context (a trivariate study on larynx, pharynx and oral cancer) this proposal is somewhat limited for spatial modeling in general. The number of components in the mixture is considered unknown, so sampling from that mixture model requires the use of reversible jump MCMC algorithms. As a consequence, neither `WinBUGS` nor `INLA` can be used for making inference on this model and a specific ad-hoc coding in another programming environment is therefore required.

Moraga and Lawson (2012) propose a multivariate version of a first-order spatial moving average process (Stern and Cressie, 1999; Botella-Rocamora et al., 2012). This multivariate moving average model considers J spatially independent patterns, although correlated between diseases. Later on, a local moving average of those underlying processes is considered for each disease. Thus, the underlying process induces dependence between diseases and the moving average induces spatial dependence on the estimated risks. In this sense, this proposal would be similar to that of Gelfand and Vounatsou (2003), which can be seen as a multivariate process where spatial dependence is induced as a second step (Martinez-Beneito, 2013). The multivariate Gaussian component mixture, as named by the authors, is implemented in WinBUGS. A three-variate study illustrates also the performance of this model on a simulated data set.

We have seen throughout this chapter that covariance between diseases may be estimated in multivariate studies when dealing with several spatial patterns together. In a similar manner, we could think of estimating the spatial covariance structure when several spatial patterns are available. This set of spatial patterns could help us know the degree of dependence of risks for nearby spatial units. Several works have proposed the joint estimation of both dependence structures, between and within diseases, at the same time. Thus, Ma and Carlin (2007) propose an adaptation of Wombling (see Section 6.5) to the multivariate context. Starting from a given neighbourhood structure, and therefore a given adjacency matrix for the spatial structure, Wombling assigned a binary 0/1 variable to all the original edges and pruned that original adjacency graph. This process is made within the model itself. Now, for the multivariate case, a more complex Wombling spatial process is considered which weighs the edges of the original graph, while a multivariate structure between diseases is also estimated. This process was applied for a shared component model where Wombling was used to enhance the spatial structure of the shared component term and on an intrinsic MCAR multivariate distribution. The Wombled shared component model gave slightly better results on a multivariate study of three cancers. This model was implemented in WinBUGS and, according to our knowledge, it cannot be implemented in INLA.

Dobra et al. (2011) make another proposal on the joint estimation of the between and within diseases covariance structures. These authors assume a $\mathcal{G}$-Wishart prior distribution for the precision matrices of both spatial structures. That distribution has as domain the cone of symmetric, positive definite matrices with non-zero cells (i, j) belonging to a graph $\mathcal{G}$. For inducing spatial dependence, the mean of the corresponding $\mathcal{G}$-Wishart prior would be a precision matrix reflecting the spatial dependence structure of the region of study, such as a typical PCAR precision matrix $(\boldsymbol{D} - \rho \boldsymbol{W})$ with unknown ρ. This prior distribution would estimate a spatial precision matrix resembling $(\boldsymbol{D} - \rho \boldsymbol{W})$, for a suitable value of ρ, with non-zero cells only for those pairs of units being neighbours in the corresponding adjacency graph. Regarding covariance between diseases, another $\mathcal{G}$-Wishart prior distribution is assumed for Σ_b^{-1}, but in this case we do not have any prior guess on a suitable dependence graph for the different causes considered. As a consequence, reversible jump MCMC is used for estimating the graph $\mathcal{G}$ which determines the non-zero cells of Σ_b^{-1}. Thus, interestingly, Dobra et al.'s approach estimates the non-zero cells of the between and within disease precision matrices in multivariate models, but also induces sparsity on Σ_b^{-1}, which is an interesting additional property of this model. Smith et al. (2015) follow also this approach but by using truncated $\mathcal{G}$-Wishart prior distributions, which enforce positive conditional correlations for all neighbouring nodes of $\mathcal{G}$. This assumption seems very sensible for modeling spatial data. Sampling from $\mathcal{G}$-Wishart prior distribution is not possible from within WinBUGS, so specific coding has to be developed in other programming languages for making inference on these models.

Exercises

1. The MV.Rdata file, available at the online material of the book (https://github.com/MigueBeneito/DisMapBook/tree/master/Exercises), contains two R objects: MV and MV.age. As always, the information in these objects has been slightly modified in order to preserve data confidentiality. The first of these objects contains the observed mortality, for each of the Valencia city census tracts, for lung cancer, prostate cancer, COPD and cirrhosis in men. The second of these objects contains the age-specific observed counts for each of these causes of death for the whole Valencia city.

   • Compute, by using internal standardization, the expected deaths for each census tract and for all 4 causes of death. For this task, you will need the age-specific population for each census tract available at the COPD.Rdata file, also available with the rest of online material.

   • Fit an LCAR multivariate M-model for these 4 causes of death.

   • Which of the variables in this model are identifiable, and which are not? Check the convergence of the identifiable variables in the model. Compute the deviance (you can find how to do it at any of the examples that compute the DIC for any WinBUGS model) for each simulation, and draw a history plot for checking the convergence of this parameter.

- Draw two choropleth maps for the $sSMR$s and $P(sSMR > 1)$, respectively, for the COPD mortality. Compare these two choropleth maps with the corresponding univariate COPD choropleth maps made as exercises for Chapter 4.

- Explore the variance-covariance and correlation matrices between diseases for this model. Draw choropleth maps for the $sSMR$s for all 4 causes of death studied. Check how those causes of death with a higher correlation between diseases show, visually, the most similar geographical patterns.

- Change the univariate LCAR distributions used in the M-model by an alternative spatial distribution. Assess the change obtained in the $sSMR$s for this new model.

9

Multidimensional modeling

We are going to conclude this book by introducing multidimensional modeling in disease mapping studies, the most complex form of disease mapping models that integrate several, but always more than 2, sources of dependence. In the previous chapter, we have seen how multivariate modeling profits from additional unstructured sources of dependence, beyond spatial correlation, in order to improve risk estimates. On the other hand, spatio-temporal modeling profited from an additional structured factor, time, in order to split the original observed cases into several disjoint time periods allowing to visualize the temporal changes in risks. Multidimensional disease mapping models integrate spatial dependence with several structured, such as time or age, or unstructured factors, such as causes of death, sex, race, etc. into a single model.

Multidimensional models are able to achieve two goals. On one hand, they allow us to disaggregate information in disease mapping studies into smaller statistical units, such as several time periods that were previously merged into single observations or several age groups when all age groups were previously merged, while keeping the reliability of the risk estimates for these new disaggregated groups. In this sense, spatio-temporal models allow us to analyze data on this collection of smaller statistical units with similar reliability than in the original pooled analysis. Multidimensional models allow for that same possibility. On the other hand, multivariate studies generally integrate additional sources of dependence with the purpose of improving the univariate risk estimates that did not take the new source of dependence into account. Multidimensional models are able to fulfill these two goals separately, or both together. As a consequence, multidimensional modeling is the most complete and advanced topic in disease mapping studies.

The structuring of several dependence structures into a single model in a sensible and computationally affordable manner is a challenging goal which makes multidimensional modeling an emerging topic with, for now, a scarce literature. The goal of this chapter is introducing this incipient branch of disease mapping which is progressively getting more attention. This chapter is divided into only two sections. Section 9.1 formulates multidimensional studies in statistical terms and reviews some of the previous proposals in the literature. Finally, Section 9.2 introduces the work by Martinez-Beneito et al. (2017) which develops a formal framework for multidimensional disease mapping studies.

9.1   A brief introduction and review of multidimensional modeling

Univariate models dealt with a single outcome per spatial unit; therefore, the set of observed deaths per unit for the region of study was arranged into a vector o. For spatio-temporal and multivariate modeling, we had several observations per spatial unit; therefore, they were arranged into a matrix O with as many rows as spatial units and as many columns as time periods or causes of death in the study. In multidimensional models, we will have at least three factors: space and two or more additional factors; therefore, we will arrange the information into an array of as many dimensions as factors we have in our study. Without any loss of generality, we will assume henceforth that our study considers just three factors and the first of them will always correspond to space, in accordance to spatio-temporal and multivariate models. If at some moment the extension of multidimensional models to 4 or more factors entailed some particularity in comparison to the three-dimensional case, we will mention it accordingly.

A statistical formulation for (three-dimensional) multidimensional modeling could be the following. Let $O = (O_{ijk})_{i,j,k=1}^{I,J,K}$ be the observed number of deaths for the i-th spatial unit for categories j and k for the second and third factors, respectively, considered in the study. In that case, it is usually assumed that

$$O_{ijk} \sim Pois(E_{ijk}\theta_{ijk})$$

where E_{ijk} and θ_{ijk} are the expected cases and relative risk, respectively, for the corresponding combinations of subindexes. Usually, $\log(\theta_{ijk})$ is decomposed as $\mu_{jk} + \theta_{ijk}$ where μ is a matrix of intercepts for each of the JK spatial patterns considered and $\Theta = (\theta_{ijk})_{i,j,k=1}^{I,J,K}$ is an array of random effects accounting for the dependence induced by all the factors in the multidimensional model. The main challenge in multidimensional models is inducing all those sources of dependence into Φ. Several proposals have been already formulated with that goal which correspond to the different proposals on multidimensional disease mapping published in the literature.

For the frequent case that one of the factors considered was age groups, the expected cases in the formulation above are usually changed by N_{ijk}, the population corresponding to that age group since the age-standardization leading to the expected cases will no longer have sense. In that case the Poisson assumption can be changed for a binomial distribution, mostly if the values of the N_{ijk}s are low. This is something common if the original data set was split into several time periods and several age groups, for example, which decreases considerably the amount of population per cell exposed in the study. In that case, a typical formulation of a multidimensional problem would be:

$$O_{ijk} \sim Bin(\theta_{ijk}, N_{ijk})$$

where now the array Θ would contain the probabilities of death for the corresponding combinations of subindexes.

Multidimensional models date back almost to the first proposals of Bayesian hierarchical models for disease mapping. The first attempts of multidimensional modeling were a bit simple. For example, Waller et al. (1997) propose a model for a 4-dimensional study including space, time, sex and race. This proposal models the effect of sex and race as fixed effects, with interaction between these factors. Additionally, space and time are also assumed to interact by assuming a different spatial pattern per time period (Type III interaction according to the classification of Knorr-Held (2000)). No interaction was assumed between sex or race with space or time, or other interactions of higher order.

Multidimensional models have also resorted to similar tools to induce dependence between observations than those used in the disease mapping literature. Thus, Sun et al. (2000) considered a three-dimensional study depending on space, time and age, that we will index in this same order. Sun et al. proposed to model interaction between periods, on one hand, and counties+age, on the other hand, as a kind of spatially varying coefficient model. More in detail, the log-risks were modeled as

$$\log(\theta_{ijk}) = \alpha_i + \beta_k + (\gamma_i + \delta_k) \cdot (t_j - \bar{t}) + \epsilon_{ijk}.$$

The third term in this expression models the effect of time in a linear manner, but that effect varies for each county and age group. Nevertheless, that interaction is a bit limited due to the linear assumption on time. Proper CAR distributions were assumed for α and γ. On the other hand, β and δ were treated as fixed effects since only 4 different levels were considered for age. Finally, ϵ considers three-way interaction between all three dimensions in the array, although independence is assumed for all their cells, which seems a restrictive assumption.

A common approach to multidimensional modeling is decomposing the variability in the log-risks as a function of main effects and interactions as in an ANOVA. The first formulation following this approach was proposed by Knorr-Held and Besag (1998). These authors pose a multidimensional real problem with 5 factors: space, time, age, gender and race, although the last two factors were combined into a single demographic factor with 4 levels. The subindexes of the following arrays correspond to these factors in this same order. In this case the binomial formulation was chosen and the logit of the probabilities of death were modeled as

$$logit(\theta_{ijkl}) = \alpha_i + \beta_j + \Gamma_{jk} + \Delta_{jl}.$$

The first of the components, α, modeling the probabilities Θ accounts for spatial dependence between counties, and a BYM structure was set for that term. In a similar manner β accounts for the temporal variability in Θ as a whole. A random walk prior is set as prior structure for this parameter. Both

α and β would model the main effects of space and time. In contrast, the age and demographic effects are assumed to vary for each year and therefore their interaction with time is modeled instead of their pure main effect. Random walk prior structures in time are set for Γ and Δ, assuming independence between age and demographic groups, respectively. Additionally, sum-to-zero constraints were imposed for the interaction terms $\Gamma_{j\cdot}$ and $\Delta_{j\cdot}$ for each time interval in order to avoid confounding between the pure temporal term β and these interactions.

Goicoa et al. (2016b) and Goicoa et al. (2018a) follow similar approaches to that of Knorr-held and Besag. Both works consider three-dimensional models for space, time and age and in a similar manner to the model above they model the main effects and different interactions for that data structure. Nevertheless, the interaction terms considered in these two works are much more comprehensive than those introduced above. Specifically, the most complex proposal in Goicoa et al. (2016b) models the log-risks as:

$$\log(\theta_{ijk}) = \alpha + \beta_i + \gamma_j + \delta_k + \Lambda_{ij}^1 + \Lambda_{ik}^2 + \Lambda_{jk}^3 + \Lambda_{ijk}^4.$$

In this expression β accounts for spatial variability and an LCAR prior distribution is assumed for this vector. The vectors γ and δ account for temporal and age-related variability, respectively, and random walk priors are considered for these terms. Matrices Λ^i, $i = 1, ..., 3$ model pairwise interaction terms for the factors in the model. All these terms are modeled as Normal random effects with separable precision matrices. These precision matrices of these terms are the product of the precision matrix of an ICAR distribution, for those interaction terms considering spatial dependence, and the precision matrix of the corresponding random walk prior. For interaction between time and age the precision matrix Λ^3 is the product of two random walk precision matrices. Finally, the three-way interaction in Λ^4 is also modeled as an array of random effects with separable structure integrating the corresponding spatial (ICAR), temporal (random walk) and age-specific (random walk) precision into a common precision matrix.

Note that, as mentioned in Chapter 6, a random walk can be considered as an equivalent of the ICAR distribution for ordinal variables. Additionally, ICAR precision matrices have a single parameter controlling variability therefore the precision matrices of the interaction terms above are all of the form $\sigma^{-2}Q$ for a given known matrix Q. This allows us to fit the model above in INLA by coding these interaction terms with the `model="generic0"` option of this software. This modeling option allows us to fit random effects where the precision term is known up to a constant term controlling the variability of the random effect. Therefore INLA can be used for fitting the interaction terms in this model. Goicoa et al. (2018a) considers basically the same models as those posed in Goicoa et al. (2016b) but modeling the effects of time and age, and the corresponding interaction terms, by means of P-spline instead of correlated random effects. INLA was also used to fit the P-spline models in this latter work.

Both modeling proposals introduced in the previous paragraphs were applied to the study of prostate and breast cancer mortality in Spain, splitting the period of study in separate years and age in quinquennial groups. For both studies, several alternative models were considered, ranging from the simplest option which included just the main effects for space, time and age, to the most complex proposals described above with all possible interaction terms. Interestingly, for both studies, the most appropriate model among the 9 possible models considered was the most complex model described above including all the interaction terms. This suggests the convenience of including high order interactions when analyzing multidimensional problems. In general, simpler models do not seem able to reproduce important features in the data required to explain them properly.

Multidimensional modeling by decomposing the log-risks as a combination of main effects and interactions requires, in general, the use of sum-to-zero restrictions. Those restrictions avoid the terms in that decomposition to be confounded and therefore favour their identifiability. The satisfactory handling of sum-to-zero restrictions by `INLA` makes it a very competitive option for making inference on models of this kind.

The use of models decomposing the log-risks into main effects and their interactions has also been proposed in conjunction with other general modeling tools in disease mapping. Thus, Richardson et al. (2006) consider also a three-dimensional model with space, time and sex. They do not include main effects in the linear component, but they use a shared component model for the interaction between space-sex and time-sex. ICAR prior distributions were used for the spatial and temporal structures of these interaction terms. Additionally, the authors include a random effect term for the three-way interaction of all three factors, considering dependence just between sexes. Tzala and Best (2008) develop a similar proposal for a multidimensional problem considering space, time and different causes of death. In this study, the authors consider 6 causes of death instead of 2 sexes, in contrast to Richardson et al. (2006), so the shared component model is now changed by factor spatial models, which generalize the first to more than 2 levels. The most complex proposal in Tzala and Best (2008) models the log-risks as:

$$\log(\theta_{ijk}) = \lambda_k \Lambda_{ij} + \Gamma_{ik} + \Delta_{jk} + \Upsilon_{ijk}$$

where $\boldsymbol{\lambda}$ models the weights of the common spatio-temporal pattern $\boldsymbol{\Lambda}$ on each cause of death. Additional space-cause ($\boldsymbol{\Gamma}$) and time-cause ($\boldsymbol{\Delta}$) interaction terms are also considered in order to model specific features that could not be captured by the first factor term. These features would be common for all time and space units, respectively, for each cause of death. Finally, a completely unstructured three-dimensional interaction term is considered accounting for the remaining variability that could not be fitted by the previous components. The main goal for these works, in contrast to the rest of proposal above, is estimating the common component (and its evolution in time) underlying both sexes in one case and all causes of death in the other case. These factors are of great interest from an epidemiological point of view. Model selection is carried out also in these studies comparing the models described with simpler alternatives. Interestingly, once again, the most complex models were preferred in both cases, pointing out the convenience of considering complex models with complex interactions in order to appropriately describe the variability in these intricate data sets with so many sources of dependence. All the models proposed in these two works were coded and run in `WinBUGS`.

Zhang et al. (2006) consider a 4-dimensional study including space, time, sex and age group (we will subindex these factors in this same order). In contrast to the previous works, which decomposed the log-risks as a sum of main effects and interaction terms, Zhang et al. model them as the sum of two arrays, one structured and another one fully unstructured providing additional flexibility that could not be reproduced by the first term. The structured term mentioned ($\mathbf{\Omega}$) is defined as an array of Normal random effects and dependence is induced into that array by the direct modeling of the covariance matrix of its cells. Thus, if $vec(\mathbf{\Omega}) = (\Omega_{1\ldots1}, \Omega_{2\ldots1}, ..., \Omega_{I\ldots1}, ..., \Omega_{IJKL})$, then this vector is assumed to follow a $N_{I\cdot J\cdot K\cdot L}(\mathbf{0}, \mathbf{\Sigma}_{\mathbf{\Omega}})$ prior distribution. Two possibilities were considered for $\mathbf{\Sigma}_{vec(\mathbf{\Omega})}$. First, a separable model was considered by setting $\mathbf{\Sigma}_{vec(\mathbf{\Omega})} = \mathbf{\Sigma}_D \otimes \mathbf{\Sigma}_T \otimes \mathbf{\Sigma}_S$ where $\mathbf{\Sigma}_D$, $\mathbf{\Sigma}_T$ and $\mathbf{\Sigma}_S$ denote demographic (sex+age), temporal and spatial covariance matrices, respectively. Regarding $\mathbf{\Sigma}_D$, it is defined as the block diagonal matrix $Bdiag(\{(\mathbf{\Sigma}_D)_l\}_{l=1}^L)$ where the 2×2 matrices in the diagonal model the covariance between sexes for each age group, which are assumed to be different. $\mathbf{\Sigma}_T$ is assumed to be the covariance matrix of a second-order random walk process in time and $\mathbf{\Sigma}_S$ is the covariance matrix corresponding to a PCAR process depending on a spatial parameter (ρ). Note that this model is a separable structure of demography, time and space but the demographic component, which integrates sex and age, is not separable since the covariance matrices between sexes vary for each age group. Therefore, we cannot talk about a single covariance matrix between sexes. Note also that the proposed model does not consider dependence of any kind between age groups.

Zhang et al. (2006) consider a second alternative modeling proposal. In this case $\mathbf{\Sigma}_{vec(\mathbf{\Omega})} = Bdiag(\{\mathbf{\Sigma}_l\}_{l=1}^L)$, where $\mathbf{\Sigma}_l = (\mathbf{\Sigma}_D)_l \otimes \mathbf{\Sigma}_T \otimes (\mathbf{\Sigma}_S)_l$, $l = 1, ..., L$ for suitable demographic, temporal and spatial covariance matrices. This new proposal considers once again independence between age groups and, in contrast to the previous model, the spatial covariance matrix $(\mathbf{\Sigma}_S)_l$ varies also between age groups. Specifically, these matrices correspond to covariance matrices of PCAR distributions with correlation parameters ρ_l varying between age groups. Obviously, this new covariance structure is no longer separable as there is not a common spatial covariance structure for all age groups considered. Zhang et al. compare both models in their paper and find that different spatial patterns (of different correlation parameters) and different correlations between sexes are required for each age group in order to appropriately describe the data set considered. Therefore, once again, the model comparison performed points towards the most complex option in a multidimensional context. This result advises the use of complex, even inseparable, modeling options since simpler models may not be enough for explaining the intricate entanglement of dependence structures in this setting. The authors report the full conditionals of the parameters in the model used to build the MCMC, although they do not make available the code used to run the models in the paper.

Multidimensional studies usually face a particular computational challenge since the number of units of study increases explosively for these models. For example, in the feasible setting of having a three-dimensional model depending on space, time and age with 10 time periods and 10 age groups we would have a problem 100 times larger than the corresponding univariate spatial problem. Moreover, all the units of study in this problem show three separate sources of dependence, which makes the computational problems in the multidimensional setting particularly challenging. As a consequence, computational issues in multidimensional studies have recently focussed considerable attention on the literature. Thus, Bradley et al. (2018) propose a multidimensional model which was successfully applied to a problem with above $4 \cdot 10^6$ observations. Bradley et al. build a conjugate log-gamma process for the log-risks instead of using a typical mixed Poisson generalized linear model with logarithmic link. This process, jointly with the rest of the assumptions made in the model, makes the conditional posterior distributions of the parameters conjugate and very convenient therefore for MCMC sampling, which makes possible the fit of such a large data set. The main focus in this work relies on computational issues instead of on the particular structuring of covariance for the units of study. Additionally, Quick et al. (2018) consider also a three-dimensional model for space, time and demographic groups (race+sex). They apply their model to a study of over $2.3 \cdot 10^5$ observations. For making this possible, they model the observed rates per 100,000 people as Normal variables making the prior distribution of the random effects in this model conjugate. Quick et al. propose two models in their paper, first a separable model for all three dependence structures in the problem is assumed. Additionally, they consider a non-separable model with covariance matrices between demographic groups varying for each time period and temporal correlations varying also for each demographic group. Once again the most complex proposal in this work is found to be more adequate than its simpler (separable) alternative. The implementation of these two works have required the ad-hoc coding of the corresponding (efficient) MCMC algorithms.

9.2   A formal framework for multidimensional modeling

The previous section has depicted a heterogeneous panorama for multidimensional disease mapping. There are already a few works in this area published, but their approaches are quite heterogeneous, interactions are considered or discarded, for example, in an ad hoc manner. Therefore, a unifying and comprehensive framework for multidimensional modeling would be very welcome. The previous works in the literature yield two main messages. First, a general multidimensional modeling framework should allow enough complexity as for modeling high order interactions between the factors considered. We have seen how the previous approaches generally prefer the most complex alternatives with complex interactions so that complexity is generally required for the modeling of data of this type. Second, the computational challenge posed by multidimensional studies is a non-negligible issue and this should be always borne in mind when formulating general (and hopefully scalable) modeling proposals. If inference on these proposals was suitable in widely used inference packages for disease mapping practitioners, such as `WinBUGS` or `INLA`, this would be also a very convenient feature of that proposal, making it accessible to a large number of potential users.

In this section, we are going to introduce the multidimensional modeling proposal in Martinez-Beneito et al. (2017). This work introduces a general modeling framework for multidimensional disease mapping. This proposal fulfills the requirements mentioned in the previous paragraph: a complex enough modeling framework, computational convenience and being implementable in `WinBUGS`. However, besides these practical advantages, the multidimensional framework of Martinez-Beneito et al. provides a theoretical study of the models proposed therein. For those models, the covariance matrix for the set of observations in the study can be easily derived, which makes it possible to explore and to classify those models. Additionally, that framework deploys a set of mathematical tools to induce dependence between factors in the model and even a nomenclature for the models generated by combining those tools. Thus, that framework provides a theoretical (and practical) basis for developing lots of proposals for multidimensional disease mapping.

The proposal in Martinez-Beneito et al. (2017) is based on the development of M-models by Botella-Rocamora et al. (2015), which are a particular case of multivariate coregionalization models, as mentioned in Chapter 8. Surely, similar general multidimensional frameworks could be also derived by following the conditional approach also introduced in Chapter 8. Currently, that generalization of the conditional approach to the multidimensional setting has not been undertaken. Possibly, this is due to the extreme flexibility of that approach that in the multidimensional setting would be difficult to summarize to useful (and computationally affordable) proposals. For this reason, we are introducing the coregionalization multidimensional approach of Martinez-Beneito et al.

9.2.1 Some tools and notation

Firstly, we are going to introduce some array algebra tools and some notation that will be extensively used for the rest of this section. We did not introduce this notation in Chapter 1, since it is going to be exclusively used in this section so there was no need to set it at the beginning of the book.

We define an N-th order *tensor*, or *array*, of dimensions $(L_1, L_2, \ldots, L_N)$ as any element in the set $\{\boldsymbol{X} : \boldsymbol{X} \in \mathbb{R}^{L_1 \times L_2 \times \ldots \times L_N}\}$. We will not make any difference in terms of notation between matrices and arrays, we will denote both of them in uppercase bold letters. Vectors and matrices will be also considered as arrays of first and second order, respectively.

The *vector unfolding* of an array $\boldsymbol{X}$, noted by $vec(\boldsymbol{X})$ as for matrices, is the result of the rearranging of the elements of $\boldsymbol{X}$ into a vector in the following way $vec(\boldsymbol{X}) = (X_{1\ldots1}, X_{2\ldots1}, \ldots, X_{L_1\ldots1}, \ldots, X_{L_1,\ldots,L_N})'$. Similarly, the reordering of the elements of $\boldsymbol{X}$ into a matrix will be called *matrix unfolding*. Thus, the *n-dimension matrix unfolding* of $\boldsymbol{X}$, denoted by $\boldsymbol{X}^{(n)}$, is just the $L_n \times \prod_{i=1,i\neq n}^{N} L_i$ matrix

$$[\boldsymbol{X}_{1\ldots1\cdot1\ldots1} : \boldsymbol{X}_{2\ldots1\cdot1\ldots1} : \ldots : \boldsymbol{X}_{L_1\ldots1\cdot1\ldots1} : \ldots : \boldsymbol{X}_{L_1\ldots L_{n-1}\cdot L_{n+1}\ldots L_N}],$$

where $\boldsymbol{X}_{i_1\ldots i_{n-1}\cdot i_{n+1}\ldots i_N}$, with "$\cdot$" in the n-th index position, is the $L_n \times 1$ vector $(X_{i_1\ldots i_{n-1},j,i_{n+1}\ldots i_N})_{j=1}^{L_n}$.

More generally, let $\boldsymbol{r} = (1, 2, \ldots, n_r)$ with $n_r < N$. The $\boldsymbol{r}$-*matrix unfolding* of the array $\boldsymbol{X}$, denoted by $\boldsymbol{X}^{(\boldsymbol{r})}$, is the $(\prod_{i\in\{1,\ldots,n_r\}} L_i) \times (\prod_{j\in\{n_r+1,\ldots,N\}} L_j)$ matrix formed by stacking the column-vectors

$$\{vec(\boldsymbol{x}_{\ldots\cdot i_{n_r+1}\ldots i_N}); \ i_{n_r+1} = 1, \ldots, L_{n_r+1}; \ldots; i_N = 1, \ldots, L_N\}.$$

The $\boldsymbol{r}$-matrix unfolding of arrays can be further generalized to any set of indices (not just for $\boldsymbol{r} = (1, \ldots, n_r)$) by simply permuting the indices $\{1, \ldots, N\}$ of the array before applying the above definition. We will refer to the inverse process of unfolding an array as *folding*. In summary: $vec(\boldsymbol{X}), \boldsymbol{X}^{(1)}, \ldots, \boldsymbol{X}^{(N)}$ and $\boldsymbol{X}^{(\boldsymbol{r})}$ just recast the array $\boldsymbol{X}$ into vector and matrices, respectively, in several alternative ways.

We are going to introduce now some array operations that will be extensively used throughout this section. The *n-dimensional product* (with $1 \leq n \leq N$) of an array $\boldsymbol{X}$ with an $L_n \times L_n$ matrix $\boldsymbol{A}$ is defined as the array $\boldsymbol{Y}$ resulting from folding $\boldsymbol{A} \cdot \boldsymbol{X}^{(n)}$ into an array of the same dimensions as $\boldsymbol{X}$. In that case, we denote $\boldsymbol{Y} = \boldsymbol{A} \circ_n \boldsymbol{X}$ or, in other words,

$$\boldsymbol{Y} = \boldsymbol{A} \circ_n \boldsymbol{X} \longleftrightarrow \boldsymbol{Y}^{(n)} = \boldsymbol{A}\boldsymbol{X}^{(n)}. \tag{9.1}$$

Note that the n-dimensional product of $\boldsymbol{A}$ and $\boldsymbol{X}$ simply premultiplies the vectors $X_{i_1 \ldots i_{n-1} \cdot i_{n+1} \ldots i_N}$, for all suitable values of the subindexes, by $\boldsymbol{A}$. Therefore, despite its apparent complexity, this operation is conceptually and mathematically very easy to compute in practice. In fact, it can be easily coded in WinBUGS. As an example, the following lines show the coding of the product $\boldsymbol{A} \circ_2 \boldsymbol{X}$ for an array $\boldsymbol{X}$ of order 3:

```
for(i in 1:L1){
  for(k in 1:L3){
    for(j in 1:L2){
      Y[i,j,k]<-inprod2(A[j,],X[i,,k])
    }
  }
}
```

The code in this example is easily generalizable to arrays of higher orders or other dimensions of the array $\boldsymbol{X}$. This operation modifies the array $\boldsymbol{X}$ by transforming each vector $\boldsymbol{X}_{i \cdot k}$ in that array into $\boldsymbol{Y}_{i \cdot k} = \boldsymbol{A}\boldsymbol{X}_{i \cdot k}$. This operation makes the cells of $\boldsymbol{Y}$ dependent, as all of them will be linear combinations of common elements, the cells of a particular dimension of $\boldsymbol{X}$. Specifically, $\boldsymbol{Y}_{ijk} = \boldsymbol{A}_{j \cdot} \boldsymbol{X}_{i \cdot k}$ and $\boldsymbol{Y}_{ij'k} = \boldsymbol{A}_{j' \cdot} \boldsymbol{X}_{i \cdot k}$ are both linear combinations of the same elements of $\boldsymbol{X}$. These are the projections of $\boldsymbol{X}_{i \cdot k}$ into different vectors ($\boldsymbol{A}_{j \cdot}$ and $\boldsymbol{A}_{j' \cdot}$, respectively) that will be correlated unless the j-th and j'-th rows of $\boldsymbol{A}$ be orthogonal. Note that, for given i and k, the degree of dependence of the different $\boldsymbol{Y}_{ijk}$ and $\boldsymbol{Y}_{ij'k}$ will depend on the corresponding rows $\boldsymbol{A}_{j \cdot}$ and $\boldsymbol{A}_{j' \cdot}$ of $\boldsymbol{A}$, specifically if they are more or less orthogonal. Thus, in the particular case above, matrix $\boldsymbol{A}$, in particular its rows, will be in charge of inducing dependence in the elements of $\boldsymbol{Y}$ along its second dimension.

The following property of n-dimensional product is also enlightening:

$$vec(\boldsymbol{A} \circ_n \boldsymbol{X}) = (\boldsymbol{I}_{L_N} \otimes \ldots \otimes \boldsymbol{I}_{L_{n+1}} \otimes \boldsymbol{A} \otimes \boldsymbol{I}_{L_{n-1}} \otimes \ldots \otimes \boldsymbol{I}_{L_1})vec(\boldsymbol{X}). \quad (9.2)$$

This is a direct consequence of the interpretation above of n-dimensional products, which multiply the elements the n-th dimension of $\boldsymbol{X}$ by the structure matrix $\boldsymbol{A}$. Although this is an equivalent reformulation of the original n-dimensional product, the original formulation avoids the use of Kronecker products, which makes possible its implementation in software packages that do not have specific functions for handling and taking advantage of those operations. Nevertheless, this new reformulation may be very interesting for exploring theoretical properties of data structures built as n-dimensional products, for instance:

$$
\begin{aligned}
\boldsymbol{\Sigma}_{vec(\boldsymbol{A} \circ_n \boldsymbol{X})} &= (\boldsymbol{I}_{L_N} \otimes \ldots \otimes \boldsymbol{I}_{L_{n+1}} \otimes \boldsymbol{A} \otimes \boldsymbol{I}_{L_{n-1}} \otimes \ldots \otimes \boldsymbol{I}_{L_1}) \cdot \boldsymbol{\Sigma}_{vec(\boldsymbol{X})} \\
&\quad \cdot (\boldsymbol{I}_{L_N} \otimes \ldots \otimes \boldsymbol{I}_{L_{n+1}} \otimes \boldsymbol{A}' \otimes \boldsymbol{I}_{L_{n-1}} \otimes \ldots \otimes \boldsymbol{I}_{L_1}),
\end{aligned}
$$

that, in the particular case that $\boldsymbol{\Sigma}_{vec(\boldsymbol{X})} = \boldsymbol{I}_{L_1 \cdot \ldots \cdot L_N}$ yields:

$$\boldsymbol{\Sigma}_{vec(\boldsymbol{A} \circ_n \boldsymbol{X})} = (\boldsymbol{I}_{L_N} \otimes \ldots \otimes \boldsymbol{I}_{L_{n+1}} \otimes \boldsymbol{A}\boldsymbol{A}' \otimes \boldsymbol{I}_{L_{n-1}} \otimes \ldots \otimes \boldsymbol{I}_{L_1}).$$

This expression makes evident the close relationship between the matrix $\boldsymbol{A}$, structuring the dependence for the n-th dimension of the array, and the covariance matrix corresponding to that dimension.

We may also generalize the n-dimensional product in parallel to how we defined the $\boldsymbol{r}$-matrix unfolding as follows. Given a vector of indices $\boldsymbol{r} = (1, ..., n_r)$, if $\boldsymbol{A}$ is a $(\prod_{i \in \{1,...,n_r\}} L_i) \times (\prod_{i \in \{1,...,n_r\}} L_i)$ matrix, then the tensor $\boldsymbol{Y}$ obtained from folding $\boldsymbol{A}\boldsymbol{X}^{(r)}$ into a vector with the same dimensions as of $\boldsymbol{X}$ will be referred to as the $\boldsymbol{r}$-*product of an array* $\boldsymbol{X}$ with $\boldsymbol{A}$. We denote this product as $\boldsymbol{A} \circ_{\boldsymbol{r}} \boldsymbol{X}$, which can be further generalized for $\boldsymbol{r}$ containing sets of indexes different to $(1, ..., n_r)$. Note that in the n-dimensional product, for any n, the matrix $\boldsymbol{A}$ combined the information in the cells of $\boldsymbol{X}$ along its n-th dimension. Now, the $\boldsymbol{r}$-product of an array $\boldsymbol{X}$ with $\boldsymbol{A}$ jointly combines the information in the cells of $\boldsymbol{X}$ along all the dimensions considered in $\boldsymbol{r}$. Therefore, this operation induces multivariate dependence in the resulting array for all the dimensions considered in the vector $\boldsymbol{r}$. Nevertheless, as we will see in the next subsections, the $\boldsymbol{r}$-product for a particular vector $\boldsymbol{r}$ induces a more general dependence structure than the concatenation of n-dimensional products for all $n \in \boldsymbol{r}$. In other words, $\boldsymbol{A}\circ_{\boldsymbol{r}}$ reproduces more general covariance structures than $\boldsymbol{A}_1 \circ_{r_1} ... \boldsymbol{A}_{n_r} \circ_{n_r}$ for suitable matrices $\boldsymbol{A}$ and $\boldsymbol{A}_1, ..., \boldsymbol{A}_{n_r}$ without any particular structure.

In a similar manner to n-dimensional products, we can also derive the following properties for $\boldsymbol{r}$-products. First,

$$vec(\boldsymbol{A} \circ_{\boldsymbol{r}} \boldsymbol{X}) = (\boldsymbol{I}_{L_N} \otimes ... \otimes \boldsymbol{I}_{L_{n_r+1}} \otimes \boldsymbol{A})vec(\boldsymbol{X}),$$

where $\boldsymbol{A}$ is now a square matrix of dimension $\prod_{i=1}^{n_r} L_i$. As a consequence,

$$\begin{aligned}\boldsymbol{\Sigma}_{vec(\boldsymbol{A}\circ_{\boldsymbol{r}}\boldsymbol{X})} &= (\boldsymbol{I}_{L_N} \otimes ... \otimes \boldsymbol{I}_{L_{n_r+1}} \otimes \boldsymbol{A}) \cdot \boldsymbol{\Sigma}_{vec(\boldsymbol{X})} \\ &\cdot (\boldsymbol{I}_{L_N} \otimes ... \otimes \boldsymbol{I}_{L_{n_r+1}} \otimes \boldsymbol{A}'),\end{aligned}$$

that, in the particular case that $\boldsymbol{\Sigma}_{vec(\boldsymbol{X})} = \boldsymbol{I}_{L_1 \cdot ... \cdot L_N}$ yields:

$$\boldsymbol{\Sigma}_{vec(\boldsymbol{A}\circ_{\boldsymbol{r}}\boldsymbol{X})} = (\boldsymbol{I}_{L_N} \otimes ... \otimes \boldsymbol{I}_{L_{n_r+1}} \otimes \boldsymbol{A}\boldsymbol{A}').$$

This expression makes it clear that now the first n_r dimensions of $\boldsymbol{A} \circ_{\boldsymbol{r}} \boldsymbol{X}$ will not have a separable covariance unless $\boldsymbol{A}$ has a particular Kronecker product structure that made that relationship possible.

Although $\boldsymbol{r}$-products are combinations of simple mathematical operations, their WinBUGS implementation is not as easy as that of n-dimensional products. That implementation requires the stacking of the dimensions of the array corresponding to $\boldsymbol{r}$ into a matrix or, preferably, a programming shortcut that allows us to circumvent that process. That shortcut could be done by decomposing the products for each row in $\boldsymbol{A}\boldsymbol{X}^{(r)}$ into smaller matrix products. Thus, let us assume that we had an $(L_1 L_2) \times (L_1 L_2)$ matrix $\boldsymbol{A}$, composed of $L_2 \times L_2$ blocks $\boldsymbol{A}_{jj'}$ of dimension $L_1 \times L_1$. Let us also assume $\boldsymbol{X}$ to be a three-dimensional array of dimensions (L_1, L_2, L_3) and $\boldsymbol{X}^{(r)}$, for $\boldsymbol{r} = (1, 2)$, a $L_2 \times 1$ block-matrix of blocks $\boldsymbol{X}_{j1}^{(r)} = \boldsymbol{X}_{\cdot j}$ for $j = 1, ..., L_2$. Then,

$$\boldsymbol{Y}_{\cdot j} = \boldsymbol{Y}_{j1}^{(r)} = \boldsymbol{A}_{j\cdot}\boldsymbol{X}^{(r)} = \sum_{j'=1}^{L_2} \boldsymbol{A}_{jj'}(\boldsymbol{X}_{j'1}^{(r)}) = \sum_{j'=1}^{L_2} \boldsymbol{A}_{jj'}\boldsymbol{X}_{\cdot j'}.$$

and then

$$\boldsymbol{Y}_{ijk} = \sum_{j'=1}^{L_2} (\boldsymbol{A}_{jj'})_{i\cdot}\boldsymbol{X}_{\cdot j'k} \ .$$

This formulation can be coded in WinBUGS in the following way, where the most inner loop calculates each of the summands in the latest expression:

```
for(i in 1:L1){
  for(j in 1:L2){
    for(k in 1:L3){
      for(j2 in 1:L2){
        Y.aux[i,j,k,j2]<-inprod2(A[(j-1)*L1+i,
                                 ((j2-1)*L1+1):(j2*L1)],
                                 X[,j2,k])
      }
      Y[i,j,k]<-sum(Y.aux[i,j,k,])
    }
  }
}
```

Similar alternative formulations can be coded into WinBUGS for multidimensional models of order higher than 3 or for $\boldsymbol{r} \neq (1, 2)$. On the contrary, to our knowledge, these complex array operations cannot be coded into INLA since it does not allow us to specifically deal with arrays.

9.2.2   Separable modeling

The multidimensional modeling in Martinez-Beneito et al. (2017) is able to reproduce both separable and inseparable covariance structures. We will start by introducing the construction of separable models within this framework and we will extend them afterwards to inseparable structures.

The starting point of the multidimensional framework in Martinez-Beneito et al. (2017) is Expression (8.9). In summary, that expression modeled the multivariate dependence for an $I \times J$ matrix $\boldsymbol{\Phi}$ as $\boldsymbol{\Phi} = \tilde{\boldsymbol{\Sigma}}_1 \boldsymbol{\Lambda} \tilde{\boldsymbol{\Sigma}}_2'$ where $\boldsymbol{\Lambda}$ was a matrix, with the same dimensions as $\boldsymbol{\Phi}$ with independent Normal cells. On the other hand, matrices $\tilde{\boldsymbol{\Sigma}}_1$ and $\tilde{\boldsymbol{\Sigma}}_2$ are in charge of inducing spatial and multivariate dependence, respectively, on $\boldsymbol{\Phi}$. Note that $\Phi_{ij} = (\tilde{\boldsymbol{\Sigma}}_1)_{i\cdot}(\boldsymbol{\Lambda}\tilde{\boldsymbol{\Sigma}}_2)_{\cdot j}$, so the rows of $\tilde{\boldsymbol{\Sigma}}_1$ combine the information of the elements of each column of $\boldsymbol{\Lambda}\tilde{\boldsymbol{\Sigma}}_2$, that is, the information of each of the spatial units inducing therefore spatial dependence. In a similar manner $\tilde{\boldsymbol{\Sigma}}_2$ mixes up the information in the columns of $\mathbf{\Lambda}$, inducing therefore multivariate dependence for the different outcomes. Therefore, inducing different sources of dependence in matrices can be seen as a sequence of matrix products, each of them inducing dependence along one of the dimensions of the array. Maybe this idea could be also extrapolated to arrays.

Expression (8.9) can be also formulated as a sequence of n-dimensional products of arrays. Thus, note that any matrix $\mathbf{X}$ can be alternatively expressed as $\mathbf{X}^{(1)}$; therefore,

$$\mathbf{\Phi}^{(1)} = \mathbf{\Phi} = \tilde{\mathbf{\Sigma}}_1 \mathbf{\Lambda} \tilde{\mathbf{\Sigma}}_2' = \tilde{\mathbf{\Sigma}}_1 (\mathbf{\Lambda} \tilde{\mathbf{\Sigma}}_2')^{(1)} \leftrightarrow \mathbf{\Phi} = \tilde{\mathbf{\Sigma}}_1 \circ_1 (\mathbf{\Lambda} \tilde{\mathbf{\Sigma}}_2').$$

In a similar manner $\mathbf{X}^{(2)} = \mathbf{X}'$, therefore

$$(\mathbf{\Lambda} \tilde{\mathbf{\Sigma}}_2')^{(2)} = (\mathbf{\Lambda} \tilde{\mathbf{\Sigma}}_2')' = \tilde{\mathbf{\Sigma}}_2 \mathbf{\Lambda}' = \tilde{\mathbf{\Sigma}}_2 \mathbf{\Lambda}^{(2)} \leftrightarrow \mathbf{\Lambda} \tilde{\mathbf{\Sigma}}_2' = \tilde{\mathbf{\Sigma}}_2 \circ_2 \mathbf{\Lambda}$$

and putting both expressions together we have

$$\tilde{\mathbf{\Sigma}}_1 \mathbf{\Lambda} \tilde{\mathbf{\Sigma}}_2' = \mathbf{\Phi} = \tilde{\mathbf{\Sigma}}_1 \circ_1 \tilde{\mathbf{\Sigma}}_2 \circ_2 \mathbf{\Lambda}. \qquad (9.3)$$

These expressions have direct consequences, as for example:

$$\tilde{\mathbf{\Sigma}}_1 \circ_1 \tilde{\mathbf{\Sigma}}_2 \circ_2 \mathbf{\Lambda} = \tilde{\mathbf{\Sigma}}_1 (\mathbf{\Lambda} \tilde{\mathbf{\Sigma}}_2') = (\tilde{\mathbf{\Sigma}}_1 \mathbf{\Lambda}) \tilde{\mathbf{\Sigma}}_2' = \tilde{\mathbf{\Sigma}}_2 \circ_2 \tilde{\mathbf{\Sigma}}_1 \circ_1 \mathbf{\Lambda},$$

so $\circ_i$ and $\circ_j$ for $i \neq j$ are commutative operations and the order in which these two operations are carried out have no relevance.

Expression (9.3) suggests the way for generalizing the multivariate approaches in Martinez-Beneito (2013) and Botella-Rocamora et al. (2015) to the multidimensional case. That expression shows that for multivariate modeling, inducing successive n-dimensional products ($n = 1, 2$) into an unstructured matrix induces (spatial and multivariate) dependence for both dimensions in the study. The obvious direct generalization of this procedure to the multidimensional case would be to make those n-dimensional products for all the dimensions in the corresponding multidimensional case. Thus, for a trivariate case that procedure would reduce to assume

$$\mathbf{\Phi} = \tilde{\mathbf{\Sigma}}_3 \circ_3 \tilde{\mathbf{\Sigma}}_2 \circ_2 \tilde{\mathbf{\Sigma}}_1 \circ_1 \mathbf{\Lambda}$$

for $\mathbf{\Lambda}$ an array of order 3 and for $\tilde{\mathbf{\Sigma}}_1, \tilde{\mathbf{\Sigma}}_2, \tilde{\mathbf{\Sigma}}_3$ square matrices of suitable dimensions. Expression (9.2) allows rewriting the latest expression as:

$$\begin{aligned} vec(\mathbf{\Phi}) &= (\tilde{\mathbf{\Sigma}}_3 \otimes \mathbf{I}_{L_2} \otimes \mathbf{I}_{L_1}) \cdot (\mathbf{I}_{L_3} \otimes \tilde{\mathbf{\Sigma}}_2 \otimes \mathbf{I}_{L_1}) \cdot (\mathbf{I}_{L_3} \otimes \mathbf{I}_{L_2} \otimes \tilde{\mathbf{\Sigma}}_1) \\ &\cdot vec(\mathbf{\Lambda}) = (\tilde{\mathbf{\Sigma}}_3 \otimes \tilde{\mathbf{\Sigma}}_2 \otimes \tilde{\mathbf{\Sigma}}_1) \cdot vec(\mathbf{\Lambda}) \end{aligned}$$

and, therefore, the covariance matrix of $vec(\mathbf{\Phi})$ yields

$$\mathbf{\Sigma}_{vec(\mathbf{\Phi})} = \tilde{\mathbf{\Sigma}}_3 \tilde{\mathbf{\Sigma}}_3' \otimes \tilde{\mathbf{\Sigma}}_2 \tilde{\mathbf{\Sigma}}_2' \otimes \tilde{\mathbf{\Sigma}}_1 \tilde{\mathbf{\Sigma}}_1',$$

which is obviously separable. Moreover, as shown above, this covariance structure does not depend at all on the order used for the n-dimensional products to induce dependence on $\mathbf{\Phi}$. Note that the covariance matrix for the k-th dimension in the Kronecker product defining the whole separable covariance structure is $\tilde{\mathbf{\Sigma}}_k \tilde{\mathbf{\Sigma}}_k'$. Therefore, as for the multivariate case, we can interpret the tilde in $\tilde{\mathbf{\Sigma}}_k$ as the operator on any matrix $\mathbf{A}$ that returns the matrix $\tilde{\mathbf{A}}$ accomplishing $\mathbf{A} = \tilde{\mathbf{A}}\tilde{\mathbf{A}}'$, so $\tilde{\mathbf{\Sigma}}_k$ is a kind of square root of the covariance matrix $\mathbf{\Sigma}_k$.

One final issue remains for putting this approach into practice, the definition of the $\tilde{\mathbf{\Sigma}}_i$ matrices. For this goal we are going to distinguish between two separate cases: first, if the corresponding dimension models an unstructured factor (such as cause of death, gender, etc.) or, on the contrary, it models a structured factor (such as space, time or age group). Following Botella-Rocamora et al. (2015), for unstructured factors we could model $\tilde{\mathbf{\Sigma}}_k$ as a matrix of independent $N(0, \sigma_k^2)$ cells, where σ_k is also estimated within the model. Regretfully, assuming $(\tilde{\mathbf{\Sigma}}_k)_{ij} \sim N(0, \sigma_k^2)$ for all unstructured factors in a multidimensional study induces identifiability problems into the model. Thus, for the simple case of a trivariate model with two unstructured dimensions (dimensions 2 and 3), the joint covariance matrix when dependence for these two factors is induced results:

$$\tilde{\mathbf{\Sigma}}_3 \tilde{\mathbf{\Sigma}}_3' \otimes \tilde{\mathbf{\Sigma}}_2 \tilde{\mathbf{\Sigma}}_2' \otimes \mathbf{I}_{L_1} = (\sigma_3^2 \tilde{\mathbf{\Sigma}}_3^* (\tilde{\mathbf{\Sigma}}_3^*)') \otimes (\sigma_2^2 \tilde{\mathbf{\Sigma}}_2^* (\tilde{\mathbf{\Sigma}}_2^*)') \otimes \mathbf{I}_{L_1},$$

where $(\Sigma_3^*)_{ij} \sim N(0,1)$ and $(\Sigma_2^*)_{ij} \sim N(0,1)$. This expression is equivalent to

$$((\lambda^{-1}\sigma_2)^2 \tilde{\mathbf{\Sigma}}_2^* (\tilde{\mathbf{\Sigma}}_2^*)') \otimes ((\lambda\sigma_1^2) \tilde{\mathbf{\Sigma}}_1^* (\tilde{\mathbf{\Sigma}}_1^*)') \otimes \mathbf{I}_{L_1}$$

for any $\lambda \neq 0$, which is equivalent to consider $(\Sigma_1)_{ij} \sim N(0, (\lambda\sigma_1)^2)$ and $(\Sigma_2)_{ij} \sim N(0, (\lambda^{-1}\sigma_2)^2)$. As a consequence σ_1 and σ_2 will not be identifiable since a multiplicative modification of λ units in any of them can be compensated with a corresponding modification of λ^{-1} for the other one. For fixing this issue, Martinez-Beneito et al. (2017) propose to set the variances of the cells in the matrices $\tilde{\mathbf{\Sigma}}_i$, for all i, to a common value σ^2. In this manner, the compensation mentioned between the different variance terms in the $\tilde{\mathbf{\Sigma}}_i$ matrices would be avoided.

In the case of structured factors, $\tilde{\mathbf{\Sigma}}_k$ should induce the specific covariance structure of that factor into the model. Since $\mathbf{\Sigma}_k = \tilde{\mathbf{\Sigma}}_k \tilde{\mathbf{\Sigma}}_k'$ and now $\mathbf{\Sigma}_k$ should have a specific structure, then $\tilde{\mathbf{\Sigma}}_k$ should also have a particular structure that we would have to impose on the model. Specifically, $\tilde{\mathbf{\Sigma}}_k$ could be given by the Cholesky decomposition of the assumed $\mathbf{\Sigma}_k$. For example, if we wanted to model time into a multidimensional model with a first-order auto-regressive structure, the corresponding covariance matrix should be of the form

$$(\Sigma_k)_{ij} = \sigma^2 \frac{\rho^{|i-j|}}{1 - \rho^2}.$$

The lower triangle of the Cholesky decomposition of that matrix is

$$
\boldsymbol{\sigma}
\begin{pmatrix}
(1-\rho^2)^{-1/2} & 0 & 0 & \cdots & 0 \\
\rho(1-\rho^2)^{-1/2} & 1 & 0 & \cdots & 0 \\
\rho^2(1-\rho^2)^{-1/2} & \rho & 1 & \cdots & 0 \\
& & & \ddots & \\
\cdots & \cdots & \cdots & & \cdots \\
\rho^{L_k-1}(1-\rho^2)^{-1/2} & \rho^{L_k-2} & \rho^{L_k-3} & \cdots & 1
\end{pmatrix}.
$$

Thus, for modeling a first-order auto-regressive process in time we could simply assume $\tilde{\boldsymbol{\Sigma}}_k$ to have this structure.

Although space is also a structured factor, its length is usually much longer than that of the rest of the factors in multidimensional models, which makes the dimension of $\tilde{\boldsymbol{\Sigma}}_k$ also much longer. Moreover, the Cholesky decomposition of spatial covariance matrices corresponding to irregular lattices will generally yield unaffordable analytic expressions. As a consequence, it is usually much more convenient to assume that the original matrix $\boldsymbol{\Lambda}$ has spatial structure from scratch, instead of imposing that structure with the corresponding n-dimensional product. In that case, we will denote the $\boldsymbol{\Lambda}$ array that already has spatial structure as $\boldsymbol{\Lambda}^*(=\tilde{\boldsymbol{\Sigma}}_1 \circ_1 \boldsymbol{\Lambda})$ in order to distinguish it from the completely unstructured array $\boldsymbol{\Lambda}$. Therefore, we will assume that the vectors $\boldsymbol{\Lambda}^*_{\cdot jk}$ follow spatial distributions such as ICAR, PCAR, etc. for $j = 1, ..., L_2$ and $k = 1, ..., L_3$ and will induce later the rest of the sources of dependence in $\boldsymbol{\Phi}$ by successive n-dimensional products $(n > 1)$ for the rest of the dimensions of $\boldsymbol{\Lambda}^*$.

The first dimension of the array $\boldsymbol{\Phi}$ has been assumed during all this section to correspond to the spatial component in the model. This has been done in accordance to multivariate models, where the first dimension also corresponded to that component. Nevertheless, this has some practical inconveniences for implementing these models in `WinBUGS` since for the array $\boldsymbol{\Lambda}^*$, `WinBUGS` only allows us to assume spatial dependence for the last dimension of that array. This requires us to work with a transposed version of $\boldsymbol{\Lambda}^*$ in `WinBUGS` which will be afterwards transposed when dependence of one of the subsequent factors is induced. Several examples of this coding procedure can be found at the online supplementary material of Example 9.1.

9.2.3   Inseparable modeling

Although separable models are interesting by themselves, separability may be a restrictive assumption in some occasions. This assumption may be particularly hard to hold if the number of categories is large for some of the factors in a multidimensional model. In that case, assuming that the covariance structures are identical for all the levels of each of those factors may be excessively restrictive. Zhang et al. (2006) already showed an example where inseparability was required for appropriately explaining the variability in a four-dimensional data set. Fortunately, Martinez-Beneito (2013) showed how to reproduce inseparable multivariate models within his framework and those ideas could be also used for the multidimensional setting.

Inseparable models consider different covariance structures for the different levels of the same factor. We are going to propose two different ways to achieve this goal, what we call *nested* and *factorial* designs. For introducing these inseparable models, we are going to assume that we had to perform a trivariate study and we wanted to impose inseparability for the second and third factors in the problem. We will keep the first factor as separable, that is, we will consider the (spatial) covariance structure of this factor to be common for any level of the second and third factor.

We will introduce first nested inseparable designs. For the separable case, we induced dependence by making

$$vec(\boldsymbol{\Phi}) = \tilde{\boldsymbol{\Sigma}}_3 \circ_3 \tilde{\boldsymbol{\Sigma}}_2 \circ_2 \tilde{\boldsymbol{\Sigma}}_1 \circ_1 vec(\boldsymbol{\Lambda}) = \tilde{\boldsymbol{\Sigma}}_3 \circ_3 \tilde{\boldsymbol{\Sigma}}_2 \circ_2 vec(\boldsymbol{\Lambda}^*).$$

We can also put this latest expression as

$$vec(\boldsymbol{\Phi}) = (\tilde{\boldsymbol{\Sigma}}_3 \otimes \boldsymbol{I}_{L_2} \otimes \boldsymbol{I}_{L_1})(\boldsymbol{I}_{L_3} \otimes \tilde{\boldsymbol{\Sigma}}_2 \otimes \boldsymbol{I}_{L_1})vec(\boldsymbol{\Lambda}^*).$$

This expression puts the same covariance $\boldsymbol{\Sigma}_3$ for each level of the second factor and $\boldsymbol{\Sigma}_2$ for each level of the third factor. Nevertheless, this may be changed by allowing the matrices $\tilde{\boldsymbol{\Sigma}}_2$ and $\tilde{\boldsymbol{\Sigma}}_3$ to vary for each level of the other factor by making

$$vec(\boldsymbol{\Phi}) = (\tilde{\boldsymbol{\Sigma}}_3 \otimes \boldsymbol{I}_{L_2} \otimes \boldsymbol{I}_{L_1})(Bdiag(\{\tilde{\boldsymbol{\Sigma}}_2(k)\}_{k=1}^{L_3}) \otimes \boldsymbol{I}_{L_1})vec(\boldsymbol{\Lambda}^*), \qquad (9.4)$$

or

$$vec(\boldsymbol{\Phi}) = \left(\left(\sum_{j=1}^{L_2} \tilde{\boldsymbol{\Sigma}}_3(j) \otimes (e_j^{L_2})(e_j^{L_2})'\right) \otimes \boldsymbol{I}_{L_1}\right) (\boldsymbol{I}_{L_3} \otimes \tilde{\boldsymbol{\Sigma}}_2 \otimes \boldsymbol{I}_{L_1})vec(\boldsymbol{\Lambda}^*),$$
$$(9.5)$$

where $e_j^{L_2}$ is an L_2-vector with all its cells equal to 0, except for its j-th position which is equal to 0. For Expression (9.4), the resulting covariance matrix will be

$$\boldsymbol{\Sigma}_{vec(\boldsymbol{\Phi})} = ((\tilde{\boldsymbol{\Sigma}}_3 \otimes \boldsymbol{I}_{L_2})Bdiag(\{\boldsymbol{\Sigma}_2(k)\}_{k=1}^{L_3})(\tilde{\boldsymbol{\Sigma}}_3' \otimes \boldsymbol{I}_{L_2})) \otimes \boldsymbol{\Sigma}_1, \qquad (9.6)$$

which is obviously inseparable for its second and third dimensions. Moreover, this expression makes it clear that the commutativity of the covariance structures for the second and third dimensions of $\boldsymbol{\Phi}$ no longer holds. If, in that same case, dependence was induced first for the third factor and afterwards for the second factor, then the corresponding model would yield, in contrast, the following covariance matrix

$$\boldsymbol{\Sigma}_{vec(\boldsymbol{\Phi})} = (Bdiag(\{\tilde{\boldsymbol{\Sigma}}_2(k)\}_{k=1}^{L_3})(\boldsymbol{\Sigma}_3 \otimes \boldsymbol{I}_{L_2})Bdiag(\{\tilde{\boldsymbol{\Sigma}}_2'(k)\}_{k=1}^{L_3})) \otimes \boldsymbol{\Sigma}_1.$$

Similar results could be derived for Expression (9.5). Thus, nesting may generate 4 different models where the second and third factors of a model interact.

These 4 models depend on the order in which the different kinds of dependence are induced and if the covariance matrix for one of the factors varies for each level of the other factor, or vice versa.

Nesting may be also easily generalized to interactions of three or more factors. For example, we can make the covariance matrix of the second factor in a multidimensional study vary for each level of the third and fourth factors in that study by changing the second term on the right-hand side of Expression (9.4) by $(Bdiag(\{\tilde{\Sigma}_2(k,l)\}_{k,l=1}^{L_3,L_4})$. This shows how to generalize nested designs to the interaction of more than two factors.

The implementation of nested designs in `WinBUGS` is not difficult to achieve. In the previous section, we showed the implementation of separable dependence structures in `WinBUGS`, which was done by premultiplying one of the dimensions of the array by a specific structure matrix inducing the corresponding covariance structure. Nested models have the particularity that the structure matrix changes for each level of another factor(s) in the model. We can easily code that feature in `WinBUGS`. Thus, if we wanted the covariance matrix for the second factor to vary for each level of the third, we could simply do

```
for(i in 1:L1){
    for(k in 1:L3){
        for(j in 1:L2){
            Y[i,j,k]<-inprod2(A[k,j,],X[i,,k])
        }
    }
}
```

where now the different $A_{k..}$, for $k = 1, ..., L_3$, represent the different $\tilde{\Sigma}_2(k)$ intervening in that nested design.

Although nesting induces interaction between two or more factors in multidimensional models, that interaction produces structured covariance matrices that could not be flexible enough in some settings. Thus, Expression (9.6) corresponds to a covariance matrix where L_3 smaller covariance matrices for the second factor are combined as a function of a single additional matrix $\tilde{\Sigma}_3$. This makes all the blocks composing that covariance matrix linear combinations of the set of matrices $\{\Sigma_2(k)\}_{k=1}^{L_3}$, which could be a restrictive assumption. Factorial designs are an alternative, and more general, way of inducing inseparability in multidimensional studies. For the trivariate example above, where interaction was pursued for the second and third factor, a factorial design could be formulated as:

$$\Phi = \tilde{\Sigma}_{(2,3)} \circ_{(2,3)} \Lambda^*$$

or, equivalently,

$$vec(\Phi) = (\tilde{\Sigma}_{(2,3)} \otimes I_{L_1})vec(\Lambda^*)$$

where now $\tilde{\Sigma}_{(2,3)}$ is a general square matrix of dimension $L_2 \cdot L_3$. This factorial design yields the following covariance matrix

$$\Sigma_{vec(\Phi)} = \Sigma_{(2,3)} \otimes \Sigma_1$$

where now $\boldsymbol{\Sigma}_{(2,3)}$ is an unstructured symmetric positive definite matrix, in contrast to the nested designs above for the second and third factors. Therefore, factorial models yield more general covariance structures, with more general interactions between factors than nested designs. The generalization of factorial designs to the interaction of more than three factors is completely straightforward. In fact, the factorial design above would be equivalent to considering a single factor of $L_2 \cdot L_3$ levels, instead of the second and third factor in the multidimensional model above, and proposing a general multivariate M-model, with a general $\boldsymbol{M}(= \tilde{\boldsymbol{\Sigma}}_{(2,3)})$ matrix for that setting.

In contrast to nested designs, factorial designs are univocally defined for any set of factors. Thus, as we showed above, for two interacting factors, 4 nested designs were possible as a function of their order and which factor depends on the other one. For the factorial design above, the $\circ_{(2,3)}$ operator is equivalent to the $\circ_{(3,2)}$ producing identical models. Moreover, when a factorial $\circ_{(2,3)}$ operator is used, it has no sense to induce further dependence in the model by using the $\circ_2$ or $\circ_3$ operators since the dependence on the second and third dimensions of the model is implicit in $\circ_{(2,3)}$.

Note that nested designs can be seen as a particular case of factorial designs by considering a particular structure for the matrix inducing joint dependence for the interacting factors, $\tilde{\boldsymbol{\Sigma}}_{(2,3)}$ in the example above. Thus, if we considered the factorial design above with

$$\tilde{\boldsymbol{\Sigma}}_{(2,3)} = (\tilde{\boldsymbol{\Sigma}}_3 \otimes \boldsymbol{I}_{L_2})Bdiag(\{\tilde{\boldsymbol{\Sigma}}_2(k)\}_{k=1}^{L_3}),$$

instead of a general $(L_2 \cdot L_3)$-matrix, we could reproduce the nested design in Expression (9.4) and so forth. Nevertheless, despite that this fact could make nested designs seem minor inseparable families of models, as compared to factorial designs, they are extremely useful for modeling structured factors. In that case, we will have a particular structure for one of the factors that we would like to preserve in the joint covariance matrix so that it reflects the ordinal, temporal, spatial, etc. dependence of that factor. In such settings, factorial designs with general matrices for structuring dependence between factors are too flexible, and they will not induce the particular covariance for the structured factor that we would like to induce. Thus, for the modeling of inseparable relationships entailing structured factors, nesting will be the default modeling tool. In that case, the interaction of a structured term, such as the first-order auto-regressive temporal term above with an unstructured term, could be done in two different ways. First, the correlation parameter of the auto-regressive time series could be allowed to vary for each level of the second factor and, alternatively, the unstructured covariance matrix for the second factor could be different for each time period. These two nested designs would preserve the temporal structure that we wanted to induce into the model, while also allowing the two factors considered to interact in different manners.

Finally, Martinez-Beneito et al. (2017) proposes also a nomenclature for the models generated within this multidimensional framework. That nomenclature is extremely useful, as it allows to classify and identify all the multidimensional models in this framework and many of those proposed in the literature. This nomenclature of models is based on the different array operations needed to generate each model within this framework. Thus, they propose to denote as $i\cdot$ the operation inducing a separable dependence structure for the i-th factor in the model. They also denote as $i(j)\cdot$ if a nested dependence is induced for factor i, whose covariance matrix depends on each level of factor j. In this case more than two factors could be put into the parentheses if the nested design induced dependence for more than two factors. Finally, they denote as $ij\cdot$ if a factorial design was considered for factors i and j. This notation could be also easily extended to the interaction of more than two factors. Thus, they propose to denote each model as the concatenation of the operations that produce that model. For example, $1\cdot2\cdot3$ denotes a trivariate separable model and $1\cdot2\cdot3(2)$ denotes a model where the first two factors are modeled in a separable way and the third factor is nested into the second (the covariance matrix of the third factors varies for each level of the second). Note that for this last model the order of the operations matters for the resulting covariance matrix, so we will read the notation of models from left to right assuming that that is the order in which the corresponding operations are carried out. Thus, for the model above, dependence is induced for the first, second and third factor in this order. As a final example, the model $1(2)\cdot23$ would denote a model where the parameters of spatial dependence (first factor) vary for each level of the second factor and factors 2 and 3 interact in a factorial way. Martinez-Beneito et al. (2017) show a full depiction of the suitable models for trivariate multidimensional studies. That description excludes those models that do not seem to be reasonable, such as the $3\cdot1\cdot2\cdot3\cdot$ or the $1\cdot23\cdot3\cdot$ model, where dependence for the third factor is induced twice. The rest of the models that are found to be reasonable for the trivariate case are listed in that paper, which can be understood as a full catalog of models for the trivariate setting.

Example 9.1

We are going to undertake now a 4-dimensional study in the Valencian Region at the municipal level. The factors considered for this 4-dimensional study are space, time, cause of death and sex in this order. This study is intended to follow the oral cancer study in men that we have repeatedly visited during the book. Thus, the spatial units in the analysis are the municipalities in the Valencian Region. The whole time period for this analysis is split into 5 quinquennial intervals dividing the whole period of study. We have preferred to consider quinquennial periods, in contrast to the analyses in Section 7 in order to reduce the computational burden of the analysis. We have considered two causes of death for this study, oral and lung cancer. These two diseases share an important determinant, tobacco consumption, and the goal of this analysis is to take advantage of the lung cancer geographical patterns, with much more deaths than oral cancer, to improve the estimates of the oral cancer geographical patterns. Hopefully, lung cancer could provide us with a valuable surrogate of the effect of tobacco consumption in the Valencian Region. Finally, we have also considered both sexes in our study so that if environmental factors, taking an effect on both, could be having an important role, this model would take advantage of the information provided by the other sex. Thus, as a summary, the current multidimensional study will model an array of dimensions $540 \times 5 \times 2 \times 2$, that is, a total of 20 correlated geographic (PCAR distributed) patterns with different correlations that we will try to estimate and take advantage of in our study.

We have run several multidimensional models in our study. All the models have been run for a total of 30,000 simulations per chain, whose 10,000 first iterations were used as burn-in. Convergence was assessed just for the identifiable terms in the model: relative risks, intercept, covariance matrix between sexes and diseases (if they did not change as a function of any factor in the model), etc. For the non-identifiable terms, such as temporal correlation when this parameter varies as a function of the diseases, for example, we notice that the two correlations parameters ρ_1 and ρ_2 switch in general their roles during the MCMC simulation (see the annex online material). Nevertheless, that switching is not done for each iteration of the MCMC but, on the contrary, the roles of ρ_1 and ρ_2 are kept for a long number of iterations between switches. This makes the convergence of these parameters seem defective, although these chains are just reproducing their bimodal posterior distributions, which is a consequence of its lack of identifiability. Additionally, the spatial correlation parameter moves very close to its upper limit 1 for several of the run models, that is, they usually have most of their posterior mass over 0.99. This makes the MCMC samples of this parameter show high autocorrelation as a consequence of sampling in such a tiny range of its posterior distribution (see once again the annex online material for an illustration of this issue). Anyway we do not expect these convergence issues to have any practical impact on the sSMRs or their covariance matrix since we are talking about differences on this parameter in a range narrower than 0.01. As a summary, it would surely be wise to increase the number of iterations of the models run in order to obtain more reliable results. Nevertheless, the models run have taken considerable computing time (between 15.4 and 21.5 hours depending on the model), so we have preferred to keep the originally planned number of iterations for illustrative purposes and for making the analysis more reproducible.

We have run several models in order to assess different inseparable multidimensional covariance structures. Specifically, we have run the following models: 1.2.3.4, 1(2).2.3.4, 1(3).2.3.4, 1(4).2.3.4, 1.2(3).3.4, 1.2(4).3.4, 1.2.3(2).4, 1.2.3(4).4, 1.2.3.4(2) and 1.2.3.4(3). The lowest DIC for these models has been obtained for the 1.2.3.4(2) model, with a DIC of 22664.24. Nevertheless, there are also some alternative models with similar DICs, such as the 1.2.3.4, 1(3).2.3.4, 1.2(3).3.4 and 1.2.3(4).4 models, all of them with DICs lower than 22668; therefore, these models in terms of their overall fit should be very similar. We have not fitted any model with factorial interaction between two of the factors in the study because we have not seen any substantial benefit, in terms of DIC, when considering simpler nested interactions. Therefore, we have not seen the necessity of fitting more complex interactions. From now on, we will focus our attention on model 1.2.3.4(2) since, besides having the lowest DIC, it allows us to illustrate and discuss the interaction of two factors in the model: time and sex. Specifically, this model allows for dependence between sexes to vary in time.

The 1.2.3.4(2) model shows substantial spatial and temporal dependence, with the corresponding spatial and temporal dependence parameters having posterior means above 0.99 in both cases. Additionally, correlation between diseases is also high, being its posterior mean equal to 0.9 and 95% credible interval equal to $[0.80, 0.96]$. Therefore, dependence between the spatial patterns of both diseases, regardless of the sex or period is evident and the $sSMR$s will be clearly benefited of the joint study of both causes of death. Nevertheless, correlations between sexes for these two diseases vary between periods of study. Thus, these correlations are for the five periods considered, respectively: 0.82 $[0.41,1]$, 0.54 $[0.10,0.88]$, 0.32 $[-0.04,0.70]$, 0.11 $[-0.24, 0.43]$, and 0.21 $[-0.10,0.50]$. Therefore, correlations between sexes vanish as the period of study evolves. This result could be explained according to Zurriaga et al. (2008), who report an increase in the risk for lung cancer mortality in women on the coast of the Alicante province (see Figure 1.2) at the south-eastern side of the Valencian Region. This increase would be due to the settlement of north European elder people in this touristic area. Tobacco consumption between north European women was much more usual than between Spanish women for cohorts born around the middle of the twentieth century. This makes lung cancer, and supposedly oral cancer in women, more prevalent in foreign people settling in this region than in the native population. Therefore, this makes mortality ratios for women in this area increase during the period of study since foreign women are steadily setting there for the whole period of study. Nevertheless, this effect is not seen in men since there were not such important differences in tobacco consumption between north European and Spanish men during the twentieth century. As a consequence, the spatial patterns for these two diseases diverge for both sexes as the period of study evolves due to, at least in part according to Zurriaga et al. (2008), the increase in mortality between women at the south-eastern side of the Valencian Region. The current example yields further insight about that result.

Table 9.1 shows the mean posterior correlation between the fitted $sSMR$s for 12 different geographical patterns, out of the 20 patterns studied in the 1.2.3.4(2) model. The remaining geographical patterns for periods 2 and 4 have been removed from that table for reasons of space. This table shows several interesting results, for example, focussing our attention on the diag-

		Oral, Men			Oral, Women			Lung, Men			Lung, Women		
		Per. 1	Per. 3	Per. 5	Per. 1	Per. 3	Per. 5	Per. 1	Per. 3	Per. 5	Per. 1	Per. 3	Per. 5
Oral, Men	Per. 1	1.00	0.89	0.75	0.85	0.76	0.82	0.89	0.73	0.58	0.78	0.71	0.76
	Per. 3	0.89	1.00	0.95	0.58	0.44	0.53	0.83	0.87	0.79	0.57	0.44	0.52
	Per. 5	0.75	0.95	1.00	0.39	0.24	0.34	0.73	0.86	0.86	0.40	0.25	0.35
Oral, Women	Per. 1	0.85	0.58	0.39	1.00	0.91	0.92	0.72	0.43	0.24	0.90	0.83	0.83
	Per. 3	0.76	0.44	0.24	0.91	1.00	0.96	0.63	0.30	0.10	0.81	0.91	0.86
	Per. 5	0.82	0.53	0.34	0.92	0.96	1.00	0.69	0.38	0.19	0.83	0.87	0.90
Lung, Men	Per. 1	0.89	0.83	0.73	0.72	0.63	0.69	1.00	0.88	0.74	0.82	0.72	0.79
	Per. 3	0.73	0.87	0.79	0.43	0.30	0.38	0.88	1.00	0.96	0.53	0.37	0.48
	Per. 5	0.58	0.79	0.86	0.24	0.10	0.19	0.74	0.96	1.00	0.33	0.16	0.27
Lung, Women	Per. 1	0.78	0.57	0.40	0.90	0.81	0.83	0.82	0.53	0.33	1.00	0.90	0.91
	Per. 3	0.71	0.44	0.25	0.83	0.91	0.87	0.72	0.37	0.16	0.90	1.00	0.95
	Per. 5	0.76	0.52	0.35	0.83	0.86	0.90	0.79	0.48	0.27	0.91	0.95	1.00

Table 9.1
Correlations between some of the geographical patterns fitted for the 1.2.3.4(2) model.

		Oral, Men			Oral, Women			Lung, Men			Lung, Women		
		Per. 1	Per. 3	Per. 5	Per. 1	Per. 3	Per. 5	Per. 1	Per. 3	Per. 5	Per. 1	Per. 3	Per. 5
Oral, Men	Per. 1	1.00	0.93	0.85	0.47	0.46	0.44	0.88	0.79	0.68	0.46	0.45	0.42
	Per. 3	0.93	1.00	0.92	0.40	0.42	0.41	0.85	0.86	0.76	0.40	0.42	0.40
	Per. 5	0.85	0.92	1.00	0.32	0.34	0.38	0.78	0.82	0.85	0.32	0.34	0.37
Oral, Women	Per. 1	0.47	0.40	0.32	1.00	0.93	0.85	0.36	0.26	0.16	0.89	0.82	0.74
	Per. 3	0.46	0.42	0.34	0.93	1.00	0.92	0.34	0.27	0.18	0.82	0.88	0.80
	Per. 5	0.44	0.41	0.38	0.85	0.92	1.00	0.34	0.28	0.22	0.76	0.82	0.88
Lung, Men	Per. 1	0.88	0.85	0.78	0.36	0.34	0.34	1.00	0.93	0.84	0.43	0.42	0.41
	Per. 3	0.79	0.86	0.82	0.26	0.27	0.28	0.93	1.00	0.93	0.34	0.36	0.36
	Per. 5	0.68	0.76	0.85	0.16	0.18	0.22	0.84	0.93	1.00	0.25	0.27	0.32
Lung, Women	Per. 1	0.46	0.45	0.42	0.89	0.82	0.76	0.43	0.34	0.25	1.00	0.92	0.85
	Per. 3	0.45	0.42	0.40	0.82	0.88	0.80	0.42	0.36	0.27	0.92	1.00	0.92
	Per. 5	0.42	0.40	0.37	0.74	0.80	0.88	0.41	0.36	0.32	0.85	0.92	1.00

Table 9.2
Correlations between some of the geographical patterns fitted for the 1.2.3.4 model.

onal of the blocks composing that matrix, we can note how the correlations between patterns corresponding to different sexes decrease with time. Thus, at the first period of study, correlations between geographical patterns of the same disease are comparable to those of patterns of the same sex. This is not true for the 5th period, where correlations are much higher for patterns of the same sex, which are similar to those in the first period, than for patterns of different sexes. Therefore, Table 9.1 suggests diverging temporal patterns for men and women that, at the beginning of the period of study, had closely similar patterns although, however, at the end are substantially different. This diverging performance has been reproduced in part because of the different correlations between sexes assumed by the 1.2.3.4(2) model. Table 9.2 shows the same correlations but for the full separable 1.2.3.4 model. For this model, the diverging pattern for both sexes is harder to notice since this model puts much more similar correlations between sexes for all the periods considered. Specifically, correlations between sexes are smaller for this model for the first period of study in order to reduce the differences in those correlations for the different periods of study. The non-separable 1.2.3.4(2) model is less restrictive than the separable 1.2.3.4 model regarding correlations between sexes, which for the first option are allowed to vary in time. Thus, the differences found between both models could be a sign of the excessive simplicity of the separable model, that could be constraining the diverging patterns found for the 1.2.3.4(2) model.

Table 9.1 shows also a second interesting result. If we pay attention to the diagonal blocks in that table, we can notice that the correlations between periods for the patterns corresponding to men show a substantially higher decrease than for women. This would mean that the units of study with higher/lower risks would vary in time much more for men than for women. That is, in the previous paragraph, we mentioned that the patterns studied diverged for both sexes during the period of study; now we can interpret that such divergence is mainly due to the evolution of the spatio-temporal pattern of the mortality causes corresponding to men. This different time trend within the mortality causes considered is completely attenuated for the separable model (Table 9.2), thus considering different correlations between sexes for the different time periods surely helps also reproducing different temporal trends per sexes.

Figure 9.1 shows the temporal component (posterior mean for each period), as defined in Chapter 7, of the spatio-temporal pattern fitted for each combination of sex and cause of death. We show this component separately in Figure 9.1 because otherwise this time trend would mask the spatio-temporal changes that have occurred for each sex and cause of death during the whole period of study. As we can see, the time trends fitted depend mostly on the corresponding sex. Thus, time trends for men (for both diseases) reach a peak around the second or third period of study, as a consequence of the temporal inflexion of the smoking habit in men produced in Spain at the end of the twentieth century. In contrast, the time trends for both causes of death related

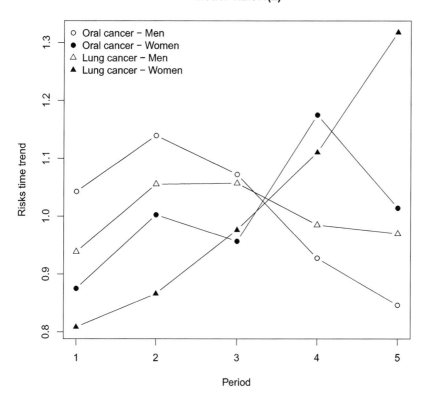

Figure 9.1
Time trends for the temporal component of the risks for each sex and cause
of death considered.

to women show upwards trends, with an increase in mortality for lung cancer higher than 50% for the 5th period in comparison to the first. The time trend for oral cancer in women is similar to that of lung cancer, although the trend for oral cancer is more wiggly as a consequence of the low number of deaths observed for this cause in women, the lowest number for all 4 combinations of causes and sexes considered.

Figures 9.2 and 9.3 show the temporal evolution of the geographical patterns for men and women, respectively, for both diseases. The temporal component has been removed for all these maps for avoiding each period to show mainly the temporal fluctuation corresponding to that period. These figures show interesting results. For example, Figure 9.2 shows how the geographical patterns studied for men get a bit flatter as the period of study progresses. Additionally, we notice some important spatio-temporal interaction for these two causes of death. Thus, if we pay attention to the set of municipalities between the two clusters mentioned during all the book (between Gandía and Alicante according to Figure 1.2), we can see that, at the first period, this area showed a slight protective effect while for the 5th period it shows a risk substantially lower than the Valencian Region as a whole. We can also notice important differences between the first and 5th period for the most southern municipalities in the Valencian Region where the mortality risks improve with the advance of the period of study. We see also in general a high agreement for the maps of these two causes of death, even for their time trends. This makes these two diseases highly benefit of this multidimensional study since they share their information which, as we can see, is highly correlated. Nevertheless, despite that high correlation, we can see how each cause of death is able to show its particular features that are not necessarily shared with the other cause. Thus, both clusters for oral cancer placed at the southern coastal area of the Valencian Region show substantial differences between causes of death. These two clusters are far milder for lung cancer than for oral cancer, having the southern part of the Valencian Region an evident lower risk (as compared to the whole Region) for lung than for oral cancer.

Regarding the temporal evolution of the spatial patterns for women, we see how both diseases show also similar spatial patterns for all the periods and these patterns stay more or less constant in time, at least more constant than for men. This is a consequence of the high temporal correlation found for the spatial patterns for oral and lung cancer in women, which makes the municipalities with high risks at the start of the period of study have also high risks at the end of that period. Nevertheless, we see how, in contrast to men, the geographical patterns are flatter for the first period of study. This is due in part to the temporal increase in mortality in the southern coast of the Valencian Region, as described for lung cancer by Zurriaga et al. (2008). We see now that such performance holds also for oral cancer in women. Note that the geographical patterns fitted for women are all similar regardless of the disease and period, and they are also similar to the spatial patterns fitted for men at the first period of study. Since the geographical pattern in

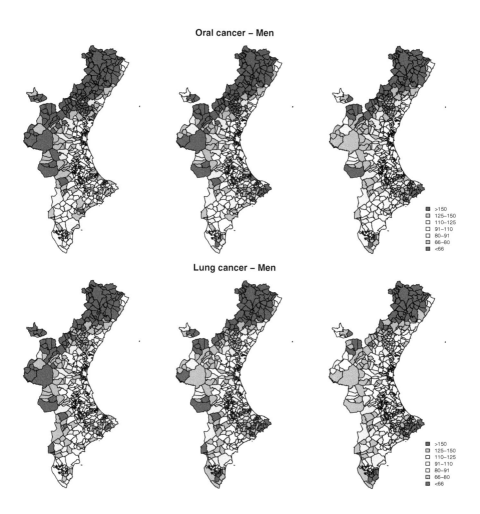

Figure 9.2
Spatio-temporal evolution (with temporal component removed) of risks for oral and lung cancer in men.

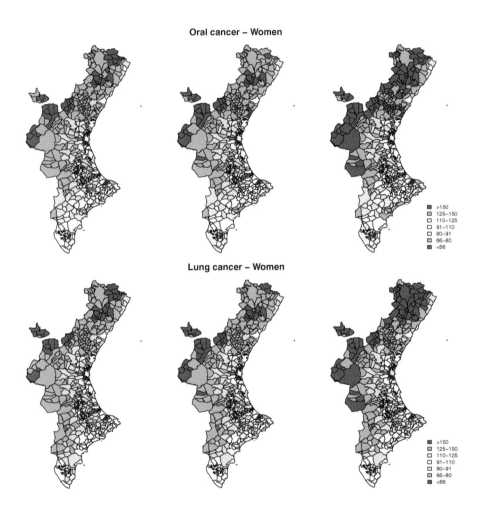

Figure 9.3
Spatio-temporal evolution (with temporal component removed) of risks for
oral and lung cancer in women.

men evolves with the period of study, the geographical pattern in the latest periods is less similar for both sexes than in the first period. The model has been able to capture this feature due to the interaction between sexes and period considered in the 1.2.3.4(2) model. Finally, note that the two clusters observed for oral cancer in men throughout the book are also present for the geographical patterns in women. Nevertheless, the time trends for risks for these two clusters seems quite different, which seems to discard the effect of an environmental risk factor taking an effect on both sexes, at least with the same temporal lag. These results encourage a more detailed exploration of this issue.

This example illustrates the most complex kind of analysis that we have introduced throughout this book. If you have followed the whole book from its beginning and you look back at the first analyses introduced there, you will notice the large gap between the original analysis and those that you should be able to undertake now. That gap is huge. The maps drawn with multivariate or multidimensional techniques show much more detail than univariate smoothed maps and they have no comparison at all with the original *SMR*s maps that hardly showed any useful information. Additionally, multivariate and multidimensional analyses allow us to draw an overall view of the geographical patterns of interest as elements of a common set and disentangle, and therefore know, their relationships. The theory for doing this task is already developed, although more developments will be made in the future for sure. Now this methodology should be widely applied in order to provide useful knowledge of interest for epidemiologists, health professionals or population in general. Let's do it, otherwise all this effort made in order to develop this set of statistical methods for disease mapping will be useless.

Exercises

1. The `MultiD.Rdata` file, available in the online material of the book (`https://github.com/MigueBeneito/DisMapBook/tree/master/Exercises`), contains two R objects: `MultiD` and `MultiD.e`, with the observed and expected deaths for several combinations of factors. As always, the information in these objects has been slightly modified in order to preserve data confidentiality. The `MultiD` object is an array of dimensions $528 \times 4 \times 2 \times 3$, where the first dimension corresponds to the Valencia city census tracts; the second dimension corresponds to each of 4 quinquennial intervals comprising the whole period of study (1996-2015); the third dimension corresponds

to both sexes; and the fourth dimension corresponds to different causes of death. For the causes of death we have considered lung cancer, COPD and cirrhosis, that is, the same as for the exercises of Chapter 8 except for prostate cancer which showed no (positive) correlation with the rest of the causes. The `MultiD.e` object has the same dimensions as `MultiD` and contains the expected cells corresponding to each of the cells of `MultiD`.

- Fit a separable multidimensional model for the observed deaths in `MultiD`. Compare the COPD $sSMR$s geographical pattern for men during 1996-2000 with that corresponding to a univariate analysis of that particular selection. Do you find a large improvement by making a multidimensional study?

- Draw a history plot of the deviance of the multidimensional model in order to explore its convergence. Beyond the deviance, which other quantities in the model do you find convenient to watch in order to monitor convergence?

- Explore and interpret the estimated correlations for all 4 factors considered in this study. Do you find a large temporal correlation? Do you find large correlations between diseases? Are the correlations found between disease larger or smaller, in general, than correlations between sexes?

- Consider some alternatives to the separable model above, such as the 1(2).2.3.4, 1(3).2.3.4, etc. models. Do you find any non-separable proposal outperforming the original separable model? In that case, assess the effect of the corresponding non-separability in the correlation matrices of that new alternative model.

Appendix 1

Theorem 1 *The Poisson-lognormal model below*

$$o_i \sim Pois(exp(\mu + \psi_i)e_i), \; i = 1, ..., I$$
$$\boldsymbol{\psi} \sim N(\mathbf{0}, \tau^{-1}\boldsymbol{I}_I)$$
$$\tau \sim Gamma(\alpha, 0)$$
$$\mu \sim Uniform(-\infty, \infty)$$

yields an improper posterior distribution for $\alpha \geq 0$.

Proof. We start by deriving the expression of the posterior distribution of the parameters in the model

$$P(\boldsymbol{\psi}, \mu, \tau | \boldsymbol{o}) \propto L(\boldsymbol{o} | \boldsymbol{\psi}, \mu) \cdot \left(\tau^{I/2} \exp\left(-\tau \frac{\boldsymbol{\psi}'\boldsymbol{\psi}}{2} \right) \right) \tau^{\alpha - 1}$$
$$= L(\boldsymbol{o} | \boldsymbol{\psi}, \mu) \cdot \tau^{I/2 + \alpha - 1} \exp\left(-\tau \frac{\boldsymbol{\psi}'\boldsymbol{\psi}}{2} \right),$$

where $L(\boldsymbol{o} | \boldsymbol{\psi}, \mu)$ denotes the likelihood function of the model, that we do not develop as it will be irrelevant for the rest of the proof. Since $P(\boldsymbol{\psi}, \mu, \tau | \boldsymbol{o})$, as a function of τ, follows a gamma distribution we can easily integrate out that parameter from the posterior distribution. In that case, we have

$$P(\boldsymbol{\psi}, \mu | \boldsymbol{o}) \propto \int_0^{\infty} P(\boldsymbol{\psi}, \mu, \tau | \boldsymbol{o}) d\tau \propto L(\boldsymbol{o} | \boldsymbol{\psi}, \mu) \cdot (\boldsymbol{\psi}'\boldsymbol{\psi})^{-(I/2 + \alpha)}$$

We propose now the following change of variable $\boldsymbol{\psi} \rightarrow (\rho, \boldsymbol{\phi})$, where $\boldsymbol{\phi} = (\phi_1, ..., \phi_{I-1})$ and $\psi_1 = \rho f_1(\boldsymbol{\phi}), ..., \psi_I = \rho f_I(\boldsymbol{\phi})$ for:

$$f_1(\boldsymbol{\phi}) = \cos(\phi_1),$$

$$f_i(\boldsymbol{\phi}) = \prod_{j=1}^{i-1} \sin(\phi_j) \cos(\phi_i) \; i = 2, ..., I - 1,$$

$$f_I(\boldsymbol{\phi}) = \prod_{j=1}^{I} \sin(\phi_j).$$

For this change of variable, the Jacobian is:

$$
\left| \frac{\partial \psi}{\partial(\rho, \phi)} \right| = \left| \begin{pmatrix} f_1(\phi) & f_2(\phi) & f_3(\phi) & \cdots & f_I(\phi) \\ \rho\frac{\partial f_1(\phi)}{\partial \phi_1} & \rho\frac{\partial f_2(\phi)}{\partial \phi_1} & \rho\frac{\partial f_3(\phi)}{\partial \phi_1} & \cdots & \rho\frac{\partial f_I(\phi)}{\partial \phi_1} \\ 0 & \rho\frac{\partial f_2(\phi)}{\partial \phi_2} & \rho\frac{\partial f_3(\phi)}{\partial \phi_2} & \cdots & \rho\frac{\partial f_I(\phi)}{\partial \phi_2} \\ 0 & 0 & \rho\frac{\partial f_3(\phi)}{\partial \phi_3} & \cdots & \rho\frac{\partial f_I(\phi)}{\partial \phi_3} \\ \vdots & \vdots & \vdots & \ddots & \vdots \end{pmatrix} \right| = \rho^{I-1} f(\phi)
$$

where $f_1(\phi), f_2(\phi), ..., f_I(\phi)$ and $f(\phi)$ are several functions of ϕ being products and sums of trigonometric functions. We will not develop $f(\phi)$ further as it will be irrelevant for the rest of the proof. Therefore,

$$
\int P(\psi, \mu | o) d\psi = \int P(\rho, \phi, \mu | o) \left| \frac{\partial \psi}{\partial(\rho, \phi)} \right| d\rho d\phi =
$$

$$
\propto \int L(o | \rho, \phi, \mu) \cdot (\rho^2)^{-(I/2+\alpha)} \rho^{I-1} f(\phi) d\rho d\phi
$$

$$
= \int \left(\int_0^\infty L(o|\rho, \phi, \mu) \cdot \rho^{-2\alpha-1} d\rho \right) f(\phi) d\phi
$$

We focus now on the latter inner integral, with respect to ρ, in that case we have:

$$
\int_0^\infty L(o|\rho, \phi, \mu) \cdot \rho^{-2\alpha-1} d\rho \geq \int_0^\epsilon L(o|\rho, \phi, \mu) \cdot \rho^{-2\alpha-1} d\rho
$$

for ϵ being a positive and low value. Since the likelihood function is a continuous function of ρ, for ρ in $[0, \epsilon]$, $L(o|\rho, \phi, \mu)$ will be close to $L(o|0, \phi, \mu)$ which takes a positive value. So, for ϵ small enough, there is a positive value K for which $L(o|\rho, \phi, \mu) \geq K$ for any ρ in $[0, \epsilon]$. In that case

$$
\int_0^\epsilon L(o|\rho, \phi, \mu) \cdot \rho^{-2\alpha-1} d\rho \geq K \int_0^\epsilon \rho^{-2\alpha-1} d\rho = \frac{K}{-2\alpha} \rho^{-2\alpha} \Big|_0^\epsilon,
$$

which diverges to infinite for any $\alpha > 0$. Note, moreover, that for $\alpha = 0$

$$
K \int_0^\epsilon \rho^{-2\alpha-1} = K \log(\rho)|_0^\epsilon
$$

which is also infinite. Thus, the posterior distribution is improper for all $\alpha \geq 0$ as we wanted to show. $\qquad \square$

Bibliography

Abellán, J., Fecht, D., Best, N., Richardson, S., and Briggs, D. J. (2007). Bayesian analysis of the multivariate geographical distribution of the socio-economic environment in england. *Environmetrics*, 18:745–758.

Adín, A., Martinez-Beneito, M. A., Botella-Rocamora, P., Goicoa, T., and Ugarte, M. D. (2017). Smoothing and high risk areas detection in space-time disease mapping: a comparison of P-splines, autoregressive and moving average models. *Stochastic and Environmental Research and Risk Assessment*, 31:403–415.

Agarwal, D. K., Gelfand, A. E., and Citron-Pousty, S. (2002). Zero-inflated models with application to spatial count data. *Environmental and Ecological Statistics*, 9:341–355.

Akaike, H. (1973). Information theory and an extension of the maximum likelihood principle. In Petrov, B. N. and Csaki, F., editors, *Proc. 2nd International Symposium on Information Theory*, pages 267–281.

Alexander, F. E. and Boyle, P., editors (1996). *Methods for Investigating Localized Clustering of Disease*. Number 135 in IARC Scientific Publications. IARC, Lyon.

Allaire, J., Xie, Y., McPherson, J., Luraschi, J., Ushey, K., Atkins, A., Wickham, H., Cheng, J., and Chang, W. (2018). *RMarkdown: Dynamic Documents for R*. R package version 1.9.

Arab, A. (2015). Spatial and spatio-temporal models for modeling epidemiological data with excess zeros. *International Journal of Environmental Research and Public Health*, 12(9):10536–10548.

Assunção, R. M., Potter, J. E., and Cavenaghi, S. M. (2002). A Bayesian space varying parameter applied to estimating fertility schedules. *Statistics in Medicine*, 21:2057–2075.

Assunção, R. M., Reis, I. A., and Oliveira, C. L. (2001). Diffusion and prediction of leishmaniasis in a large metropolitan area in Brazil with a Bayesian space-time model. *Statistics in Medicine*, 20:2319–2335.

Assunçao, R. M. (2003). Space varying coefficient models for small area data. *Environmetrics*, 14:453–473.

Assunçao, R. M. and Krainski, E. (2009). Neighborhood dependence in Bayesian spatial models. *Biometrical Journal*, 51:851–869.

Baath, R. (2014). Bayesian first aid. http://www.sumsar.net/blog/2014/01/bayesian-first-aid/.

Balderama, E., Gardner, B., and Reich, B. J. (2016). A spatial-temporal double-hurdle model for extremely over-dispersed avian count data. *Spatial Statistics*, 18:263–275.

Banerjee, S. and Carlin, B. P. (2003). Semiparametric spatio-temporal frailty modeling. *Environmetrics*, 14(5):523–535.

Banerjee, S. and Carlin, B. P. (2004). Parametric spatial cure rate models for interval-censored time-to-relapse data. *Biometrics*, 60(1):268–275.

Banerjee, S., Carlin, B. P., and Gelfand, A. E. (2014). *Hierarchical modelling and analysis for spatial data, Second edition.* Chapman & Hall/CRC.

Banerjee, S. and Gelfand, A. E. (2006). Bayesian Wombling: Curvilinear gradient assessment under spatial process models. *Journal of the American Statistical Association*, 101(476):1487–1501.

Banerjee, S., Gelfand, A. E., and Sirmans, C. (2003a). Directional rates of change under spatial process models. *Journal of the American Statistical Association*, 98:946–954.

Banerjee, S., Wall, M. M., and Carlin, B. P. (2003b). Frailty modeling for spatially correlated survival data, with application to infant mortality in Minnesota. *Biostatistics*, 4(1):123–42.

Bauer, C., Wakefield, J., Rue, H., Self, S., Feng, Z., and Wang, Y. (2016). Bayesian penalized spline models for the analysis of spatio-temporal count data. *Statistics in Medicine*, 35(11):1848–1865.

Bayarri, M. J., Berger, J., and Datta, G. S. (2008). Objective Bayes testing of Poisson versus inflated Poisson models. In *Pushing the Limits of Contemporary Statistics: Contributions in Honor of Jayanta K. Ghosh*, volume 3, pages 105–121. Institute of Mathematical Statistics.

Bayarri, M. J., Berger, J. O., Forte, A., and García-Donato, G. (2012). Criteria for Bayesian model choice with application to variable selection. *The Annals of Statistics*, 40(3):1550–1577.

Berger, J. (2006). The case for objective Bayesian analysis. *Bayesian Analysis*, 1:385–402.

Berger, J. O. (1985). *Statistical Decision Theory and Bayesian Inference.* Springer-Verlag, Berlin.

Berger, J. O. and Pericchi, L. R. (2001). *Objective Bayesian Methods for Model Selection: Introduction and Comparison*, Volume 38 of *Lecture Notes–Monograph Series*, pages 135–207. Institute of Mathematical Statistics, Beachwood, OH.

Berke, O. (2004). Exploratory disease mapping: kriging the spatial risk function from regional count data. *International Journal of Health Geographics*, 3:18.

Bernardinelli, L., Clayton, D., and Montomoli, C. (1995a). Bayesian estimates of disease maps: How important are priors? *Statistics in Medicine*, 14:2411–2431.

Bernardinelli, L., Clayton, D., Pascutto, C., Montomoli, C., Ghislandi, M., and Songini, M. (1995b). Bayesian analysis of space-time variation in disease risk. *Statistics in Medicine*, 14:2433–2443.

Besag, J. (1974). Spatial interaction and the statistical analysis of lattice systems. *Journal of the Royal Statistical Society: Series B (Statistical Methodology)*, 36:192–236.

Besag, J. (1975). Statistical analysis of non-lattice data. *The Statistician*, 24(3):179–195.

Besag, J., Green, P., Higdon, D., and Mengersen, K. (1995). Bayesian computation and stochastic systems. *Statistical Science*, 10(1):3–41.

Besag, J. and Kooperberg, C. (1995). On conditional and intrinsic autoregressions. *Biometrika*, 82(4):733–746.

Besag, J. and Newell, J. (1991). The detection of clusters in rare diseases. *Applied Statistics*, 154(1):143–155.

Besag, J., York, J., and Mollié, A. (1991). Bayesian image restoration, with two applications in spatial statistics. *Annals of the Institute of Statistical Mathemathics*, 43:1–21.

Best, N., Ickstadt, K., Wolpert, R. L., and Briggs, D. J. (2000a). Combining models of health and exposure data: The SAVIAH Study. In Elliott, P., Wakefield, J. C., Best, N., and Briggs, D. J., editors, *Spatial Epidemiology-Methods and Applications*, pages 393–414. Oxford University Press.

Best, N., Ickstadt, K., Wolpert, R. L., and Briggs, D. J. (2000b). Spatial Poisson regression for health and exposure data measured at disparate resolutions. *Journal of the American Statistical Association*, 95:1076–1088.

Best, N., Richardson, S., and Thomson, A. (2005). A comparison of Bayesian spatial models for disease mapping. *Statistical Methods in Medical Research*, 14:35–59.

Best, N. G., Arnold, Arnold, R., Thomas, A., Waller, L. A., and Conlon, E. M. (1999). Bayesian models for spatially correlated disease and exposure data. In *Bayesian Statistics 6*. Oxford University Press.

Biggeri, A. and Lagazio, C. (1999). Case-control analysis of risk around putative sources. In Lawson, A., Biggeri, A., Bohning, D., Lesaffre, E., Viel, J. F., and Bertollini, R., editors, *Disease Mapping and Risk Assessment for Public Health*. Wiley.

Billheimer, D., Cardoso, T., Freeman, E., Guttorp, P., Hiu-Wan, K., and Silkey, M. (1997). Natural variability of benthic species composition in the Delaware Bay. *Environmental and Ecological Statistics*, 5:95–115.

Bithell, J. (1995). The choice of test for detecting raised disease risk near a point source. *Statistics in Medicine*, 14:2309–2322.

Bivand, R., Pebesma, E. J., and Gómez-Rubio, V. (2008). *Applied Spatial Data Analysis with R*. Springer-Verlag.

Blangiardo, M. and Cameletti, M. (2015). *Spatial and Spatio-Temporal Bayesian Models with R-INLA*. Wiley.

Blangiardo, M., Cameletti, M., Baio, G., and Rue, H. (2013). Spatial and spatio-temporal models with R-INLA. *Spatial and Spatio-Temporal Epidemiology*, 4:33–49.

Böhning, D. and Schlattmann, P. (1999). Disease mapping with hidden structure using mixture models. In Lawson, A., Biggeri, A., Böhning, D., Lesaffre, E., Viel, J.-F., and Bertollini, R., editors, *Disease Mapping and Risk Assessment for Public Health*, pages 49–60. Wiley.

Böhning, D., Schlattmann, P., and Lindsay, B. (1992). Computer-assisted analysis of mixtures (C.A.MAN): statistical algorithms. *Biometrics*, 48(1):283–303.

Borrell, C., Cano Serral, G., Martínez-Beneito, M. A., Dell'Olmo, M., Marc, Rodriguez Sanz, M., and Grupo MEDEA (2009). *Atlas de mortalidad en ciudades de España (1996-2003)*.

Borrell, C., Marí Dell'Olmo, M., Serrall, G., Martínez-Beneito, M. A., and Gotséns, M. (2010). Inequalities in mortality in small areas of eleven Spanish cities (the multicenter MEDEA Project). *Health & Place*, 16:703–711.

Botella-Rocamora, P., López-Quílez, A., and Martinez-Beneito, M. A. (2012). Spatial moving average risk smoothing. *Statistics in Medicine*, 32:2595–2612.

Botella-Rocamora, P., Martinez-Beneito, M. A., and Banerjee, S. (2015). A unifying modeling framework for highly multivariate disease mapping. *Statistics in Medicine*, 34(9):1548–1559.

Box, G. E. P. and Draper, N. R. (1987). *Empirical Model-Building and Response Surfaces*. John Wiley & Sons.

Bradinath, P., Day, N. E., and Stockton, D. (1995). Geographical culustering of acute adult leukaemia in the East Anglian region of the United Kingdom: a registry-based analysis. *Journal of Epidemiology and Community Health*, 53:317–318.

Bradley, J. R., Holan, S. H., and Wikle, C. K. (2018). Computationally efficient multivariate spatio-temporal models for high-dimensional count-valued data (with discussion). *Bayesian Analysis*, 13(1):253–310.

Brewer, C. A., MacEachern, A. M., Pickle, L. W., and Herrman, D. J. (1997). Mapping mortality: Evaluating color schemes for choropleth maps. *Annals of the Association of American Geographers*, 87(3):411–438.

Brezger, A., Fahrmeir, L., and Hennerfeind, A. (2007). Adaptive Gaussian Markov random fields with applications in human brain mapping. *Applied Statistics*, 56(3):327–345.

Brinks, R. (2008). On the convergence of derivatives of B-splines to derivatives of the Gaussian function. *Computational & Applied Mathematics*, 27: 79–92.

Brook, D. (1964). On the distinction between the conditional probability and joint probability approaches in the specification of nearest neighbour systems. *Biometrika*, 51(3):481–483.

Brooks, S. P. and Gelman, A. (1998). General methods for monitoring convergence of iterative simulations. *Journal of Computational & Graphical Statistics*, 7:434–455.

Carlin, B. P. and Banerjee, S. (2003). Hierarchical multivariate CAR models for spatio-temporally correlated survival data. In Bernardo, J. M., Bayarri, M. J., Berger, J. O., Dawid, A. P., Heckerman, D., Smith, A. F. M., and West, M., editors, *Bayesian Statistics 7*, pages 45–64. Oxford University Press.

Carlin, B. P., Gelfand, A. E., and Smith, A. F. M. (1992). Hierarchical Bayesian analysis of changepoint problems. *Applied Statistics*, 41(2): 389–405.

Carlin, B. P., Gelman, A., and Neal, R. M. (1998). Markov chain Monte Carlo in practice: A roundtable discussion. *The American Statistician*, 52(2): 93–100.

Carlin, B. P. and Louis, T. A. (2000). *Bayes and Empirical Bayes Methods for Data Analysis*. Chapman & Hall/CRC.

Celeux, G., Forbes, F., Robert, C. P., and Titterington, D. M. (2006). Deviance information criteria for missing data models (with discussion). *Bayesian Analysis*, 1(30):651–706.

Chilès, J. P. and Delfiner, P. (2012). *Geostatistics: Modeling Spatial Uncertainty. Second edition*. Wiley, New Jersey.

Choo, L. and Walker, S. G. (2008). A new approach to investigating spatial variations of disease. *Journal of the Royal Statistical Society: Series A (Statistics in Society)*, 171(2):395–405.

Christensen, O. F. and Waagepetersen, R. (2002). Bayesian prediction of spatial count data using generalized linear mixed models. *Biometrics*, 58:280–286.

Christensen, W. F. and Amemiya, Y. (2002). Latent variable analysis of multivariate spatial data. *Journal of the American Statistical Association*, 97(457):302–317.

Clayton, D., Bernardinelli, L., and Montomoli, C. (1993). Spatial correlation in ecological analysis. *International Journal of Epidemiology*, 22:1193–1202.

Clayton, D. and Hills, M. (1993). *Statistical Models in Epidemiology*. Oxford University Press, Oxford.

Clayton, D. and Kaldor, J. (1987). Empirical Bayes estimates of age-standardized relative risks for use in disease mapping. *Biometrics*, 43(3):671–681.

Congdon, P. (2002). A life table approach to small area health need profiling. *Statistical Modelling*, 2:63–88.

Congdon, P. (2007a). Bayesian modelling strategies for spatially varying regression coefficients: A multivariate perspective for multiple outcomes. *Computational Statistics & Data Analysis*, 51:2586–2601.

Congdon, P. (2007b). Mixtures of spatial and unstructured effects for spatially discontinuous health outcomes. *Computational Statistics & Data Analysis*, 51:3197–3212.

Congdon, P. (2008). A spatially adaptive conditional autoregressive prior for area health data. *Statistical Methodology*, 5:552–563.

Cook, D. and Pocock, S. (1983). Multiple regression in geographic mortality studies with allowance for spatially correlated errors. *Biometrics*, 39:361–371.

Corpas-Burgos, F., Botella-Rocamora, P., and Martinez-Beneito, M. A. (2019). On the convenience of heteroscedasticity in highly multivariate disease mapping. *TEST*.

Corpas-Burgos, F., García-Donato, G., and Martinez-Beneito, M. A. (2018). Some findings on zero-inflated and hurdle Poisson models for disease mapping. *Statistics in Medicine*, 37(23):3325–3337.

Cressie, N. (1996). Change of support and the modifiable areal unit problem. *Geographical Systems*, 3(2-3):159–180.

Cressie, N. and Chan, N. H. (1989). Spatial modeling of regional variables. *Journal of the American Statistical Association*, 84:393–401.

Cressie, N. and Kapat, P. (2008). Some diagnostics for Markov random fields. *Journal of Computational and Graphical Statistics*, 17(3):726–749.

Cressie, N. and Wikle, C. K. (2011). *Statistics for Spatio-Temporal Data*. John Wiley & Sons.

Cressie, N. A. (1993). *Statistics for Spatial Data. Revised edition.* John Wiley & Sons.

Crook, A. M., Knorr-Held, L., and Hemingway, H. (2003). Measuring spatial effects in time to event data: a case study using months from angiography to coronary artery bypass graft (CABG). *Statistics in Medicine*, 22(18):2943–2961.

Cui, Y., Hodges, J. S., Kong, X., and Carlin, B. P. (2010). Partitioning degrees of freedom in hierarchical and other richly-parameterized models. *Technometrics*, 52:124–136.

Cuzick, J. and Edwards, R. (1990). Spatial clustering for inhomogeneous populations (with discussion). *Journal of the Royal Statistical Society: Series B (Statistical Methodology)*, 52:73–104.

Daniels, M. J. and Kass, R. E. (1999). Nonconjugate Bayesian estimation of covariance matrices and its use in hierarchical models. *Journal of the American Statistical Association*, 94:1254–1263.

Dean, C. B., Ugarte, M. D., and Militino, A. F. (2001). Detecting interaction between random region and fixed age effects in disease mapping. *Biometrics*, 57:197–202.

Denison, D. G. and Holmes, C. C. (2001). Bayesian partitioning for estimating disease risk. *Biometrics*, 57:143–149.

Diggle, P. J. (1990). A point process modelling approach to raised incidence of a rare phenomenon in the vicinity of a prespecified point. *Journal of the Royal Statistical Society, Series A*, 153:340–362.

Diggle, P. J., Elliott, P., Morris, S. E., and Shaddick, G. (1997). Regression modelling of disease risk in relation to point sources. *Journal of the Royal Statistical Society, Series A*, 160:491–505.

Diggle, P. J., Morris, S. E., and Wakefield, J. C. (2000). Point source modeling using matched case-control data. *Biostatistics*, 1:89–105.

Diggle, P. J., Tawn, J. A., and Moyeed, R. A. (1998). Model based geostatistics (with discussion). *Applied Statistics*, 47(3):299–350.

Dobra, A., Lenkoski, A., and Rodriguez, A. (2011). Bayesian inference for general Gaussian graphical models with application to multivariate lattice data. *Journal of the American Statistical Association*, 106(496):1418–1433.

Dwyer-Lindgren, L., Flaxman, A. D., Ng, M., Hansen, G. M., Murray, C. J., and Mokdad, A. H. (2015). Drinking patterns in US counties from 2002 to 2012. *American Journal of Public Health*, 105(6):1120–1127. PMID: 25905846.

Earnest, A., Beard, J. R., Morgan, G., Lincoln, D., Summerhayes, R., Donoghue, D., Dunn, T., Muscatello, D., and Mengersen, K. (2010). Small area estimation of sparse disease counts using shared component models-application to birth defect registry data in New South Wales, Australia. *Health & Place*, 16:684–693.

Earnest, A., Morgan, G., Mengersen, K., Louise, R., Richard, S., and Beard, J. (2007). Evaluating the effect of neighbourhood weight matrices on smoothing properties of conditional autoregressive (CAR) models. *International Journal of Health Geographics*, pages 6–54.

Eberly, L. E. and Carlin, B. P. (2000). Identifiability and convergence issues for Markov chain Monte Carlo fitting of spatial models. *Statistics in Medicine*, 19:2279–2294.

Eilers, P. H. C. and Marx, B. D. (1996). Flexible smoothing with B-splines and penalties. *Statistical Science*, 11(2):89–102.

Elliott, P., Wakefield, J. C., Best, N., and Briggs, D. J., editors (2000). *Spatial Epidemiology*. Oxford University Press.

Esteve, J., Benhamou, E., and Raymond, L. (1994). *Descriptive Epidemiology*. IARC Scientific publications.

Fan, J. and Zhang, W. (1999). Statistical estimation in varying coefficient models. *The Annals of Statistics*, 27:1491–1518.

Faraway, J. J. (2016). *Extending the Linear Model with R: Generalized Linear, Mixed Effects and Nonparametric Regression Models, Second Edition*. CRC Press.

Fernández, C. and Green, P. (2002). Modelling spatially correlated data via mixtures: a Bayesian approach. *Journal of the Royal Statistical Society: Series B (Statistical Methodology)*, 64(4):805–826.

Ferrándiz, J., Abellán, J., Gómez-Rubio, V., López-Quílez, A., Sanmart'in, P., Abellán, C., Martínez-Beneito, M. A., Melchor, I., Vanaclocha, H., Zurriaga, O., Ballester, F., Gil, J. M., Pérez-Hoyos, S., and Ocaña, R. (2004). Spatial analysis of the relationship between mortality from cardiovascular and cerebrovascular disease and drinking water hardness. *Environmental Health Perspectives*, 112(9):1037–1044.

Ferrándiz, J., López-Quílez, A., Gómez-Rubio, V., Sanmartín, P., Martínez-Beneito, M. A., Melchor, I., Vanaclocha, H., Zurriaga, O., Ballester, F., Gil, J. M., Pérez-Hoyos, S., and Abellán, J. J. (2003). Statistical relationship between hardness of drinking water and cerebrovascular mortality in Valencia: a comparison of spatiotemporal models. *Environmetrics*, 14(5):491–510.

Fleiss, J. L., Levin, B., and Cho Paik, M. (2003). *Statistical Methods for Rates and Proportions. Third edition.* John Wiley & Sons.

Franco-Villoria, M., Ventrucci, M., and Rue, H. (2018). Bayesian varying coefficient models using PC priors. arXiv:1806.02084v1.

Freedman, D. A. (2001). Ecological inference and the ecological fallacy. In *International Encyclopedia of the Social & Behavioral Sciences*, volume 6, pages 4027–4030. Pergamon, Oxford, UK.

Gamerman, D. and Lopes, H. F. (2006). *Markov Chain Monte Carlo: Stochastic Simulation for Bayesian Inference.* Chapman & Hall/CRC.

Gamerman, D., Moreira, A., and Rue, H. (2003). Space-varying regression models: specifications and simulation. *Computational Statistics and Data Analysis*, 42:513–533.

Gelfand, A. E., Kim, J., Sirmans, C., and Banerjee, S. (2003). Spatial modeling with spatially varying coefficient processes. *Journal of the American Statistical Association*, 98(462):387–396.

Gelfand, A. E., Sahu, S. K., and Carlin, B. P. (1995a). Efficient parametrizations for generalized linear mixed models (with discussion). In Bernardo, Jose M. Berger, J. O., Dawid, A. P., and Smith, A. F. M., editors, *Bayesian Statistics 5*. Oxford University Press.

Gelfand, A. E., Sahu, S. K., and Carlin, B. P. (1995b). Efficient parametrizations for Normal linear mixed models. *Biometrika*, 82(3):479–488.

Gelfand, A. E., Schmidt, A. M., Banerjee, S., and Sirmans, C. F. (2004). Nonstationary multivariate process modeling through spatially varying coregionalization. *Test*, 13(2):263–312.

Gelfand, A. E. and Smith, A. F. M. (1990). Sampling-based approaches to calculating marginal densities. *Journal of the American Statistical Association*, 85(410):398–409.

Gelfand, A. E. and Vounatsou, P. (2003). Proper multivariate conditional autoregressive models for spatial data analysis. *Biostatistics*, 4(1):11–25.

Gelman, A. (2005a). Analysis of variance — why it is more important than ever (with discussion). *The Annals of Statistics*, 33:1–53.

Gelman, A. (2005b). Prior distributions for variance parameters in hierarchical models. *Bayesian Analysis*, 1(3):515–533.

Gelman, A., Carlin, J. B., Stern, H. S., and Rubin, D. B. (2003). *Bayesian Data Analysis*. Chapman & Hall/CRC, Boca Raton, 2nd edition.

Gelman, A. and Rubin, D. B. (1992). Inference from iterative simulation using multiple sequences. *Statistical Sciences*, 7:457–511.

Gentle, J. E. (2007). *Matrix Algebra. Theory, Computations, and Applications in Statistics*. Springer-Verlag.

Gerber, F. and Furrer, R. (2015). Pitfalls in the implementation of Bayesian hierarchical modeling of areal count data: An illustration using BYM and Leroux models. *Journal of Statistical Software*, 63(1):1–32.

Geyer, C. (1992). Practical Markov Chain Monte Carlo. *Statistical Science*, 7(4):473–511.

Gilks, W. R., Richardson, S., and Spiegelhalter, D. J., editors (1996). *Markov Chain Monte Carlo in Practice*. Chapman & Hall/CRC.

Gneiting, T. and Raftery, A. E. (2007). Strictly proper scoring rules, prediction, and estimation. *Journal of the American Statistical Association*, 102:359–378.

Goicoa, T., Adin, A., Etxeberria, J., Militino, A., and Ugarte, M. (2018a). Flexible bayesian p-splines for smoothing age-specific spatio-temporal mortality patterns. *Statistical Methods in Medical Research*, 0(0):0962280217726802. PMID: 28847210.

Goicoa, T., Adin, A., Ugarte, M. D., and Hodges, J. S. (2018b). In spatio-temporal disease mapping model, identifiability constraints affect PQL and INLA. *Stochastic Environmental Research and Risk Assessment*, 32(3):749–770.

Goicoa, T., Etxeberria, J., and Ugarte, M. D. (2016a). Splines in disease mapping. In *Handbook of Spatial Epidemiology*, chapter 12, pages 225–238. CRC Press.

Goicoa, T., Ugarte, M. D., Etxebarria, J., and Militino, A. F. (2016b). Age-space-time CAR models in Bayesian disease mapping. *Statistics in Medicine*, 35:2391–2405.

Goicoa, T., Ugarte, M. D., Etxeberria, J., and Militino, A. F. (2012). Comparing CAR and P-spline models in spatial disease mapping. *Environmental and Ecological Statistics*, 19:573–599.

Goovaerts, P. (2006). Geostatistical analysis of disease data: accounting for spatial support and population density in the isopleth mapping of cancer mortality risk using area-to-point Poisson kriging. *International Journal of Health Geographics*, 5:52.

Goovaerts, P. and Gebreab, S. (2008). How does Poisson Kriging compare to the popular BYM model for mapping disease risks? *International Journal of Health Geographics*, 7:6.

Goulard, M. and Voltz, M. (1992). Linear coregionalization model: Tools for estimation and choice of cross-variogram matrix. *Mathematical Geology*, 24:269–286.

Greco, F. P. and Trivisano, C. (2009). A multivariate CAR model for improving the estimation of relative risks. *Stat. Med.*, 28(12):1707–1724.

Green, P. and Richardson, S. (2002). Hidden Markov models and disease mapping. *Journal of the American Statistical Association*, 97(460):1–16.

Green, P. J. (1995). Reversible Jump Markov chain Monte Carlo computation and Bayesian model determination. *Biometrika*, 82(4):711–732.

Greenland, S. (1992). Divergent biases in ecological and individual-level studies. *Statistics in Medicine*, 11:1209–1223.

Gschlößl, S. and Czado, C. (2008). Modelling count data with overdispersion and spatial effects. *Statistical Papers*, 49(3):531–552.

Gómez-Rubio, V., Ferrándiz-Ferragud, J., and Lopez-Quílez, A. (2005). Detecting clusters of disease with R. *Journal of Geographical Systems*, 7(2):189–206.

Haining, R., Li, G., Maheswaran, R., Blangiardo, M., Law, J., Best, N., and Richardson, S. (2010). Inference from ecological models: Estimating the relative risk of stroke from air pollution exposure using small area data. *Spatial and Spatio-Temporal Epidemiology*, 1:123–131.

Hanks, E. M., Schliep, E. M., Hooten, M. B., and Hoeting, J. A. (2015). Restricted spatial regression in practice: geostatistical models, confounding and robustness under model misspecification. *Environmetrics*, 26:243–254.

Harrower, M. A. and Brewer, C. A. (2003). Colorbrewer.org: An online tool for selecting color schemes for maps. *The Cartographic Journal*, 40(1):27–37.

Harville, D. A. (1997). *Matrix Algebra from a Statistician's Perspective*. Springer.

Hastie, T. and Tibshirani, R. (1993). Varying-coefficient models. *Journal of the Royal Statistical Society, Series B*, 55(4):757–796.

Held, L., Natário, I., Fenton, S. E., Rue, H., and Becker, N. (2005). Towards joint disease mapping. *Statistical Methods in Medical Research*, 14:61–82.

Henderson, H. V. and Searle, S. R. (1979). Vec and vech operators for matrices, with some uses in Jacobians and multivariate statistics. *The Canadian Journal of Statistics*, 7:65–81.

Higdon, D. (2002). Space and space-time modeling using process convolutions. In Anderson, C., Barnett, V., Chatwin, P. C., and El Shaarawai, A. H., editors, *Quantitative Methods for Current Environmental Issues*, pages 37–54. Springer-Verlag, London.

Hodges, J. (2013). *Richly Parameterized Linear Models: Additive, Time Series and Spatial Models Using Random Effects*. Chapman & Hall-CRC.

Hodges, J. S., Carlin, B. P., and Fan, Q. (2003). On the precision of the conditionally autoregressive prior in spatial models. *Biometrics*, 59:317–322.

Hodges, J. S., Cui, Y., Sargent, D. J., and Carlin, B. P. (2007). Smoothing balanced single-error-term analysis of variance. *Technometrics*, 49:12–25.

Hodges, J. S. and Reich, B. J. (2010). Adding spatially-correlated errors can mess up the fixed effect you love. *The American Statistician*, 64(4):325–334.

Hoffmann, W. and Schlattmann, P. (1999). Geographical distribution of leukaemia incidence in the vicinity of a suspected point source: A case study. In Lawson, A., Biggeri, A., Bohning, D., Lesaffre, E., Viel, J. F., and Bertollini, R., editors, *Disease Mapping and Risk Assessment for Public Health*. Wiley.

Hoffmann, W., Terschueren, C., and Richardson, D. B. (2007). Childhood leukaemia in the vicinity of the Geesthacht nuclear establishment near Hamburg, Germany. *Environmental Health*, 115:947–952.

Hogan, J. W. and Tchernis, R. (2004). Bayesian factor analysis for spatially correlated data, with application to summarizing area-level material deprivation from census data. *Journal of the American Statistical Association*, 99:314–324.

Huang, J., Wu, C., and Zhou, L. (2002). Varying-coefficient models and basis function approximations for the analysis of repeated measurements. *Biometrika*, 89(1):111–128.

Hughes, J. and Haran, M. (2013). Dimension reduction and alleviation of confounding for spatial generalized linear mixed models. *Journal of the Royal Statistical Society: Series B (Statistical Methodology)*, 75(1):139–159.

Ibañez Beroiz, B., Librero-López, J., Peiró-Moreno, S., and Bernal-Delgado, E. (2011). Shared component modelling as an alternative to assess geographical variations in medical practice: gender inequalities in hospital admissions for chronic diseases. *BMC Medical Research Methodology*, 11:172.

Ibrahim, J. G. and Laud, P. W. (1991). On Bayesian analysis of generalized linear models using Jeffreys's prior. *Journal of the American Statistical Association*, 86:981–986.

Ickstadt, K. and Wolpert, R. L. (1999). Spatial regresion for marked point processes. In Bernardo, J. M., Berger, J. O., Dawid, A. P., and Smith, A. F. M., editors, *Bayesian Statistics 6*, pages 323–341. Oxford University Press.

Ioannidis, J. P. A. (2005). Contradicted and initially stronger effects in highly cited clinical research. *Journal of the American Medical Association*, 294(2):218–228.

Jin, X., Banerjee, S., and Carlin, B. P. (2007). Order-free co-regionalized areal data models with application to multiple-disease mapping. *Journal of the Royal Statistical Society: Series B (Statistical Methodology)*, 69(5):817–838.

Jin, X., Carlin, B. P., and Banerjee, S. (2005). Generalized hierarchical multivariate CAR models for areal data. *Biometrics*, 61:950–961.

Karlis, D. and Meligkotsidou, L. (2007). Finite mixtures of multivariate Poisson distributions with application. *Journal of Statistical Planning and Inference*, 137(6):1942–1960.

Kelsall, J. E. and Wakefield, J. (1999). Discussion to: "Bayesian models for spatially correlated disease and exposure data". In *Bayesian Statistics 6*, pages 131–156. Oxford University Press.

Kelsall, J. E. and Wakefield, J. (2002). Modeling spatial variation in disease risk: A geostatistical approach. *Journal of the American Statistical Association*, 97:692–701.

Kim, H., Sun, D., and Tsutakawa, R. K. (2001). A bivariate Bayes method for improving the estimates of mortality rates with a twofold conditional autoregressive model. *J. Amer. Statist. Assoc.*, 96(456):1506–1521.

Kim, H.-J., Fay, M. P., Feuer, E. J., and Midthune, D. N. (2000). Permutation tests for joinpoint regression with applications to cancer rates. *Statistics in Medicine*, 19:335–351.

Kim, H.-J., Yu, B., and Feuer, E. (2009). Selecting the number of change-points in segmented line regression. *Statistica Sinica*, 19:597–609.

Knorr-Held, L. (2000). Bayesian modelling of inseparable space-time variation in disease risk. *Statistics in Medicine*, 19:2555–2567.

Knorr-Held, L. and Besag, J. (1998). Modelling risk from a disease in time and space. *Statistics in Medicine*, 17:2045–2060.

Knorr-Held, L. and Best, N. (2001). A shared component model for detecting joint and selective clustering of two diseases. *Journal of the Royal Statistical Society: Series A (Statistics in Society)*, 164(13):73–85.

Knorr-Held, L. and Rainer, E. (2001). Projections of lung cancer mortality in West Germany: a case study in Bayesian prediction. *Biostatistics*, 2(1):109–129.

Knorr-Held, L. and Raßer, G. (2000). Bayesian detection of clusters and discontinuities in disease maps. *Biometrics*, 56(13-21):2045–2060.

Knox, E. G. (1994). Leukaemia clusters in childhood: geographical analysis in britain. *Journal of Epidemiology and Community Health*, 48(4):369–376.

Kottas, A., Duan, J. A., and Gelfand, A. E. (2007). Modeling disease incidence data with spatial and spatio-temporal Dirichlet process mixtures. *Biometrical Journal*, 49:1–14.

Krainski, E. T., Gómez-Rubio, V., Bakka, H., Lenzi, A., Castro-Camilo, D., Simpson, D., Lindgren, F., and Rue, H. (2018). *Advanced Spatial Modeling with Stochastic Partial Differential Equations Using R and INLA*. CRC Press.

Kulldorff, M. (1999). Statistical evaluation of disease cluster alarms. In Lawson, A. B., Biggeri, A., Bohning, D., Lesaffre, E., Viel, J. F., and Bertollini, R., editors, *Disease Mapping and Risk Assessment for Public Health*, pages 143–149. John Wiley & Sons.

Kunsch, H. R. (1987). Intrinsic autoregressions and related models on the two-dimensional lattice. *Biometrika*, 74:517–524.

Kyung, M., Gilly, J., Ghosh, M., and Casella, G. (2010). Penalized regression, standard errors and Bayesian lassos. *Bayesian Analysis*, 5(2):369–412.

Lagazzio, C., Biggeri, A., and Dreassi, E. (2003). Age-period-cohort models and disease mapping. *Environmetrics*, 14:475–490.

Lambert, D. (1992). Zero-inflated Poisson regression, with an application to detects on manufacturing. *Technometrics*, 34:1–14.

Lambert, P. C., Sutton, A. J., Burton, P. R., Abrams, K. R., and Jones, D. R. (2005). How vague is vague? a simulation study of the impact of the use of vague prior distributions in MCMC using WinBUGS. *Statistics in Medicine*, 24:2401–2428.

Lang, S. and Brezger, A. (2004). Bayesian P-splines. *Journal of Computational and Graphical Statistics*, 13(1):183–212.

Langford, I. H., Leyland, A. H., Rasbash, J., and Goldstein, H. (1999). Multi-level modelling of the geographical distributions of diseases. *Applied Statistics*, 48(2):253–268.

Lasserre, V., Guihenneuc-Jouyaux, C., and Richardson, S. (2000). Biases in ecological studies: utility of including within area distribution of confounders. *Statistics in Medicine*, 19:45–59.

Lavine, M. L. and Hodges, J. S. (2012). On rigorous specification of ICAR models. *The American Statistician*, 66(1):42–49.

Lawson, A., , Song, H.-R., Cai, B., Hossain, M. M., and Huang, K. (2010). Space-time latent component modeling of geo-referenced health data. *Statistics in Medicine*, 29(19):2012–2027.

Lawson, A., Biggeri, A., Bohning, D., Lesaffre, E., Viel, J. F., and Bertollini, R., editors (1999). *Disease Mapping and Risk Assessment for Public Health*. Wiley.

Lawson, A. and Williams, F. (1994). Armadale: a case-study in environmental epidemiology. *Journal of the Royal Statistical Society, Series A*, 157:285–298.

Lawson, A. B. (1993). On the analysis of mortality events associated with a prespecified fixed point. *Journal of the Royal Statistical Society, Series A*, 156:363–377.

Lawson, A. B. (2006). *Statistical Methods in Spatial Epidemiology (2nd. edition)*. John Wiley & Sons.

Lawson, A. B. (2018). *Bayesian Disease Mapping: Hierarchical Modeling in Spatial Epidemiology (3rd edition)*. CRC Press.

Lawson, A. B., Banerjee, S., Haining, R. P., and Ugarte, M. D., editors (2016). *Handbook of Spatial Epidemiology*. CRC Press.

Lawson, A. B., Biggeri, A., Boehning, D., Lesaffre, E., Viel, J.-F., Clark, A., Schlattmann, P., and Divino, F. (2000). Disease mapping models: an empirical evaluation. *Statistics in Medicine*, 19(17/18):2217–2242.

Lawson, A. B., Browne, W. J., and Vidal Rodeiro, C. L. (2003). *Disease Mapping with WinBUGS and MLwiN*. John Wiley & Sons.

Lawson, A. B. and Clark, A. (2002). Spatial mixture relative risk models applied to disease mapping. *Statistics in Medicine*, 21:359–370.

Lee, D. (2011). A comparison of conditional autoregressive models used in bayesian disease mapping. *Spatial and Spatio-temporal Epidemiology*, 2: 79–89.

Lee, D. and Durban, M. (2011). P-spline anova-type interaction models for spatio-temporal smoothing. *Statistical Modelling*, 11(1):49–69.

Lee, D.-J. and Durban, M. (2009). Smooth-CAR mixed models for spatial count data. *Computational Statistics & Data Analysis*, 53(8):2968–2979.

Leroux, B. G. (2000). Modelling spatial disease rates using maximum likelihood. *Statistics in Medicine*, 19:2321–2332.

Leroux, B. G., Lei, X., and Breslow, N. (1999). Estimation of disease rates in small areas: a new mixed model for spatial dependence. In Halloran, M. E. and Berry, D., editors, *Statistical Models in Epidemiology, the Environment and Clinical Trials*. Springer, Berlin Heidelberg New York.

LeSage, J. P. and Pace, R. K. (2007). A matrix exponential spatial specification. *Journal of Econometrics*, 140(1):190–214.

Li, Y. and Ryan, L. (2002). Modeling spatial survival data using semiparametric frailty models. *Biometrics*, 58(2):287–297.

Lindgren, F., Rue, H., and Lindstrom, J. (2011). An explicit link between Gaussian fields and Gaussian Markov random fields: The stochastic partial differential equation approach. *Journal of the Royal Statistical Society, Series B*, 73(4):423–498.

López-Abente, G., Aragonés, N., García-Pérez, J., and Fernández-Navarro, P. (2014). Disease mapping and spatio-temporal analysis: Importance of expected-case computation criteria. *Geospatial Health*, 9(1):27–35.

López-Abente, G., Aragonés, N., Pérez-Gómez, B., Pollán, M., García-Pérez, J., Ramis, R., and Fernández-Navarro, P. (2014). Time trends in municipal distribution patterns of cancer mortality in Spain. *BMC Cancer*, 14(1):535.

López-Abente, G., Ramis, R., Pollán, M., Aragonés, N., Pérez-Gómez, B., Gómez-Barroso, D., Carrasco, J. M., Lope, V., García-Pérez, J., Boldo, E., and García-Mendizábal, M. J. (2006). *Atlas municipal de mortalidad por cáncer en España, 1989-1998*. Instituto de Salud Carlos III.

Lu, H. and Carlin, B. P. (2005). Bayesian areal Wombling for geographical boundary analysis. *Geographical Analysis*, 35:265–285.

Lu, H., Reilly, C. S., Banerjee, S., and Carlin, B. P. (2007). Bayesian areal Wombling via adjacency modelling. *Environmental and Ecological Statistics*, 14:433–452.

Lunn, D., Jackson, C., Best, N., Thomas, A., and Spiegelhalter, D. (2013). *The BUGS Book: A Practical Introduction to Bayesian Analysis*. CRC Press, Boca Raton.

Lunn, D., Thomas, A., Best, N., and Spiegelhalter, D. (2000). WinBUGS – a Bayesian modelling framework: concepts, structure, and extensibility. *Statistics and Computing*, 10:325–337.

Lynch, J. and Smith, G. D. (2005). A life course approach to chronic disease epidemiology. *Annual Review of Public Health*, 26:1–35.

Ma, H. and Carlin, B. P. (2007). Bayesian multivariate areal Wombling for multiple disease boundary analysis. *Bayesian Analysis*, 2(2):281–302.

MacNab, Y., Kemetic, A., Gustafson, P., and Sheps, S. (2006). An innovative application of Bayesian disease mapping methods to patient safety research: A Canadian adverse medical event study. *Statistical Methods in Medical Research*, 25:3960–3980.

MacNab, Y. C. (2003). Hierarchical Bayesian modeling of spatially correlated health service outcome and utilization rates. *Biometrics*, 59(2):305–315.

MacNab, Y. C. (2007). Spline smoothing in Bayesian disease mapping. *Environmetrics*, 18:727–744.

MacNab, Y. C. (2010). On Bayesian shared component disease mapping and ecological regression with errors in covariates. *Statistics in Medicine*, 29:1239–1249.

MacNab, Y. C. (2011). On Gaussian Markov random fields and Bayesian disease mapping. *Statistical Methods in Medical Research*, 20:49–68.

MacNab, Y. C. (2014). On identification in Bayesian disease mapping and ecological-spatial regression models. *Statistical Methods in Medical Research*, 23(2):134–155.

MacNab, Y. C. (2016a). Linear models of coregionalization for multivariate lattice data: a general framework for coregionalized multivariate CAR models. *Statistics in Medicine*, pages 3827–3850.

MacNab, Y. C. (2016b). Linear models of coregionalization for multivariate lattice data: Order-dependent and order-free cMCARs. *Statistical Methods in Medical Research*, 25(4):1118–1144.

MacNab, Y. C. (2018). Some recent work on multivariate Gaussian Markov random fields. *TEST*, 27(3):497–541.

MacNab, Y. C. and Dean, C. B. (2000). Parametric bootstrap and penalized quasi-likelihood inference in conditional autoregressive models. *Statistics in Medicine*, 19:2421–2435.

MacNab, Y. C. and Dean, C. B. (2001). Autoregressive spatial smoothing and temporal spline smoothing for mapping rates. *Biometrics*, 57:949–956.

MacNab, Y. C. and Dean, C. B. (2002). Spatio-temporal modelling of rates for the construction of disease maps. *Statistics in Medicine*, 21(3):347–358.

MacNab, Y. C. and Gustafson, P. (2007). Regression B-spline smoothing in Bayesian disease mapping: With an application to patient safety surveillance. *Statistics in Medicine*, 26:4455–4474.

Maiti, T. (1998). Hierarchical Bayes estimation of mortality rates for disease mapping. *Journal of Statistical Planning and Inference*, 69:339–348.

Mardia, K. V. (1988). Multidimensional multivariate Gaussian Markov random fields with application to image processing. *J. Multivariate Anal.*, 24(2):265–284.

Marí-Dell'Olmo, M., Gotséns, M., Borrell, C., Martinez-Beneito, M. A., Palència, L., Pérez, G., Cirera, L., Daponte, A., Domínguez-Berjón, F., Esnaola, S., Gandarillas, A., Lorenzo, P., Martos, C., Nolasco, A., and Rodríguez-Sanz, M. (2014). Trends in socioeconomic inequalities in ischemic heart disease mortality in small areas of nine Spanish cities from 1996 to 2007 using smoothed ANOVA. *Journal of Urban Health*, 91(1):46–61.

Marí-Dell'Olmo, M. and Martínez-Beneito, M. A. (2015). A multilevel regression model for geographical studies in sets of non-adjacent cities. *PLoS ONE*, 10(8):e0133649.

Marí-Dell'Olmo, M., Martínez-Beneito, M. A., Borrell, C., Zurriaga, O., Nolasco, A., and Dominguez-Berjon, M. F. (2011). Bayesian factor analysis to calculate a deprivation index and its uncertainty. *Epidemiology*, 22(3): 356–364.

Marí Dell'Olmo, M., Martinez-Beneito, M. A., Gotséns, M., and Palència, L. (2014). A smoothed ANOVA model for multivariate ecological regression. *Stochastic Environmental Research and Risk Assessment*, 28(3):695–706.

Marshall, E. C. and Spiegelhalter, D. (2003). Approximate cross-validatory predictive checks in disease mapping models. *Statistics in Medicine*, 22:1649–1660.

Martinez-Beneito, M. A. (2013). A general modelling framework for multivariate disease mapping. *Biometrika*, 100(3):539–553.

Martinez-Beneito, M. A. (2019). Comments on: Some recent work on multivariate Gaussian Markov random fields. *TEST*, 27(3):542–544.

Martinez-Beneito, M. A., Botella-Rocamora, P., and Banerjee, S. (2017). Towards a multidimensional approach to Bayesian disease mapping. *Bayesian Analysis*, 12:239–259.

Martinez-Beneito, M. A., García-Donato, G., and Salmerón, D. (2011). A Bayesian joinpoint regression model with an unknown number of break-points. *Annals of Applied Statistics*, 5(3):2150–2168.

Martinez-Beneito, M. A., Hodges, J. S., and Marí-Dell'Olmo, M. (2016). Smoothed ANOVA modeling. In Lawson, A. B., Banerjee, S., Haining, R. P., and Ugarte, M. D., editors, *Handbook of Spatial Epidemiology*. CRC Press.

Martínez-Beneito, M. A., López Quílez, A., Amador, A., Melchor, I., Botella Rocamora, P., Abellán, C., Abellán, J., Verdejo, F., Zurriaga, O., Vanaclocha, H., and Escolano, M. (2005). *Atlas de mortalidad de la Comunidad Valenciana, 1991-2000*. Generalitat Valenciana.

Martinez-Beneito, M. A., López-Quílez, A., and Botella-Rocamora, P. (2008). An autoregressive approach to spatio-temporal disease mapping. *Statistics in Medicine*, 27:2874–2889.

Martino, S. and Rue, H. (2008). Implementing approximate Bayesian inference using integrated nested Laplace approximation: a manual for the inla program. Technical report, Norwegian University of Science and Technology, Trondheim, Norway.

Martins, T. C., Simpson, D., Lindgren, F., and Rue, H. (2013). Bayesian computing with INLA: New features. *Computational Statistics and Data Analysis*, 67:68–83.

Meligkotsidou, L. (2007). Bayesian multivariate poisson mixtures with an unknown number of components. *Statistics and Computing*, 17:93–107.

Militino, A. F., Ugarte, M. D., and Dean, C. B. (2001). The use of mixture models for identifying high risks in disease mapping. *Statistics in Medicine*, 20(13):2035–2049.

Mohebbi, M., Wolfe, R., and Forbes, A. (2014). Disease mapping and regression with count data in the presence of overdispersion and spatial autocorrelation: A Bayesian model averaging approach. *International Journal of Environmental Research and Public Health*, 11(1):883–902.

Mollié, A. (1996). Bayesian mapping of disease. In Gilks, W. R., Richardson, S., and Spiegelhalter, D. J., editors, *Markov Chain Monte Carlo in Practice*, pages 359–380. Chapman & Hall-CRC, London.

Moraga, P. and Lawson, A. B. (2012). Gaussian component mixtures and CAR models in Bayesian disease mapping. *Computational Statistics & Data Analysis*, 56(6):1417–1433.

Morgenstern, H. (1982). Uses of ecologic analysis in epidemiologic research. *American Journal of Public Health*, 72:1336–1344.

Morgenstern, H. (1995). Ecologic studies in epidemiology: Concepts, principles, and methods. *Annual Review of Public Health*, 16:61–81.

Morris, S. E. and Wakefield, J. C. (1999). Assessment of disease risk in relation to a pre-specified source. In *Spatial Epidemiology. Methods and Applications.*, chapter 9, pages 153–184. Oxford University Press.

Mu, J., Wang, G., and Wang, L. (2018). Estimation and inference in spatially varying coefficient models. *Envirometrics*, 29(1):e2485.

Mugglin, A. S., Carlin, B. P., and Gelfand, A. E. (2000). Fully model-based approaches for spatially misaligned data. *Journal of the American Statistical Association*, 95(451):877–887.

Mullahy, J. (1986). Specification and testing of some modified count data models. *Journal of Econometrics*, 33:341–365.

Musenge, E., Freeman Chirwa, T., Kahn, K., and Vounatsou, P. (2013). Bayesian analysis of zero inflated spatiotemporal HIV/TB child mortality data through the INLA and SPDE approaches: Applied to data observed between 1992 and 2010 in rural North East South Africa. *International Journal of Applied Earth Observation and Geoinformation*, 22:86–98.

Natario, I. and Knorr-Held, L. (2003). Non-parametric ecological regression and spatial variation. *Biometrical Journal*, 45(6):670–688.

Nathoo, F. S. and Ghosh, P. (2013). Skew-elliptical spatial random effect modeling for areal data with application to mapping health utilization rates. *Statistics in Medicine*, 32:290–306.

Neelon, B., Chang, H. H., Ling, Q., and Hastings, N. S. (2014). Spatiotemporal hurdle models for zero-inflated count data: Exploring trends in emergency department visits. *Statistical Methods in Medical Research*, 25(6):2558–2576.

Neelon, B., Ghosh, P., and Loebs, P. F. (2013). A spatial Poisson hurdle model for exploring geographic variation in emergency department visits. *Journal of the Royal Statistical Society, Series A*, 176(2):389–413.

Neyens, T., Lawson, A. B., Kirby, R. S., Nuyts, V., Watjou, K., Aregay, M., Carroll, R., Nawrot, T. S., and Faes, C. (2017). Disease mapping of zero-excessive mesothelioma data in Flanders. *Annals of Epidemiology*, 27(1):59–66.

Nieto-Barajas, L. and Bandyopadhyay, D. (2013). A zero-inflated spatial gamma process model with application to disease mapping. *Journal of Agricultural, Biological, and Environmental Statistics*, 18(2):137–158.

Nobile, A. and Green, P. J. (2000). Bayesian analysis of factorial experiments by mixture modelling. *Biometrika*, 87:15–35.

Nuzzo, R. (2014). Statistical errors. *Nature*, 506:150–152.

Ocaña Riola, R. (2007). The misuse of count data aggregated over time for disease mapping. *Statistics in Medicine*, 26:4489–4504.

O'Hara, R. B. and Sillanpää, M. J. (2009). A review of Bayesian variable selection methods: What, how and which. *Bayesian Analysis*, 4(1):85–118.

Osnes, K. and Aalen, O. O. (1999). Spatial smoothing of cancer survival: a Bayesian approach. *Statistics in Medicine*, 18(16):2087–2099.

Paciorek, C. J. (2010). The importance of scale for spatial-confounding bias and precision of spatial regression estimators. *Statistical Science*, 25(1):107–125.

Papageorgiou, G., Richardson, S., and Best, N. (2015). Bayesian non-parametric models for spatially indexed data of mixed type. *Journal of the Royal Statistical Society: Series B (Statistical Methodology)*, 77(5):973–999.

Park, B., Mammen, E., Lee, Y., and Lee, D. (2015). Varying coefficient regression models: A review and new developments. *International Statistics Review*, 83(1):36–64.

Perperoglou, A. and Eilers, P. H. C. (2010). Penalized regression and individual deviance effects. *Computational Statistics*, 25(2):341–361.

Plummer, M. (2008). Penalized loss functions for Bayesian model comparison. *Biostatistics*, 9:523–539.

Plummer, M. and Clayton, D. (1996). Estimation of population exposure in ecological studies. *Journal of the Royal Statistical Society: Series B (Methodological)*, 58(1):113–126.

Prates, M. O., Assunçao, R. M., and Castilho Rodrigues, E. (2018). Alleviating spatial confounding for areal data problems by displacing the geographical centroids. *Bayesian Analysis*.

Quick, H., Waller, L. A., and Casper, M. (2018). A multivariate space-time model for analysing county level heart disease death rates by race and sex. *Applied Statistics*, 67(1):291–304.

Rao, J. N. K. (2003). *Small Area Estimation*. John Wiley & Sons.

Reich, B. J., Hodges, J. S., and Carlin, B. P. (2007). Spatial analysis of periodontial data using conditionally autoregressive priors having two class of neighbors relations. *Journal of the American Statistical Association*, 102:44–55.

Reich, B. J., Hodges, J. S., and Zadnik, V. (2006). Effects of residual smoothing on the posterior of the fixed effects in disease-mapping models. *Biometrics*, 62:1197–1206.

Richardson, S. (2003). Spatial models in epidemiological applications. In Green, P. J., Hjort, N. L., and Richardson, S., editors, *Highly Structured Stochastic Systems*, chapter 8, pages 237–259. Oxford University Press.

Richardson, S., Abellán, J., and Best, N. (2006). Bayesian spatio-temporal analysis of joint patterns of male and female lung cancer risks in Yorkshire (UK). *Statistical Methods in Medical Research*, 15:385–407.

Richardson, S. and Green, P. J. (1997). On Bayesian analysis of mixtures with an unknown number of components. *Journal of the Royal Statistical Society: Series B (Statistical Methodology)*, 59(4):731–792.

Richardson, S., Guihenneuc-Jouyaux, C., and Lasserre, V. (1996). Ecological studies-biases, missconceptions and counterexamples (letter to the editor). *American Journal of Epidemiology*, 143(5):522–523.

Richardson, S. and Monfort, C. (2000). Ecological correlation studies. In Elliott, P., Wakefield, J. C., Best, N. G., and Briggs, D. B., editors, *Spatial Epidemiology: Methods and Applications*, pages 205–220. Oxford University Press.

Richardson, S., Thomson, A., Best, N., and Elliot, P. (2004). Interpreting posterior relative risk estimates in disease-mapping studies. *Environmental Health Perspectives*, 112(9):1016–1025.

Riebler, A., Sorbye, S. H., Simpson, D., Rue, H., and Abellán, C. (2016). An intuitive Bayesian spatial model for disease mapping that accounts for scaling. *Statistical Methods in Medical Research*.

Robert, C. P. and Casella, G. (2009). *Introducing Monte Carlo Methods with R*. Springer-Verlag.

Robinson, W. S. (1950). Ecological correlation and the behaviour of individuals. *American Sociological Review*, 15:351–357.

Rodrigues, E., Assunção, R. M., and Dey, D. K. (2014). A closer look at the spatial exponential matrix specification. *Spatial Statistics*, 9:109–121.

Royle, J. A. and Berliner, L. M. (1999). A hierarchical approach to multivariate spatial modeling and prediction. *Journal of Agricultural, Biological, and Environmental Statistics*, 4(1):29–56.

Rue, H. and Held, L. (2005). *Gaussian Markov Random Fields: Theory & Applications*. Chapman & Hall/CRC.

Rue, H., Martino, S., and Chopin, N. (2009). Approximate Bayesian inference for latent Gaussian models by using integrated nested Laplace approximations. *Journal of the Royal Statistical Society: Series B (Statistical Methodology)*, 71(2):319–392.

Ruppert, D. and Carroll, R. J. (2000). Spatially-adaptive penalties for spline fitting. *Australian and New Zealand Journal of Statistics*, 42(2):205–223.

Sain, S. and Cressie, N. (2007). A spatial analysis of multivariate lattice data. *Journal of Econometrics*, 140:226–259.

Sain, S., Furrer, R., and Cressie, N. (2011). A spatial analysis of multivariate output from regional climate models. *The Annals of Applied Statistics*, 5(1):150–175.

Salway, R. and Wakefield, J. (2005). Sources of bias in ecological studies of non-rare events. *Environmental and Ecological Statistics*, 12:321–347.

Schlattmann, P. and Böhning, D. (1993). Mixture models and disease mapping. *Statistics in Medicine*, 12:1037–1044.

Schmid, V. and Held, L. (2004). Bayesian extrapolation of space-time trends in cancer registry data. *Biometrics*, 60:1034–1042.

Schrödle, B. and Held, L. (2011a). A primer on disease mapping and ecological regression using INLA. *Computational Statistics*, 26:241–258.

Schrödle, B. and Held, L. (2011b). Spatio-temporal disease mapping using INLA. *Environmetrics*, 22(6):725–734.

Schrödle, B., Held, L., Riebler, A., and Danuser, J. (2011). Using integrated nested Laplace approximations for the evaluation of veterinary surveillance data from Switzerland: a case study. *Journal of the Royal Statistical Society, Series c (Applied Statistics)*, 60(2):261–279.

Segen, J. C. (2002). *Concise Dictionary of Modern Medicine*. McGraw-Hill, New York.

Silva, G. L., Dean, C. B., Nisonyenga, T., and Vanasse, A. (2008). Hierarchical Bayesian spatiotemporal analysis of revascularization odds using smoothing splines. *Statistics in Medicine*, 27:2381–2401.

Simpson, D., Rue, H., Riebler, A., Martins, T. G., and Sørbye, S. H. (2017). Penalising model component complexity: A principled, practical approach to constructing priors. *Statistical Science*, 32(1):1–28.

Simpson, E. H. (1951). The interpretation of interaction in contingency tables. *Journal of the Royal Statistical Society: Series B*, 13:238–241.

Smith, T. R., Wakefield, J., and Dobra, A. (2015). Restricted covariance priors with applications in spatial statistics. *Bayesian Analysis*, 10(4):965–990.

Song, H.-R., Lawson, A., D'Agostino Jr, R. B., and Liese, A. D. (2011). Modeling type 1 and type 2 diabetes mellitus incidence in youth: an application of Bayesian hierarchical regression for sparse small area data. *Spatial and Spatiotemporal Epidemiology*, 2(1):23–33.

Spiegelhalter, D. (2001). Bayesian methods for cluster randomized trials with continuous responses. *Statistics in Medicine*, 20:435–452.

Spiegelhalter, D. J., Abrams, K. R., and Miles, J. P. (2004). *Bayesian Approaches to Clinical Trials and Health-Care Evalutaion*. John Wiley & Sons, Chichester.

Spiegelhalter, D. J., Best, N. G., Carlin, B. P., and Van Der Linde, A. (2002). Bayesian measures of model complexity and fit (with discussion). *Journal of the Royal Statistical Society: Series B (Statistical Methodology)*, 64:583–641.

Stephens, M. (2000a). Bayesian analysis of mixture models with an unknown number of components - an alternative to reversible jump methods. *Annals of Statistics*, 28:40–74.

Stephens, M. (2000b). Dealing with label switching in mixture models. *Journal of the Royal Statistical Society: Series B (Statistical Methodology)*, 62(4):795–809.

Stern, H. and Cressie, N. (1999). Inference for extremes in disease mapping. In Lawson, A. B., Biggeri, A., Bohning, D., Lesaffre, E., Viel, J.-F., and Bertollini, R., editors, *Disease Mapping and Risk Assessment for Public Health*. John Wiley & Sons, Chichester, UK.

Stern, H. S. and Cressie, N. (2000). Posterior predictive model checks for disease mapping models. *Statistics in Medicine*, 19:2377–2397.

Stone, R. (1988). Investigations of excess environmental risks around putative source: Statistical problems and a proposed test. *Statistics in Medicine*, 7:649–660.

Sun, D., Tsutakawa, R. K., and He, Z. (2001). Propriety of posterior with improper priors in hierarchical linear mixed models. *Statistica Sinica*, 11(77-95):77–95.

Sun, D., Tsutakawa, R. K., Kim, H., and Zhuoqiong, H. (2000). Spatio-temporal interaction with disease mapping. *Statistics in Medicine*, 19:2015–2035.

Sun, D., Tsutakawa, R. K., and Speckman, P. L. (1999). Posterior distribution of hierarchical models using CAR(1) distributions. *Biometrika*, 86(2):341–350.

Thompson, S. G., Smith, T. C., and Sharp, S. J. (1997). Investigating underlying risk as a source of heterogeneity in meta-analysis. *Statistics in Medicine*, 16:2741–2758.

Thurston, S. W., Wand, M. P., and Wiencke, J. K. (2000). Negative binomial additive models. *Biometrics*, 56:139–144.

Tierney, L. and Kadane, J. B. a. (1986). Accurate approximations for posterior moments and marginal densities. *Journal of the American Statistical Association*, 81:82–86.

Torabi, M. (2013). Spatio-temporal modeling for disease mapping using CAR and B-spline smoothing. *Envirometrics*, 24(3):180–188.

Torabi, M. and Rosychuk, R. J. (2011). Spatio-temporal modelling using B-splines for disease mapping: analysis of childhood cancer trends. *Journal of Applied Statistics*, 38(9):1769–1781.

Torres-Avilés, F. and Martinez-Beneito, M. A. (2015). STANOVA: A smooth-ANOVA-based model for spatio-temporal disease mapping. *Stochastic Environmental Research and Risk Assessment*, 29(1):131–141.

Tsutakawa, R. K. (1988). Mixed model for analyzing geographical variability in mortality rates. *Journal of the American Statistical Association*, 83(401):37–42.

Tzala, E. and Best, N. (2008). Bayesian latent variable modelling of multivariate spatio-temporal variation in cancer mortality. *Statistical Methods in Medical Research*, 17(1):97–118.

Ugarte, M. D., , Goicoa, T., , and Militino, A. F. (2010). Spatio-temporal modeling of mortality risks using penalized splines. *Environmetrics*, 21:270–289.

Ugarte, M. D., Adin, A., and Goicoa, T. (2016). Two-level spatially structured models in spatio-temporal disease mapping. *Statistical Methods in Medical Research*, 25(4):1080–1100.

Ugarte, M. D., Adin, A., and Goicoa, T. (2017). One-dimensional, two-dimensional, and three dimensional B-splines to specify space-time interactions in Bayesian disease mapping: Model fitting and model identifiability. *Spatial Statistics*, 22:451–468.

Ugarte, M. D., Adin, A., Goicoa, T., and Fernandez Militino, A. (2014). On fitting spatio-temporal disease mapping models using approximate Bayesian inference. *Statistical Methods in Medical Research*.

Ugarte, M. D., Adin, A., Goicoa, T., and López-Abente, G. (2015). Analyzing the evolution of young people's brain cancer mortality in Spanish provinces. *Cancer Epidemiology*, 39:480–485.

Ugarte, M. D., Goicoa, T., Etxebarria, J., and Militino, A. F. (2012). Projections of cancer mortality risks using spatio-temporal P-spline models. *Statistical Methods in Medical Research*, 21(5):545–560.

Ugarte, M. D., Ibañez, B., and Militino, A. F. (2004). Testing for Poisson zero inflation in disease mapping. *Biometrical Journal*, 46:526–539.

Ugarte, M. D., Ibañez, B., and Militino, A. F. (2006). Modelling risks in disease mapping. *Statistical Methods*, 15:21–35.

Van Der Broek, J. (1995). A score test for zero inflation in a Poisson distribution. *Biometrics*, 51(2):738–743.

Wackernagel, H. (1998). *Multivariate Geostatistics, Second edition*. Springer Verlag, New York.

Wackernagel, H. (2003). *Multivariate Geostatistics: An Introduction with Applications*. Springer.

Wakefield, J. (2003). Sensitivity analyses for ecologic regression. *Biometrics*, 59(1):9–17.

Wakefield, J. (2007). Disease mapping and spatial regression with count data. *Biostatistics*, 8(2):158–183.

Wakefield, J. (2008). Ecologic studies revisited. *Epidemiologic Reviews*, 29:75–90.

Wakefield, J. C., Best, N. G., and Waller, N. A. (2000). Bayesian approaches to disease mapping. In Elliot, P., Wakefield, J. C., Best, N. G., and Briggs, D., editors, *Spatial Epidemiology: Methods and Applications*, pages 104–127. Oxford University Press, Oxford.

Wakefield, J. C. and Morris, S. E. (2002). The Bayesian modelling of disease risk in relation to a point source. *Journal of the American Statistical Association*, 96:77–91.

Wall, M. M. (2004). A close look at the spatial structure implied by the CAR and SAR models. *Journal of Statistical Planning and Inference*, 121:311–324.

Waller, L. A., Carlin, B. P., Xia, H., and Gelfand, A. E. (1997). Hierarchical spatio-temporal mapping of disease rates. *Journal of the American Statistical Association*, 92:607–617.

Waller, L. A. and Gotway, C. A. (2004). *Applied Spatial Statistics for Public Health*. John Wiley & Sons.

Waller, L. A. and Lawson, A. B. (1995). The power of focused tests to detect disease clustering. *Statistics in Medicine*, 14:2291–2308.

Watanabe, S. (2010). Asymptotic equivalence of Bayes cross validation and widely applicable information criterion in singular learning theory. *Journal of Machine Learning Research*, 11:3571–3594.

Wikipedia contributors (2018a). Epidemiology — Wikipedia, the free encyclopedia. [Online; accessed 28-May-2018].

Wikipedia contributors (2018b). Statistics — Wikipedia, the free encyclopedia. [Online; accessed 28-May-2018].

Womble, W. H. (1951). Differential systematics. *Science*, 114:315–322.

Wood, S. N. (2017). *Generalized Additive Models. An Introduction with R (Second Edition)*. CRC Press.

Xia, H. and Carlin, B. P. (1998). Spatio-temporal models with errors in covariates: Mapping Ohio lung cancer mortality. *Statistics in Medicine*, 17:2025–2043.

Zellner, A. (1986). On assessing prior distributions and Bayesian regression analysis with g-prior distributions. In *Bayesian Inference and Decision Techniques: Essays in Honor of Bruno de Finetti*, pages 389–399. Edward Elgar Publishing Limited.

Zhang, H. (2004). Inconsistent estimation and asymptotically equal interpolations in model-based geostatistics. *Journal of the American Statistical Association*, 99(465):250–261.

Zhang, S., Sun, D., He, C. Z., and Schootman, M. (2006). A Bayesian semi-parametric model for colorectal cancer incidences. *Statistics in Medicine*, 25:285–309.

Zhang, Y., Hodges, J. S., and Banerjee, S. (2009). Smoothed ANOVA with spatial effects as a competitor to MCAR in multivariate spatial smoothing. *Annals of Applied Statistics*, 3(4):1805–1830.

Zurriaga, O., Martínez-Beneito, M. A., Botella-Rocamora, P., López-Quílez, A., Melchor, I., Amador, A., Vanaclocha, H., and Nolasco, A. (2010). Spatio-temporal mortality atlas of Comunitat Valenciana. (http://www.geeitema.org/AtlasET/index.jsp?idioma=I. Accessed: May, 2nd 2016).

Zurriaga, O., Vanaclocha, H., Martínez-Beneito, M. A., and Botella Rocamora, P. (2008). Spatio-temporal evolution of female lung cancer mortality in a region of Spain: is it worth taking migration into account? *BMC Cancer*, 8(35):1.

Index